THYROID CANCER - ADVANCES IN DIAGNOSIS AND THERAPY

Edited by **Hojjat Ahmadzadehfar**

Thyroid Cancer - Advances in Diagnosis and Therapy
http://dx.doi.org/10.5772/61889
Edited by Hojjat Ahmadzadehfar

Contributors

Reza Vali, Syed Mudassar, Shariq R Masoodi, Khursheed A Wani, Mahboob Ul Hussain, Mosin S Khan, Khurshid I Andrabi, Dana I Stoian, Marius Craina, Bogdan Timar, Mihaela Craciunescu, Adalbert Schiller, Romulus Timar, Robert Pichler, Irina Wimmer, Marcus Ruhlmann, Verena Ruhlmann, Walter Jentzen, Andreas Bockisch, Lei Zhang, Beverly Wang, Chao Ma, Nazan Ciledag, Burcu Savran Sahin, Elif Aktas, Gul Buyukbayraktar, Bilgin Kadri Aribas, Hidir Kaygusuz, Salvatore Ulisse, Alessandro Antonelli, Enke Baldini, Salvatore Sorrenti, Poupak Fallahi, Paolo Miccoli, Angelo Filippini, Lebriz Uslu-Beşli, Mustafa Demir, Carmen Georgescu, Ana Valea, Yadranko Ducic, Barbara Hertz

Published by InTech

Janeza Trdine 9, 51000 Rijeka, Croatia

Publishing Process Manager Edi Lipovic

Technical Editor SPi Global

Cover InTech Design team

First published September, 2016

Printed in Croatia

Additional hard copies can be obtained from orders@intechopen.com

Thyroid Cancer - Advances in Diagnosis and Therapy, Edited by Hojjat Ahmadzadehfar

p. cm.

Print ISBN 978-953-51-2588-4
Online ISBN 978-953-51-2589-1

For EU product safety concerns:
IN TECH d.o.o., Prolaz Marije Krucifikse Kozulić 3, 51000 Rijeka, Croatia,
info@intechopen.com or visit our website at intechopen.com.

Meet the editor

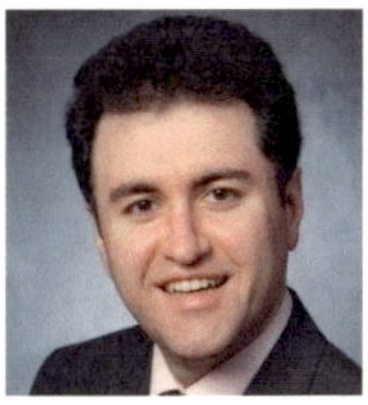

Dr. Hojjat Ahmadzadehfar, MSc, is an associate professor and head of the therapy section at the Department of Nuclear Medicine, University of Bonn. He received medical degree from the Guilan University of Medical Sciences in Iran in 1999 and did residency in nuclear medicine in Germany at the Department of Nuclear Medicine, University Hospital Bonn, between 2003 and 2008. From 2008 to 2013, he was the assistant medical director of the Department of Nuclear Medicine at the University Hospital Bonn and since 2013 has worked as the head of the therapy section. Dr. Ahmadzadehfar serves as an editor and reviewer for several international journals and has written and co-written over 80 papers and book chapters.

Contents

Preface

The approach to thyroid cancer is a real example of multidisciplinary work in medicine. Different specialities from surgery and endocrinology to oncology and nuclear medicine work together to plan the best diagnosis and therapy for these patients. This book is for medical doctors with experience in the field of thyroid cancer. It comprises different subjects, especially the advances in the diagnosis of thyroid cancer with PET imaging and elastography, as well as the new therapeutic approaches with tyrosine kinase inhibitors. Radioiodine ablation of the thyroid remnant is one of the oldest radionuclide therapies, invented by Dr. Saul Hertz 75 years ago, and has changed the prognosis of thyroid cancer patients dramatically. His daughter, Barbara Hertz, wrote the story of Saul Hertz for this book, which is a real story about one of the pioneers of nuclear medicine.

Hojjat Ahmadzadehfar, MD, Msc
Associate Professor
University Hospital Bonn
Department of Nuclear Medicine
Bonn, Germany

Chapter 1

Dr. Saul Hertz (1905–1950) Discovers the Medical Uses of Radioactive Iodine: The First Targeted Cancer Therapy

Barbara Hertz

Additional information is available at the end of the chapter

http://dx.doi.org/10.5772/64609

Abstract

Dr. Saul Hertz spontaneously posed the question "Could iodine be made radioactive artificially?" to the MIT President Karl Compton, on November 12, 1936. MGH's Dr. Hertz and his MIT collaborator, Dr. Arthur Roberts, were the first and the foremost to develop the experimental data for the medical uses of radioiodine (RAI) and apply it in the clinical setting. Dr. Hertz expanded the successful use of RAI of treating hyperthyroidism, Graves' disease, to the treatment of thyroid cancer in 1946. Dr. Saul Hertz established the Radioactive Isotope Research Institute to diagnose and treat thyroid cancer, which he believed held the key to the larger problem of cancer in general. RAI is the first and gold standard of targeted cancer therapies.

Keywords: radioiodine (RAI), Dr. Saul Hertz

1. Seminal question

Dr. Saul Hertz (**Figure 1**) attended a luncheon meeting at Harvard Medical School's Vanderbilt Hall on November 12, 1936 (**Figure 2**). Karl T. Compton, the President of Massachusetts Institute of Technology (MIT), was speaking on the topic "What Physics Can Do for Biology and Medicine."

Dr. Hertz, who was the director of the Thyroid Clinic (1931–1943) at Massachusetts General Hospital (MGH), asked President Compton the seminal question, "Could iodine be made radioactive artificially?" Hertz had been conducting studies on the use of iodine and its effect on thyroid function. Hertz's question came spontaneously as documented in MGH's Dr. James Means's letter (**Figure 3**) to Archie Woods of the Mary and John Markle Foundation that sponsored the building of the MIT Cyclotron. Dr. Arthur Roberts, Dr. Hertz's MIT collaborator, wrote to Dr. John Stanbury, the author of *A Constant Ferment: A History of MGH Thyroid Clinic and Laboratory at The Massachusetts General Hospital: 1913–1990,* as Stanbury was developing his book. Dr. Roberts in his letter dated April 3, 1991, states "Your conjecture that it was the outcome of a group discussion has no basis in fact." Stanbury's book has been in publication for many decades and has been used as a citation with false information (**Figure 4a–c**).

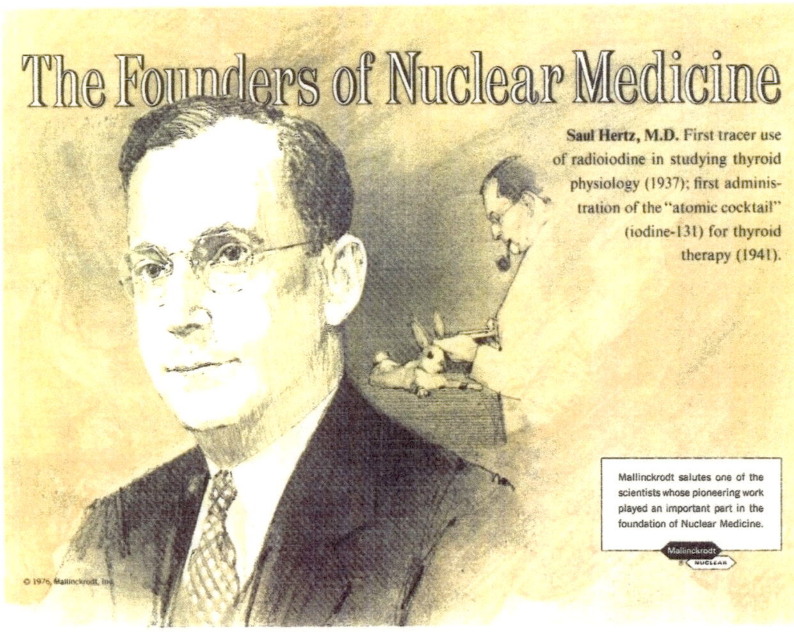
The Founders of Nuclear Medicine
Saul Hertz, M.D. First tracer use of radioiodine in studying thyroid physiology (1937); first administration of the "atomic cocktail" (iodine-131) for thyroid therapy (1941).
Mallinckrodt salutes one of the scientists whose pioneering work played an important part in the foundation of Nuclear Medicine.
Mallinckrodt
NUCLEAR

Figure 1. Mallinckrodt, a $2.1 billion global pharmaceutical company honors Dr Saul Hertz's discovery of the medical uses of radioiodine (RAI).

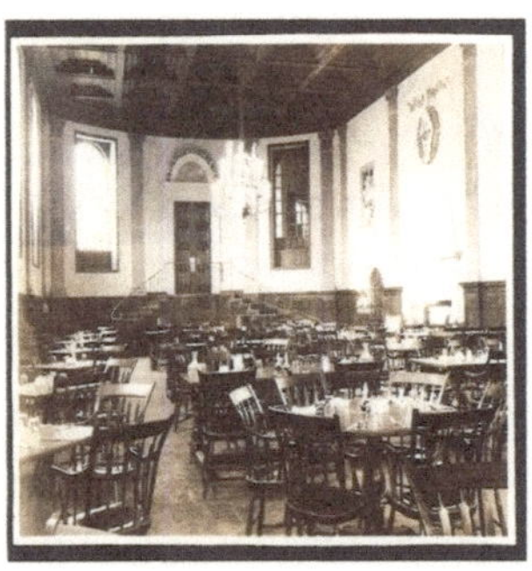

On November 12, 1936, MIT's President Karl Compton (1887-1954) spoke at Harvard Medical School's Vanderbilt Hall. President Compton's topic was "What Physics can do for Biology and Medicine." After the presentation with Dr. James H. Means, MGH's Chief of Medical Services, standing next to him; **Saul Hertz spontaneously posed the seminal question that launched the RAI research.** Dr. Hertz had been conducting studies on the effects of iodine on thyroid function.

Figure 2. Harvard Medical School's Vanderbilt Hall the site of Dr Hertz spontaneously asking MIT's President Karl Compton, "Could iodine be made radioactive artificially?".

http://dx.doi.org/10.5772/64609

April 17, 1939

Archie S. Woods, Esq.,
The John and Mary R. Markle Foundation,
14 Wall Street,
New York, New York.

Dear Mr. Woods:

With regard to the two points raised in your letter of April 13, namely the merit of the work proposed by Dr. Greenberg and his ability to direct it, I have made inquiries from several sources on both of these.

I think there is little doubt that Dr. Greenberg is qualified to direct the proposed work in a skilful manner. I don't know him personally but inquiries among biochemists disclose that he enjoys a high reputation.

The projects themselves we have thought about here somewhat and it seems to us that they are thoroughly worth while, but not highly imaginative or original. It impresses us that the man is trying to find a good use to which to put a unique method rather than finding a method to solve a burning question. I believe that it is rather different from the situation here with regard to iodine. Our primary interest was in iodine metabolism and when it became apparent that there might be radioactive isotopes of iodine, it at once occurred to Hertz that we might make use of them to solve a problem that we were already working on. Indeed, we got going on radioactive isotopes of short half length almost before we heard of such an instrument as a cyclotron. In other words, iodine was the primary item here, whereas in California the cyclotron is the primary item and they are trying to think up ways to use it. None of these opinions is intended to deter you from making the grant. Indeed, I think you should make it. I think the originators of the cyclotron deserve to have grants made toward the use of the instrument in the solving of biologic problems.

Sincerely yours,

JHM:EAL

J. H. Means

Figure 3. MGH's Chief of Medicine's letter to the Markle Foundation documenting Dr Hertz's spontaneous seminal question that launched the RAI breakthrough research.

Dr. Hertz's seminal question brought together the work established in 1896 of E. Bauman's reporting the effect of iodine on the functioning of the thyroid. Bauman found high concentrations of iodine tightly bound to proteins in extracts of the thyroid gland, thyroid extracts were standardized to contain 0.2% iodine in order to maintain equal potency of different preparations. Additionally, in the field of radioactivity, in 1896 Henri Becquerel investigated the newly discovered X-rays that led to studies of how uranium salts are affected by light. Saul Hertz's seminal question brought together the effect of iodine on the thyroid and radioactivity. Hertz's question launched the radioactive iodine (RAI) research that established the cornerstone of Nuclear Medicine.

DUMAND—Deep Underwater Muon and Neutrino Detection

Hawaii DUMAND Center
University of Hawaii
2505 Correa Rd.
Honolulu, HI 96822
808 - 948-7391

1536 Alewa Drive
Honolulu, HI 96817
Apr. 3, 1991

Dr. John B. Stanbury
43 Circuit Rd
Chestnut Hill, MA 02167

Dear Dr. Stanbury,

Mrs. Vitta Hertz has sent me a copy of Chapter V from the book I understand you will soon publish on the history of the MGH Thyroid Clinic. I have read it with great interest, since I was closely involved with the earliest history of the use of radioactive iodine in connection with thyroid physiology and therapy.

You will no doubt remember telephoning me in regard to a minor point concerning references to M.I.T. in the first paper on the use of radioiodine in rabbits. At that time I gave you a detailed description of the work at M.I.T. and of the degree of Evans' scientific participation in it – namely zero. I was unpleasantly surprised to see how completely you have ignored it.

I understood it somewhat better as I read the false and distorted picture you have given of the early work on radioiodine. I began to understand even more when I read your description of Evans: I quote "an exceptionally engaging, modest, and brilliant colleague whose contributions to the Thyroid unit were incomparable." That literally turned my stomach. Evans may have been engaging when he wanted to be, but brilliant? The great contribution to the thyroid unit was not his, but Saul Hertz's. It was Hertz who first conceived the idea of using radioactive iodine for both research and therapy in thyroid work; it was Hertz who asked the question at Comptons' lecture – though Chapman and Evans tried their best to cast doubt on this after he died. Your conjecture that it was the outcome of a group discussion has no basis in fact. Not only did Saul tell me that the idea was his alone, but Evans is on written record as confirming it; Mrs. Hertz and I have copies of his letter. There cannot be the slightest doubt on that subject.

More important, it was Hertz who conceived and carried out, with my help, all the ground-breaking work in the next seven years. The notion that you advance that it was Evans who led the "team" because he headed the laboratory in which the work was done is simply naive and absurd. He wasn't even on the "team", much less its leader. He was the owner, back in the clubhouse.

Furthermore, that was the way he wanted it. He had every opportunity, and certainly the authority, to have taken an active part in the work; but he chose not to do so. I do not know why; but it may well be, in view of his known anti-Semitism, that he could not stomach the notion of working with two Jews.

Cable Address:

I would believe nothing on this subject from Chapman, whose self- interest is obvious, and who bungled – whether deliberately or not – the follow-up on Hertz's original series when Hertz joined the Navy. (See Hertz's letter to him on this subject.) It was Hertz – with some suggestions from me – who designed the animal experiments we carried out, and the therapeutic tests on patients with Graves' disease. Evans took no part in any of this work in the five years I was connected with it. He was not excluded; he simply had no interest in doing anything other than managerial work.

You seem to attach great significance to the fact that Evans' name appears o the first few publications (as does Means's). If you think that necessarily implies a scientific contribution to the work, you don't understand how authorship on academ papers is obtained. In Evans' case, we omitted his name from the first draft of the first paper because he had made not the slightest contribution to the work, other than that involved in managing the laboratory in which we worked.

An example of his managerial contribution was providing the neutron source w used to produce the radio-iodine. Later, with the help of Means, he secured the funds with which the M.I.T. Markle cyclotron was constructed, and which provided the much more intense therapeutic quantities of radio-iodine.

The customary and proper way of crediting this sort of contribution is as an acknowledgment of assistance, such as the one you will find in the paper of Hertz and Roberts in Endocrinology, July 1941. It most emphatically is not to include th person in question among the authors, which implies participation in the scientific work.

Evans made it a condition of my employment – I wish I still had the letter that his name was to appear on all publications. Even at that time, this was unusual, and occasioned much comment. It led to the contretemps concerning the late addition of his name to our first paper. It was also on the second paper; but after that Saul and I felt sufficiently secure that we ignored him in our subsequent publications. Had he actually participated in the work, there would have been no problem in including him.

Evans was the first boss I worked under after receiving my degree at N.Y.U. was puzzled and unhappy at the way I was treated; but at the time I had no ba for comparisons. (An example: he constantly assured me my work was highly satisfactory; but in five years I never received any salary raise. As a consequence, when I joined the MIT Radiation Lab in 1943, I found my salary suddenly double He also made it clear that I could look for no advancement at M.I.T., and for no recommendations from him to any subsequent employer. Luckily the war made tha immaterial.

It was only later that I fully realized what a thoroughly unprincipled racist manipulator he was. Have you ever taken the trouble to find out what other your people who had the misfortune to work under him thought of him? His particular talent was taking all the credit for the work others had done. In the case of the radioiodine field, he had a clear field for operations after I left, and Hertz and M died. He was abetted in this by Chapman, and between them they concocted the preposterous story that you repeat. They did their best to denigrate the initial se of patients that Hertz treated, but were eventually unsuccessful, as you eventually - apparently reluctantly - admit.

Finally, your verdict (on p.77) that the credit for priorities in investigations of thyroid function and therapeutics goes to Hertz, Means, and Evans is faulty and inexact, in that implies equal credit. It omits my name entirely. Did you think I w just a glorified lab technician? I made important contributions, not only to the technology of the measurement of uptake and dosages, and for this work received a award of honor from the New England Society of Nuclear Medicine in, I think, 197 My own allocation of credit, percentage-wise, would be Hertz 80, Roberts 15, Mean and Evans 2.5 each.

It is of course possible that I am biased; if so, with good reason. In the near fifty years since I escaped from Evans's clutches I have known many unprincipled o aggressive scientists; but never again have I met anyone quite like him. The late Stan Livingston, who built the MIT cyclotron, and I became colleagues again much later, at Fermilab. Our recollections of Evans were similar. It would not take much effort on your part to confirm what I have told you, nor would the changes in yo manuscript that my objections imply be either extensive or radical. I do not ask th you paint a true picture of the man - it would take a Voltaire to do that - but only that you refrain from glorifying him. I hope you will see fit to make such changes. Otherwise your book will perpetuate a biased and untrue version of a history that deserves better.

I do not fault you for falling into the trap so carefully laid. The true story i not easily available. It would have taken some effort to dig it out, and that may have been what you had in mind. However, a historian has obligations (as I have myself discovered). I hope you will live up to them.

Sincerely yours,

Arthur Roberts

Figure 4. (a–c) Pivitol letter from MIT's Dr Arthur Roberts to the author of *A Constant Ferment*, of which the author, Dr John Stanbury, chose to ignore.

2. Rabbit studies

In early 1937, the collaboration was established between the Massachusetts Institute of Technology and Boston's Massachusetts General Hospital. The young physicist Dr. Arthur Roberts was hired by MIT, and MGH's Dr. Saul Hertz began the first studies on rabbits to evaluate the effects of a nuclear substance, radioactive iodine, on the thyroid. Dr. Roberts produced noncyclotron I-128 in small quantities based on Fermi's work. The experiment involved 48 rabbits. The RAI was administered to rabbits with altered thyroid function. Quantitative analysis showed that hyperplastic thyroid glands retained more RAI than normal thyroid glands. The studies demonstrated the principle that tracer amounts of radioactive iodine could be used to investigate thyroid gland physiology demonstrating the tracer capabilities of RAI and its effects on the thyroid gland (**Figure 5**).

The original draft of the article describing their rabbit study findings had Hertz and Roberts as the coauthors as they had done the work and written the paper. MIT's Robley Evans, who was the administrator of the lab at MIT and who had hired the physicist Arthur Roberts, insisted that his name be added to the paper while it was at the publishers. Robley Evans had done no work in the construction of the experiment, analysis of the data, or writing the paper (**Figure 4a–c**). When Roberts was hired Evans had included a condition of his employment, that his (Evans) name be added to any papers that might be forthcoming. Evans dictated a letter to the editor for Hertz to sign that Robley Evans's name be added although Evans made no contribution.

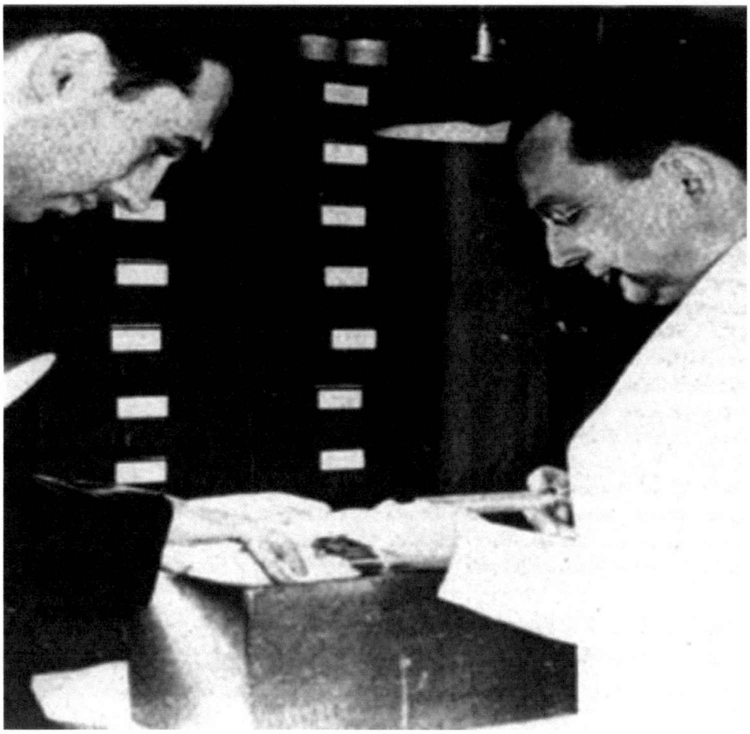

Figure 5. MIT's Dr Arthur Roberts (left) MGH's Dr Saul Hertz (right) administering non cyclotron produced I-128. These studies demonstrated the principle of using a radioactive substance as a tracer.

Hertz and Roberts were hopeful that they could go from diagnosis to treatment; however, they knew that they would need a larger quantity of RAI with a longer half-life. Cyclotron-produced RAI was needed. MGH's Chief of Medicine, Dr. James H. Means, took the train from Boston to New York City and secured a $30,000.00 check from the Mary and John Markel Foundation for the building of MIT's Cyclotron.

2.1. The first therapeutic use of RAI

The new Markel MIT Cyclotron, the first built exclusively for medical purposes, began operations in late 1940. Most of the RAI produced by this cyclotron was I-130 that has a half-life of 12 hours. Another 10% of the cyclotron product was I-131. Dr. Hertz administered the first therapeutic treatment of RAI on March 31, 1941 to Elizabeth D. at the Massachusetts General Hospital. Noted on Hertz's Data Charts (**Figure 6a** and **b**) was that this first patient received 2.1 mCi (77.7 MBq) of I-130 because its radiation was delivered rapidly to the thyroid cells over a day or two.

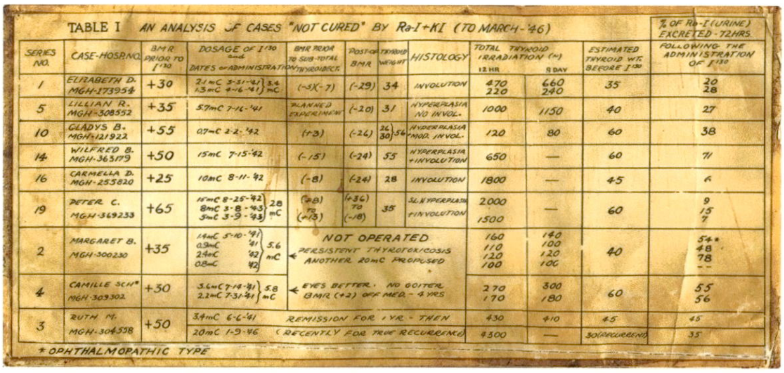

TABLE I AN ANALYSIS OF CASES "NOT CURED" BY Ra-I+KI (TO MARCH-'46)

SERIES NO.	CASE-HOSP. NO.	BMR PRIOR TO I^{130}	DOSAGE OF I^{130} and DATES of ADMINISTRATION	BMR PRIOR TO SUB-TOTAL THYROIDECT.	POST-OP BMR	THYROID WEIGHT	HISTOLOGY	TOTAL THYROID IRRADIATION (r) 12 HR	8 DAY	ESTIMATED THYROID WT. BEFORE I^{130}	% OF Ra-I (URINE) EXCRETED - 72 HRS. FOLLOWING THE ADMINISTRATION OF I^{130}
1	ELIZABETH D. MGH-173954	+30	2.1mC 3-31-'41, 1.3mC 4-16-'41 } 3.4 mC	(-5)(-7)	(-29)	34	INVOLUTION	470 220	660 240	35	20 28
5	LILLIAN R. MGH-308552	+35	5.7mC 7-16-'41	PLANNED EXPERIMENT	(-20)	31	HYPERPLASIA NO INVOL.	1000	1150	40	27
10	GLADYS B. MGH-121922	+55	0.7mC 2-2-'42	(+3)	(-26)	26, 30 } 56	HYPERPLASIA +MOD. INVOL.	120	80	60	38
14	WILFRED B. MGH-363179	+50	15mC 7-15-'42	(-15)	(-24)	55	HYPERPLASIA +INVOLUTION	650	—	60	71
16	CARMELLA D. MGH-255820	+25	10mC 8-11-'42	(-8)	(-24)	28	INVOLUTION	1800	—	45	6
19	PETER C. MGH-369233	+65	15mC 8-25-'42, 8mC 3-8-'43, 5mC 3-9-'43 } 28 mC	(+8) TO (+13)	(+36) TO (-18)	35	SL. HYPERPLASIA +INVOLUTION	2000 1500	—	60	9 15 7
2	MARGARET B. MGH-300230	+35	1.4mC 5-10-'41, 0.9mC '41, 2.4mC '42, 0.8mC '42 } 5.6 mC	← NOT OPERATED PERSISTENT THYROTOXICOSIS ANOTHER 20mC PROPOSED				160 110 120 100	140 100 120 100	40	54* 48 78 --
4	CAMILLE SCH* MGH-309302	+30	3.6mC 7-14-'41, 2.2mC 7-31-'41 } 5.8 mC	← EYES BETTER. NO GOITER. BMR (+2) OFF MED. - 4 YRS				270 170	300 180	60	55 56
3	RUTH M. MGH-304558	+50	3.4mC 6-6-'41	REMISSION FOR 1 YR. - THEN				430	410	45	45
			20mC 1-9-'46	(RECENTLY FOR TRUE RECURRENCE)				4300	—	30 (RECURRENT)	35

* OPHTHALMOPATHIC TYPE

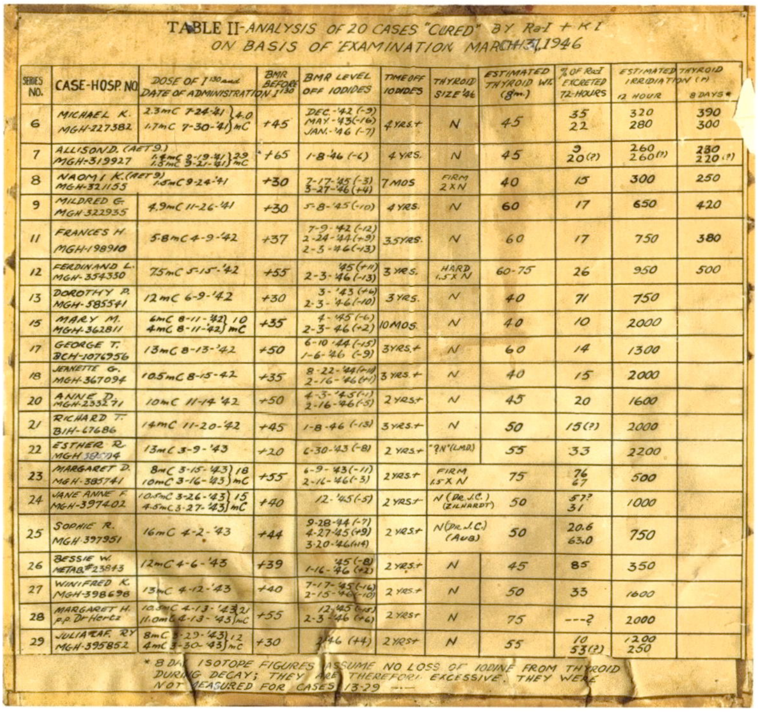

TABLE II-ANALYSIS OF 20 CASES "CURED" BY Ra-I + KI ON BASIS OF EXAMINATION MARCH 31, 1946

SERIES NO.	CASE-HOSP. NO	DOSE OF I^{130} and DATE OF ADMINISTRATION	BMR BEFORE I^{130}	BMR LEVEL OFF IODIDES	TIME OFF IODIDES	THYROID SIZE '46	ESTIMATED THYROID WT. (gm.)	% OF Ra-I EXCRETED 72-HOURS	ESTIMATED THYROID IRRADIATION (r) 12 HOUR	8 DAYS*
6	MICHAEL K. MGH-227382	2.3mC 7-24-'41, 1.7mC 7-30-'41 } 4.0 mC	+45	DEC.-'42 (-9), MAY-'43 (-16), JAN.-'46 (-7)	4 YRS.+	N	45	35 22	320 280	390 300
7	ALLISON D. (AET 9.) MGH-319927	1.4mC 9-19-'41, 1.5mC 9-21-'41 } 2.9 mC	+65	1-8-'46 (-6)	4 YRS.	N	45	9 20 (?)	260 260 (?)	280 220 (?)
8	NAOMI K. (AET 9) MGH-321155	1.5mC 9-24-'41	+30	7-17-'45 (-3), 3-27-'46 (+4)	7 MOS	FIRM 2XN	40	15	300	250
9	MILDRED G. MGH-322935	4.9mC 11-26-'41	+30	5-8-'45 (-10)	4 YRS.	N	60	17	650	420
11	FRANCES H. MGH-198910	5.8mC 4-9-'42	+37	7-9-'42 (-12), 2-24-'44 (+9), 2-3-'46 (-13)	3.5 YRS.	N	60	17	750	380
12	FERDINAND L. MGH-354330	7.5mC 5-15-'42	+55	'45 (+11), 2-3-'46 (-13)	3 YRS.	HARD 1.5XN	60-75	26	950	500
13	DOROTHY P. MGH-585541	12mC 6-9-'42	+30	3-'43 (+6), 2-3-'46 (-10)	3 YRS.	N	40	71	750	
15	MARY M. MGH-362811	6mC 8-11-'42, 4mC 8-11-'42 } 10 mC	+35	4-'45 (-6), 2-3-'46 (+2)	10 MOS.	N	40	10	2000	
17	GEORGE T. BCH-1076956	13mC 8-13-'42	+50	6-10-'44 (-15), 1-6-'46 (-9)	3 YRS.+	N	60	14	1300	
18	JEANETTE G. MGH-367094	10.5mC 8-15-42	+35	8-22-'44 (+11), 2-16-'46 (+1)	3 YRS.+	N	40	15	2000	
20	ANNE D. MGH-233271	10mC 11-14-'42	+50	4-3-'45 (-1), 2-16-'46 (-5)	2 YRS.+	N	45	20	1600	
21	RICHARD T. BIH-67686	14mC 11-20-'42	+45	1-8-46 (-13)	3 YRS.+	N	50	15 (?)	2000	
22	ESTHER R. MGH 385704	13mC 3-9-'43	+20	6-30-'43 (-8)	2 YRS.+	"?N" (LMD.)	55	33	2200	
23	MARGARET D. MGH-385741	8mC 3-15-'43, 10mC 3-16-'43 } 18 mC	+55	6-9-'43 (-11), 2-16-'46 (-3)	2 YRS.+	FIRM 1.5XN	75	76 67	500	
24	JANE ANNE F. MGH-397402	10.5mC 3-26-'43, 4.5mC 3-27-'43 } 15 mC	+40	12-'45 (-5)	2 YRS.+	N (DR. J.C.) (ZILHARDT)	50	57? 31	1000	
25	SOPHIE R. MGH-397951	16mC 4-2-'43	+44	9-28-'44 (-7), 4-27-'45 (+9), 3-20-'46 (+14)	2 YRS.+	N (DR. J.C.) (AUB)	50	20.6 63.0	750	
26	BESSIE W. METAB. #23843	12mC 4-6-'43	+39	'45 (-8), 1-16-'46 (+2)	2 YRS.+	N	45	85	350	
27	WINIFRED K. MGH-398698	13mC 4-12-'43	+40	7-17-'45 (-16), 2-15-'46 (-10)	2 YRS.+	N	50	33	1600	
28	MARGARET H. p.p. Dr Hertz	10.5mC 4-13-'43, 11.0mC 4-13-'43 } 21 mC	+55	12-'45 (-15), 2-3-'46 (+6)	2 YRS+	N	75	---?	2000	
29	JULIA ZAF. RY MGH-395852	8mC 3-29-'43, 4mC 3-30-'43 } 12 mC	+30	2-'46 (+4)	2 YRS+	N	55	10 53 (?)	1200 250	

* 8 DAY ISOTOPE FIGURES ASSUME NO LOSS OF IODINE FROM THYROID DURING DECAY; THEY ARE THEREFORE EXCESSIVE. THEY WERE NOT MEASURED FOR CASES 13-29 --.--

Figure 6. (a and b) Dr Hertz's handwritten Data Charts (1941–1946) of the very first series of patients treated successfully with a radioactive substance, RAI.

Dr. Hertz and his MIT collaborator Dr. Arthur Roberts continued to treat about one new patient per month for the rest of 1941. The total estimated RAI given to each of the eight patients ranged from 55 to 230 MBq with an average of 144 MBq. RAI was taken up by the patient's thyroid glands, and the patients did in fact get better. Hertz gave each patient a stable iodine beginning 1–3 days after the radioiodine at the insistence of his chief Dr. James Means. Means wanted to protect the patients against thyroid storm in case the RAI therapy was not effective. At the American Society for Clinical Investigation Meeting in May, 1942, Hertz presented a series of eight patients treated with RAI he had followed for at least 3 months; according to the abstract there were both "failures and successes."

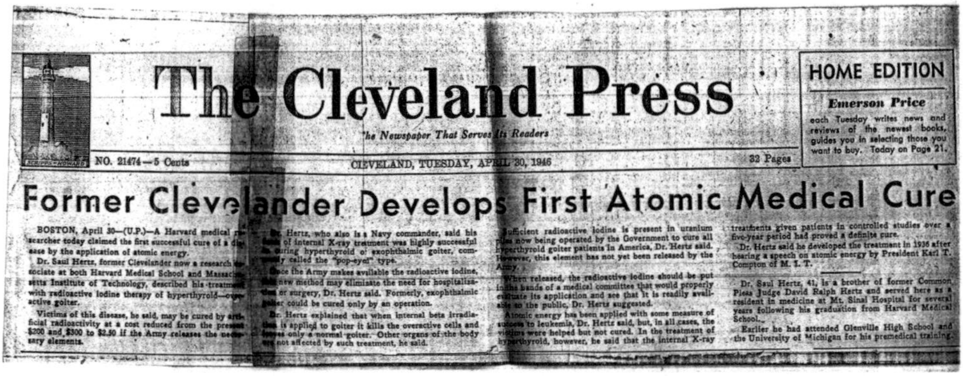

The Cleveland Press

The Newspaper That Serves Its Readers

NO. 21474—5 Cents | CLEVELAND, TUESDAY, APRIL 30, 1946 | 32 Pages

HOME EDITION

Emerson Price each Tuesday writes news and reviews of the newest books, guides you in selecting those you want to buy. Today on Page 21.

Former Clevelander Develops First Atomic Medical Cure

BOSTON, April 30—(U.P.)—A Harvard medical researcher today claimed the first successful cure of a disease by the application of atomic energy.

Dr. Saul Hertz, former Clevelander now a research associate at both Harvard Medical School and Massachusetts Institute of Technology, described his treatment with radioactive iodine therapy of hyperthyroid—overactive goiter.

Victims of this disease, he said, may be cured by artificial radioactivity at a cost reduced from the present $200 and $300 to $2.50 if the Army releases the necessary elements.

Dr. Hertz, who also is a Navy commander, said his form of internal X-ray treatment was highly successful in curing hyperthyroid or exophthalmic goiter, commonly called the "pop-eyed" type.

Once the Army makes available the radioactive iodine, this new method may eliminate the need for hospitalization or surgery, Dr. Hertz said. Formerly, exophthalmic goiter could be cured only by an operation.

Dr. Hertz explained that when internal beta irradiation is applied to goiter it kills the overactive cells and leaves only a normal goiter. Other organs of the body are not affected by such treatment, he said.

Sufficient radioactive iodine is present in uranium piles now being operated by the Government to cure all hyperthyroid goiter patients in America, Dr. Hertz said. However, this element has not yet been released by the Army.

When released, the radioactive iodine should be put in the hands of a medical committee that would properly evaluate its application and see that it is readily available to the public, Dr. Hertz suggested.

Atomic energy has been applied with some measure of success to leukemia, Dr. Hertz said, but, in all cases, the victims were helped but not cured. In the treatment of hyperthyroid, however, he said that the internal X-ray treatments given patients in controlled studies over a five-year period had proved a definite cure.

Dr. Hertz said he developed the treatment in 1936 after hearing a speech on atomic energy by President Karl T. Compton of M. I. T.

Dr. Saul Hertz, 41, is a brother of former Common Pleas Judge David Ralph Hertz and served here as a resident in medicine at Mt. Sinai Hospital for several years following his graduation from Harvard Medical School.

Earlier he had attended Glenville High School and the University of Michigan for his premedical training.

Figure 7. Cleveland Press Newspaper headline. Dr Hertz was born and grew up in Cleveland, Ohio.

Hertz continued to treat hyperthyroid patients with I-130 throughout 1942. In January 1943, Dr. Hertz joined the United States Navy to serve his country during World War II. MGH's Dr. Earl Chapman was Four "F" and was ineligible for service. Chapman, a private practice doctor who treated Boston's Beacon Hill-style affluent patients managed to carry on clinical research and worked part-time at MGH. Hertz asked Chapman to take over his RAI cases, in that he felt he (Hertz) had firmly established the work. Dr. Leonard Wartofsky stated "Chapman was probably honored to get involved in some clinical research and take on these patients [1]." Chapman saw an opportunity. Dr. Arthur Roberts, Hertz's MIT collaborator, writes "I would believe nothing on this subject from Chapman, whose self-interest is obvious and who bungled —whether deliberately or not—the follow-up on Hertz's original series when Hertz joined the Navy." Yes, Chapman tweaked the protocol and the letters between Hertz and Chapman during the war years produced tension. In March of 1946, at the end of World War II, Hertz received a cold reception at MGH. His service to his country was not honored. In Boston, The Beth Israel Hospital was emerging and welcoming "outsiders" to the establishment to be on staff. Although there remained quotas at medical schools, "Jews" were being trained and needed a place to practice. Dr. Hertz joined the staff of The Beth Israel Hospital.

Meanwhile, Chapman had established 22 patients of his own along with MIT's Robley Evans. Chapman and Evans wrote up their first paper on the subject and sent it to the *Journal of The American Medical Association* (*JAMA*). Morris Fishbein, the editor of *JAMA*, contacted Dr. Hertz sharing with him that "I have a paper here from Chapman and Evans and they are saying they have propriety of the discovery of radioiodine and your name is not even on the paper [2]." Fishbein asked Hertz and Roberts to write up their seventh paper on the medical uses of RAI. And so there appeared side by side in *JAMA* May 11, 1946, two articles from the same hospital using RAI describing the successful treatment of hyperthyroidism (**Figure 8a** and **b**) [3, 4].

Dr. James Thrall, Chairman Emeritus MGH Department of Radiologist, stated on April 5, 2016, that "Chapman and Evans had basically stolen his (Hertz's) work … the most flagrant, I think, unethical academically reprehensible behavior…worst yet, Saul Hertz died at 44 years old in 1950 and theses two gentlemen (Chapman and Evans) spent a great deal of time and effort rewriting history [5]."

Hertz strongly encouraged the U.S. Atomic Energy Commission to distribute RAI off of the atomic pile. In August 1946, this service began and I-131 was used exclusively because it was much less expensive. Going forward RAI became the preferred method of treating "Graves" disease worldwide (**Figure 7**).

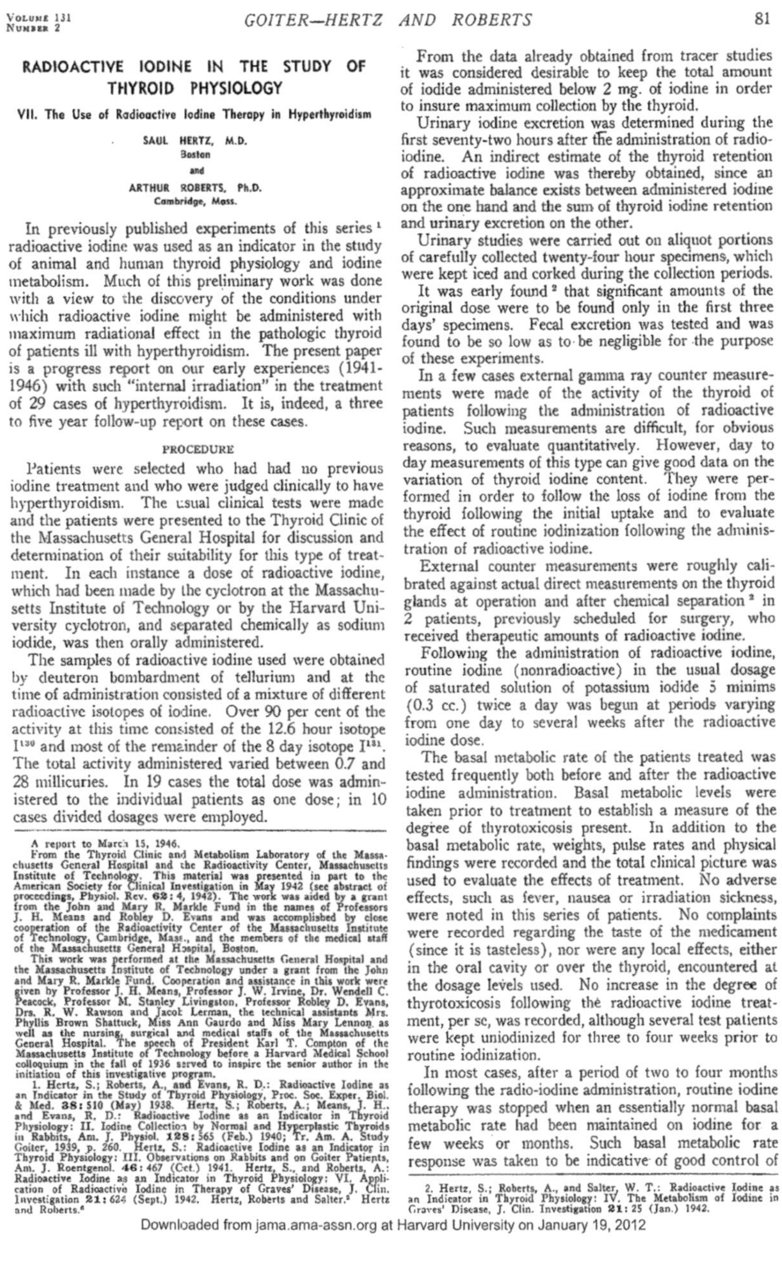

Volume 131
Number 2

RADIOACTIVE IODINE IN THE STUDY OF THYROID PHYSIOLOGY

VII. The Use of Radioactive Iodine Therapy in Hyperthyroidism

SAUL HERTZ, M.D.
Boston
and
ARTHUR ROBERTS, Ph.D.
Cambridge, Mass.

In previously published experiments of this series [1] radioactive iodine was used as an indicator in the study of animal and human thyroid physiology and iodine metabolism. Much of this preliminary work was done with a view to the discovery of the conditions under which radioactive iodine might be administered with maximum radiational effect in the pathologic thyroid of patients ill with hyperthyroidism. The present paper is a progress report on our early experiences (1941-1946) with such "internal irradiation" in the treatment of 29 cases of hyperthyroidism. It is, indeed, a three to five year follow-up report on these cases.

PROCEDURE

Patients were selected who had had no previous iodine treatment and who were judged clinically to have hyperthyroidism. The usual clinical tests were made and the patients were presented to the Thyroid Clinic of the Massachusetts General Hospital for discussion and determination of their suitability for this type of treatment. In each instance a dose of radioactive iodine, which had been made by the cyclotron at the Massachusetts Institute of Technology or by the Harvard University cyclotron, and separated chemically as sodium iodide, was then orally administered.

The samples of radioactive iodine used were obtained by deuteron bombardment of tellurium and at the time of administration consisted of a mixture of different radioactive isotopes of iodine. Over 90 per cent of the activity at this time consisted of the 12.6 hour isotope I^{130} and most of the remainder of the 8 day isotope I^{131}. The total activity administered varied between 0.7 and 28 millicuries. In 19 cases the total dose was administered to the individual patients as one dose; in 10 cases divided dosages were employed.

A report to March 15, 1946.
From the Thyroid Clinic and Metabolism Laboratory of the Massachusetts General Hospital and the Radioactivity Center, Massachusetts Institute of Technology. This material was presented in part to the American Society for Clinical Investigation in May 1942 (see abstract of proceedings, Physiol. Rev. **62**: 4, 1942). The work was aided by a grant from the John and Mary R. Markle Fund in the names of Professors J. H. Means and Robley D. Evans and was accomplished by close cooperation of the Radioactivity Center of the Massachusetts Institute of Technology, Cambridge, Mass., and the members of the medical staff of the Massachusetts General Hospital, Boston.
This work was performed at the Massachusetts General Hospital and the Massachusetts Institute of Technology under a grant from the John and Mary R. Markle Fund. Cooperation and assistance in this work were given by Professor J. H. Means, Professor J. W. Irvine, Dr. Wendell C. Peacock, Professor M. Stanley Livingston, Professor Robley D. Evans, Drs. R. W. Rawson and Jacob Lerman, the technical assistants Mrs. Phyllis Brown Shattuck, Miss Ann Gaurdo and Miss Mary Lennon as well as the nursing, surgical and medical staffs of the Massachusetts General Hospital. The speech of President Karl T. Compton of the Massachusetts Institute of Technology before a Harvard Medical School colloquium in the fall of 1936 served to inspire the senior author in the initiation of this investigative program.

1. Hertz, S.; Roberts, A., and Evans, R. D.: Radioactive Iodine as an Indicator in the Study of Thyroid Physiology, Proc. Soc. Exper. Biol. & Med. **38**: 510 (May) 1938. Hertz, S.; Roberts, A.; Means, J. H., and Evans, R. D.: Radioactive Iodine as an Indicator in Thyroid Physiology: II. Iodine Collection by Normal and Hyperplastic Thyroids in Rabbits, Am. J. Physiol. **128**: 565 (Feb.) 1940; Tr. Am. A. Study Goiter, 1939, p. 260. Hertz, S.: Radioactive Iodine as an Indicator in Thyroid Physiology: III. Observations on Rabbits and on Goiter Patients, Am. J. Roentgenol. **46**: 467 (Oct.) 1941. Hertz, S., and Roberts, A.: Radioactive Iodine as an Indicator in Thyroid Physiology: VI. Application of Radioactive Iodine in Therapy of Graves' Disease, J. Clin. Investigation **21**: 624 (Sept.) 1942. Hertz, Roberts and Salter.[2] Hertz and Roberts.[6]

From the data already obtained from tracer studies it was considered desirable to keep the total amount of iodide administered below 2 mg. of iodine in order to insure maximum collection by the thyroid.

Urinary iodine excretion was determined during the first seventy-two hours after the administration of radioiodine. An indirect estimate of the thyroid retention of radioactive iodine was thereby obtained, since an approximate balance exists between administered iodine on the one hand and the sum of thyroid iodine retention and urinary excretion on the other.

Urinary studies were carried out on aliquot portions of carefully collected twenty-four hour specimens, which were kept iced and corked during the collection periods.

It was early found [2] that significant amounts of the original dose were to be found only in the first three days' specimens. Fecal excretion was tested and was found to be so low as to be negligible for the purpose of these experiments.

In a few cases external gamma ray counter measurements were made of the activity of the thyroid of patients following the administration of radioactive iodine. Such measurements are difficult, for obvious reasons, to evaluate quantitatively. However, day to day measurements of this type can give good data on the variation of thyroid iodine content. They were performed in order to follow the loss of iodine from the thyroid following the initial uptake and to evaluate the effect of routine iodinization following the administration of radioactive iodine.

External counter measurements were roughly calibrated against actual direct measurements on the thyroid glands at operation and after chemical separation [2] in 2 patients, previously scheduled for surgery, who received therapeutic amounts of radioactive iodine.

Following the administration of radioactive iodine, routine iodine (nonradioactive) in the usual dosage of saturated solution of potassium iodide 5 minims (0.3 cc.) twice a day was begun at periods varying from one day to several weeks after the radioactive iodine dose.

The basal metabolic rate of the patients treated was tested frequently both before and after the radioactive iodine administration. Basal metabolic levels were taken prior to treatment to establish a measure of the degree of thyrotoxicosis present. In addition to the basal metabolic rate, weights, pulse rates and physical findings were recorded and the total clinical picture was used to evaluate the effects of treatment. No adverse effects, such as fever, nausea or irradiation sickness, were noted in this series of patients. No complaints were recorded regarding the taste of the medicament (since it is tasteless), nor were any local effects, either in the oral cavity or over the thyroid, encountered at the dosage levels used. No increase in the degree of thyrotoxicosis following the radioactive iodine treatment, per se, was recorded, although several test patients were kept uniodinized for three to four weeks prior to routine iodinization.

In most cases, after a period of two to four months following the radio-iodine administration, routine iodine therapy was stopped when an essentially normal basal metabolic rate had been maintained on iodine for a few weeks or months. Such basal metabolic rate response was taken to be indicative of good control of

2. Hertz, S.; Roberts, A., and Salter, W. T.: Radioactive Iodine as an Indicator in Thyroid Physiology: IV. The Metabolism of Iodine in Graves' Disease, J. Clin. Investigation **21**: 25 (Jan.) 1942.

profession, this form of treatment may well prove itself not only highly effective, safe and noninjurious but also cheap and of least inconvenience to the patient who may receive it while continuing at his normal pursuits. After a short period of hospitalization for the usual preliminary clinical studies and the administration of radio-iodine, the patient may be fully iodinized and released, to be followed as an ambulatory case.

SUMMARY

On the basis of a series of animal and clinical experiments using radioactive isotopes of iodine as a tracer in the study of thyroid physiology and iodine metabolism, the treatment of 29 cases of hyperthyroidism with internal irradiation by radioactive iodine was instituted. By careful excretion studies, external counter measurements over the thyroid gland and by planned operations in 2 cases, data were obtained which allow us to construct a formula for a procedure in treatment.

The addition of ordinary iodine therapy after the administration of radio-iodine offers many advantages in the clinical care of these patients and in the economy and safety of the procedure.

By an analysis, over a long period, of both the failures and successes in this series of 29 cases, it is shown that radioactive iodine when given in the dosage range of 5 to 25 millicuries to uniodinized patients with hyperthyroidism possessing goiters of 60 to 75 Gm. is highly effective as a cure of the disease in about 80 per cent of cases. When appreciable activity has been administered and subtotal thyroidectomy is resorted to, myxedema or hypometabolism may be expected to develop in a large fraction of the cases (100 per cent in 5 cases in this series).

THE TREATMENT OF HYPERTHYROIDISM WITH RADIOACTIVE IODINE

EARLE M. CHAPMAN, M.D.
and
ROBLEY D. EVANS, Ph.D.
Cambridge, Mass.

Roentgen treatment has been used for hyperthyroidism for many years. In 1923 Means and Holmes[1] pointed out that in this form of treatment about one third of the patients are cured, another third improved and another third not affected. Since 1923 ordinary iodine by mouth has been used as a preoperative method of quieting the hyperactive thyroid in preparation for surgery. Under iodine alone occasionally the patient and the doctor have been agreeably surprised to find that the symptoms and signs of hyperthyroidism disappeared, and a permanent remission apparently was effected. That x-ray treatment and iodine treatment sometimes cure hyperthyroidism led to the hope that some day a more effective, nonsurgical agent would be found. Then the MacKenzies[2] and Astwood[3] discovered that several chemical compounds inhibit the function of the thyroid in hyperthyroidism as well as under other circumstances. Several of these agents have been investigated, and until now thiouracil has been found to be most useful in the treatment of thyrotoxicosis.

Induced radioactivity was discovered in 1934, and that same year Fermi and his co-workers[4] in Italy prepared radioactive isotopes of iodine. Because the thyroid absorbs iodine selectively, it seemed likely that beta rays from iodine rendered radioactive would have a greater radiation effect than that derived from roentgen rays delivered through the skin and overlying tissues.

The use of radioactive iodine in the study of thyroid physiology was soon undertaken and reported first in 1938 by Hertz, Roberts and Evans.[5] Subsequently these and other investigators used various isotopes of radioactive iodine as tracers for the study of thyroid function[6] and it was found that in untreated hyperthyroidism the thyroid may take up as much as 80 per cent of a small dose (less than 2 mg.) of iodide within a few hours after oral administration.[7] This established the basis for therapeutic trials of radioactive iodine, and in 1942 Hertz and Roberts[8] published a preliminary report of the treatment in this manner of 10 patients. In this series the procedure was to give the radioactive iodine and follow this with ordinary iodine by mouth for a period of several months. However, our review in the clinic of these 10 cases of Hertz and Roberts, and an additional 18 so treated under the direction of Hertz, has led to the conclusion that it is difficult to decide whether those patients who improved were responding to the ordinary iodine, to the radioactive iodine or to their combination. The dosage of radioactive iodine given to these 28 patients averaged 5 millicuries in 1941, 10 millicuries in 1942 and 14.5 millicuries in 1943, the largest single dose being 21 millicuries. In April 1943 Dr. Hertz went on active duty in the Navy and asked us to continue with this study. The present report is on a series of 22 patients with hyperthyroidism treated only with radioactive iodine and with considerably higher doses. Although both Hertz and Roberts[8] and Hamilton and Lawrence[9] were encouraged by their therapeutic trials, the details of their findings have not yet been published.

METHODS AND DOSAGE

Selection and Care of Patients

The patients selected in the Thyroid Clinic of the Massachusetts General Hospital for radioactive iodine therapy were judged by several physicians to be thyrotoxic on the basis of classic disease pattern accompanied with constantly elevated basal metabolic rates. All patients had thyroids estimated to be at least two to three times normal in size. All but 3 were kept free from all forms of treatment, especially iodine, for at least four weeks prior to giving radioactive iodine. For the administration of the drug they were usually hospitalized for a time adequate to obtain levels of their basal metabolic rate, then given radioactive iodine by mouth—simply a drink of what tastes like rather stale water.

Aided in part by a grant from the John and Mary R. Markle Foundation.

From the Thyroid Clinic of the Massachusetts General Hospital (Dr. Chapman) and the Radioactivity Center of the Department of Physics of the Massachusetts Institute of Technology (Dr. Evans).

1. Means, J. H., and Holmes, G. W.: Further Observations on the Roentgen Ray Treatment of Toxic Goiter, Arch. Int. Med. **31**: 303 (March) 1923.
2. MacKenzie, C. G., and MacKenzie, J. B.: Effect of Sulfonamides and Thioureas on the Thyroid Gland and Basal Metabolism, Endocrinology **32**: 185 (Feb.) 1943.
3. Astwood, E. B.: Treatment of Hyperthyroidism with Thiourea and Thiouracil, J. A. M. A. **122**: 78 (May 8) 1943.
4. Fermi, E.: Radioactivity Induced by Neutron Bombardment, Nature, London **133**: 757 (May 19) 1934.
5. Hertz, S.; Roberts, A., and Evans, R. D.: Radioactive Iodine as an Indicator in the Study of Thyroid Physiology, Proc. Soc. Exper. Biol. & Med. **38**: 510 (May) 1938.
6. Rawson, R. W.: Radio Iodine: Its Use as a Tool in the Study of Thyroid Physiology, to be published. Hamilton, J. G., and Soley, M. H.: Studies in Iodine Metabolism by the Use of a New Radioactive Isotope of Iodine, Am. J. Physiol. **127**: 557 (Oct.) 1939. Le Blond, C. P.; Sue P., and Chamorre, A.: Passage de l'iode radi-oactif dans la thyroide d'animaux sans hypophyse, Compt. rend. Soc. de biol. **133**: 540, 1940.
7. Hertz, S.; Roberts, A., and Salter, W. T.: Radioactive Iodine as an Indicator in Thyroid Physiology: IV. The Metabolism of Iodine in Graves' Disease, J. Clin. Investigation **21**: 25 (Jan.) 1942.
8. Hertz, S., and Roberts, A.: Application of Radioactive Iodine in Therapy of Graves' Disease, J. Clin. Investigation **21**: 624 (Sept.) 1942.
9. Hamilton, J. G., and Lawrence, J. H.: Recent Clinical Developments in the Therapeutic Application of Radio-Phosphorus and Radio-Iodine, J. Clin. Investigation **21**: 624 (Sept.) 1942.

Figure 8. (a) JAMA: May 11, 1946 MGH's Saul Hertz/MIT's Arthur Roberts VII. The use of radioactive iodine therapy in hyperthyroidism and (b) JAMA: May 11, 1946 MGH's Earl Chapman/MIT's Robley Evans the treatment of hyperthyroidism with radioactive iodine. Documentation of unethical publishing practices…stolen intellectual property.

2.2. RAI: the first and gold standard of targeted cancer therapy

Dr. Hertz responded to MGH's Director, Dr. Paxton's letter on March 12, 1946, "It is a coincidence that my new research project is in Cancer of the Thyroid which I believe holds the key to the larger problem of Cancer in general." The next day March 13, 1946, Hertz writes to MIT President Compton, "I have certain ideas in the field of Cancer of the Thyroid which are even more intriguing from a physician's point of view than the cure of Graves' disease with Radioactive Iodine without operation....the cancer field is relatively virgin territory both from the standpoint of actual knowledge or prognostic attack." Hertz goes on in the same correspondence to make note, "Only recently a group of workers in England have reported the regular production of Cancer of the Thyroid in animals by a series of steps which are subject to analysis by means of RAI as a tracer. The relationship of this project to the one on Graves' disease will be evident to you."

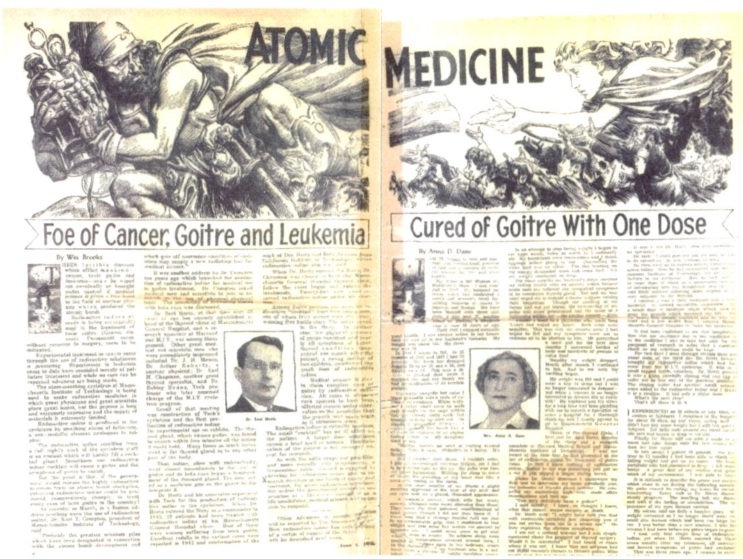
ATOMIC MEDICINE

Foe of Cancer, Goitre and Leukemia

Cured of Goitre With One Dose

Figure 9. The *American Weekly* June 2, 1946 Dr Hertz states, "...demand is expected for radioactive iodine and as research develops in the field of cancer and leukemia for other radioactive medicines.".

The American Weekly, June 2, 1946, quoted Dr. Hertz as stating, "...demand is expected for radioactive iodine and as research develops in the fields of cancer and leukemia for radioactive medicines" (**Figure 9**).

On September 9, 1946, The Radioactive Isotope Research Fund was registered in Boston, Massachusetts. The Fund established The Radioactive Isotope Research Institute with Clinical and Laboratory facilities on Commonwealth Avenue in Boston and on 5th Avenue in New York City. Dr. Hertz reached out to Montefiore Hospital's Dr. S.M. Seidlin to be the Associative Director. His brother Dr. Roy Hertz was the oncologist. Roy Hertz went on to The National Institutes of Health after his brother Saul's death to win a Lasker Award. Dr. Eugene Nelson was the Physicist (**Figure 10**).

SAUL HERTZ, M. D.
(Director of the Radioactive Isotope Research Fund*
270 Commonwealth Avenue, Boston, Massachusetts)
Announces
The Establishment of a Memorial to the
AARON DANIEL and BERTHA HERTZ Family
of Cleveland, Ohio
to be known as

The Radioactive Isotope Research Institute

with Clinical and Laboratory Facilities at
Commonwealth Avenue, Boston, Massachusetts
and
New York City Headquarters at 932 5th Avenue**

To Be Devoted to the Application of
Nuclear Physics to Medical Investigation,
Diagnosis and Treatment.

*Registered at Boston, Mass. on the 9th Day of September, 1946.
**Dr. S. M. Seidlin, Associate Director; Dr. Roy Hertz, Oncologist; Dr. Eugene Nelson, Physicist.

Figure 10. September 9, 1946 announcement of the world's first Radioactive Isotope Institute. Dr Saul Hertz established the institute and served as the director.

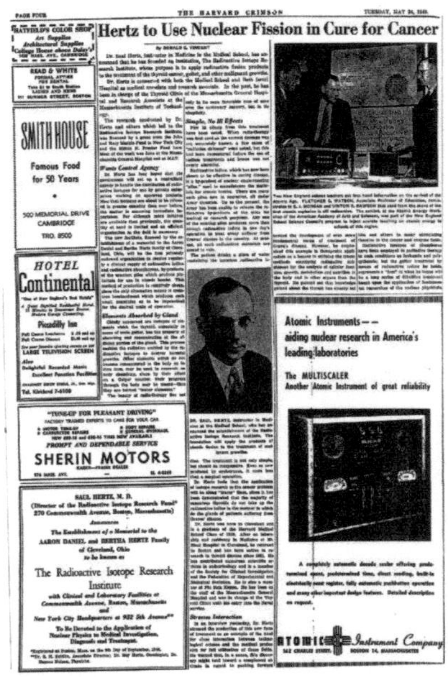
THE HARVARD CRIMSON

Hertz to Use Nuclear Fission in Cure for Cancer

SMITH HOUSE
Famous Food for 50 Years

HOTEL Continental

SHERIN MOTORS

Atomic Instruments — aiding nuclear research in America's leading laboratories

Figure 11. *The Harvard Crimson*, May 24, 1949 Hertz To Use Nuclear Fission in Cure for Cancer "&he (Hertz)emphasized this example in therapeutic application as a beacon in utilizing the tracer methods employing radioactive substances in other organs than the thyroid.".

http://dx.doi.org/10.5772/64609

Dr. Hertz while at The Beth Israel Hospital explored the use of RAI in treating thyroid cancer patients. In a radio broadcast on Boston's WEEI's Yankee Network, November 18, 1948, Hertz discussed extensively RAI treatment being used in treating thyroid cancer at The Beth Israel Hospital.

The headline of *The Harvard Crimson* May 24, 1949, reads "Hertz to Use Fission in Cure for Cancer." In the text of the article is "Dr. Hertz feels that the application of isotope research to the cancer problem will be along the 'tracer' lines, since it has been demonstrated that the majority of cancerous thyroids do not take up the radioactive iodine in the manner in which do the glands of patients suffering from Graves' disease...he (Hertz) emphasized this example in therapeutic application as a beacon in utilizing the tracer methods... (**Figure 11**).

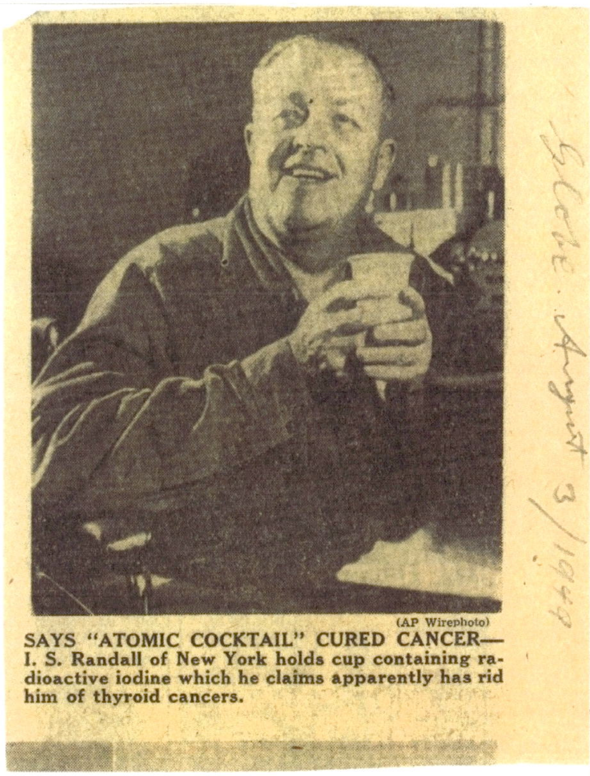
(AP Wirephoto)
SAYS "ATOMIC COCKTAIL" CURED CANCER— I. S. Randall of New York holds cup containing radioactive iodine which he claims apparently has rid him of thyroid cancers.
Globe. August 3/1949

Figure 12. Boston Globe August 3, 1949 "atomic cocktail" cured cancer.

Figure 12 shows Boston Globe photo of a man drinking an "atomic cocktail."

A patient emailed this in March 2016, *Treatment with radioactive iodine knocked the thyroid cancer (metastatic to a little bit of bone and lung) right out of me, exceeding my doctor's expectations... I am now 81. We have a large family. Many were praying for me. The cure delivered on the wings of prayer was Dr. Saul Hertz's discovery, the miracle of radioactive iodine. Few can equal such a powerful and precious gift.*

Author details

Barbara Hertz

Address all correspondence to: htziev@aol.com

Dr. Saul Hertz Archives, Greenwich, CT, USA

References

[1] Bagley D. The saga of radioiodine therapy. *Endocrine News* 2016: 27–30.

[2] Hertz BE. Response to: "radioactive Iodine: a slice of History." *Thyroid: Official Journal of the American Thyroid Association* 2014; 24: 177–178.

[3] Hertz S, Roberts A. Radioactive iodine in the study of thyroid physiology: the use of radioactive iodine therapy in hyperthyroidism. *Journal of the American Medical Association* 1946; 131: 81–86.

[4] Chapman EM, Evans RD. The treatment of hyperthyroidism with radioactive iodine. *Journal of the American Medical Association* 1946; 131: 86–91.

[5] MGH. The Story of Saul Hertz. https://youtu.be/34Qhm8CeMuc, Youtube, 2016.

Chapter 2

Molecular Alterations and Expression Dynamics in the Etiopathogenesis of Thyroid Cancer

Syed Mudassar, Mosin S. Khan, Shariq R. Masoodi,
Khursheed A. Wani, Mahboob Ul Hussain and
Khurshid I. Andrabi

Additional information is available at the end of the chapter

http://dx.doi.org/10.5772/63740

Abstract

Thyroid carcinoma is the most prevalent endocrine malignancy and accounts for 2% of all human cancers. In the past decade, knowledge of genetic alterations of thyroid cancer (TC) has rapidly expanded, which has provided new insights into thyroid cancer etiology and has offered novel diagnostic tools and prognostic markers that enable improved and personalized management of thyroid cancer patients. Alterations in key signaling effectors seem to be the hallmark of distinct forms of thyroid neoplasia. Mutations or rearrangements in genes that encode Mitogen activated protein kinase (MAPK) pathway effectors seem to be required for transformation. Mutations in *BRAF* were the most recently identified MAPK effector in thyroid cancer. *BRAF* V600E is the most common alteration in sporadic papillary carcinoma. Three *RAS* proto-oncogenes (*NRAS, HRAS* & *KRAS*) are implicated in human thyroid tumorigenesis. High incidence of thyroid cancer worldwide indicates the importance of studying genetic alterations that lead to its carcinogenesis. *BRAF* and *RAS* alterations represent a novel indicator of the progression and aggressiveness of thyroid carcinogenesis. The GSα-adenylyl cyclase-cyclic AMP (cAMP) cascade is effected in thyroid cancer. Promoter hypermethylation of multiple genes especially *TSHR* has been identified to play a role in thyroid cancers, in particular showing a close association with *BRAF* mutational status. So, the main aim of the study was to elucidate the involvement of *BRAF* and *RAS* gene mutations along with BRAF expression and thyroid-stimulating hormone receptor (TSHR) hypermethylation in North Indian patients and investigate their association with clinicopathological characteristics.

We screened exon 15 of *BRAF* gene and exons 1 and 2 of *RAS* genes (*HRAS, KRAS*, and *NRAS*) in 60 consecutive thyroid tissue (tumor and adjacent normal) samples. Overall mutations in *BRAF* were found to be 25% (15 of 60) affecting codon 600 (valine to glutamine) and restricted only to papillary thyroid cancer and well-differentiated grade.

BRAF mutations were significantly associated with well-differentiated disease and elevated thyroid-stimulating hormone (TSH) levels ($P < 0.05$). Overall, increased expression of BRAF was found in 90% (54 of 60) of thyroid cancer cases and significantly associated with nonsmokers. Totally, 86.7% (13 of 15) of *BRAF* mutation-positive patients were having BRAF protein overexpression compared to 91.2% (41 of 45) of patients with wild-type *BRAF* status ($P > 0.05$). We screened 60 consecutive thyroid tumor and adjacent normal tissues for mutations, if any, in the exons 1 and 2 of *RAS* genes (*HRAS, KRAS,* and *NRAS*) and 140 blood samples from thyroid cancer patients for *HRAS* T81C polymorphism in codon 27 in comparison with 170 cancer-free controls from a Kashmiri population. Thyroid tumor tissue samples were devoid of any mutation, but a frequent nucleotide change at position 81 (T > C) in exon 1 of *HRAS* gene was seen. In *HRAS* T81C SNP, frequencies of TT, TC, and CC genotypes among cases were 41.4, 38.6, and 20.0%, while in controls genotype frequencies were 84.1, 11.7, and 4.2%, respectively. A significant difference was observed in variant allele frequencies (TC + CC) between the cases and controls (58.6 vs. 16%) with odds ratio of 7.4 (CI = 04.3–12.7; $P < 0.05$). Interestingly, combined TC and CC genotype abundantly presented in follicular thyroid tumor ($P < 0.05$). Moreover, a significant association of the variant allele (TC + CC) was found with nonsmokers ($P < 0.05$). *TSHR* gene was found to be hypermethylated in 25% (15 of 60) of the cases with strong association with elevated TSH levels (OR = 4.0, $P = 0.02$). *TSHR* promoter was hypermethylated in 73.3% (11 of 15) of patients with *BRAF* V600E mutation compared to 26.7% (4 of 15) of patients having absence of *TSHR* promoter methylation and the association was significant ($P < 0.05$).

We conclude that both mutational events and overexpression of *BRAF* gene are highly implicated in pathogenesis of thyroid cancer and the BRAF protein overexpression is independent of the *BRAF* mutational status of thyroid cancer patients. *RAS* gene mutation does not prevail in this population. Contrary to this, *HRAS* T81C polymorphism moderately increases thyroid cancer risk with rare allele as a predictive marker for follicular tumors. Our study showed a high implication of *TSHR* gene methylation and its significant association with *BRAF* V600E mutation in thyroid tumors, depicting a positive connection between *TSHR* pathway and MAP kinase pathway.

Keywords: polymerase chain reaction, papillary thyroid cancer, thyroid-stimulating hormone, benign thyroid disease, lymph node metastasis, follicular thyroid cancer, mutation, polymorphism, gene, hypermethylation, genotype, expression

1. Introduction

Thyroid gland is the largest endocrine gland comprised of follicular cells and C cells. It synthesizes, stores, and secretes triiodothyronine (T3) and thyroxine (T4) (**Figure 1**). Follicular cells comprise most of the epithelium and are responsible for iodine uptake and thyroid hormone synthesis. C cells are dedicated to the production of the calcium-regulating hormone calcitonin [1].

http://dx.doi.org/10.5772/63740

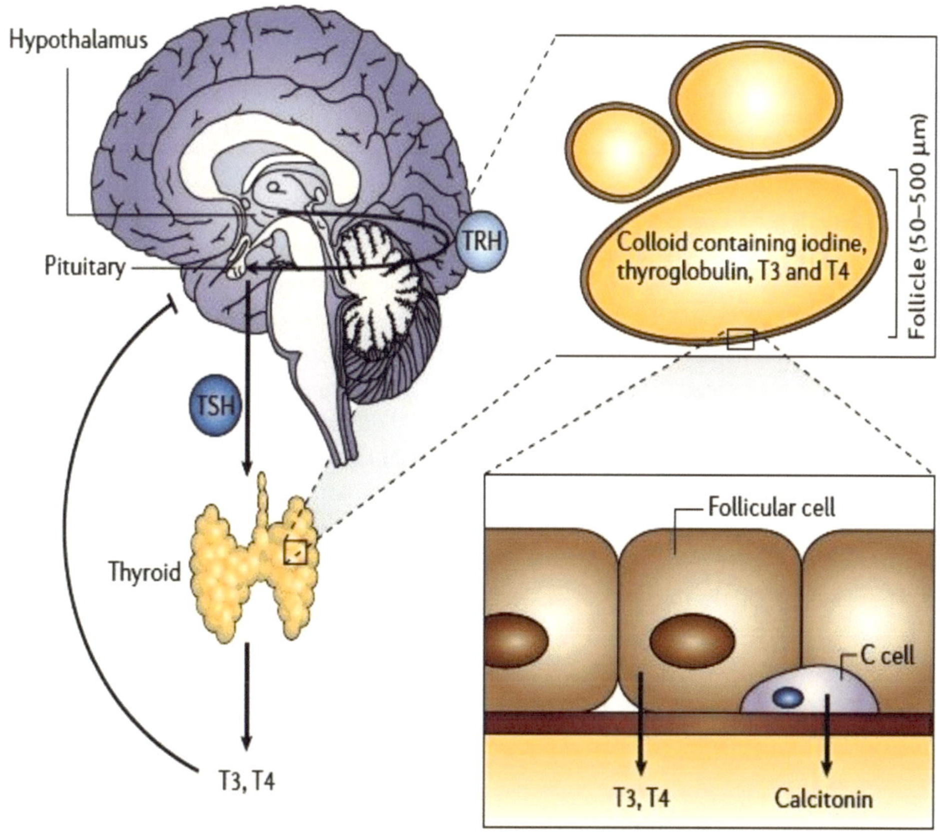

Figure 1. The thyroid gland.

At molecular level, cancer is caused by molecular defects in cell function resulting from common types of alterations to a cell's genes. Cancer is a disease of abnormal gene expression which may occur due to DNA mutation, translocation, amplification, deletion, loss of heterozygosity, etc. The overall result is an imbalance of cell replication and cell death that leads to unregulated growth and spread of cells in different parts of body [2, 3].

Thyroid cancer (TC) typically occurs in *thyroid nodules* and is relatively common, occurring in 6% of adult women and 2% of adult men which can be detected by palpation and imaging in a large proportion of adults. Approximately 90% of thyroid malignancies are well-differentiated thyroid carcinomas arising from thyroid follicular epithelial cells, which are classified as papillary or follicular based on histopathological criteria, whereas 3–5% of cancers originate from parafollicular or C cells. Follicular adenoma is a benign tumor that may serve as a precursor for some follicular carcinomas. Recurrence occurs in 20–40% of patients in spite of the fact that differentiated thyroid carcinomas are usually curable by the combination of surgery, radioiodine ablation, and thyroid-stimulating hormone suppressive therapy [4] due to cellular dedifferentiation which is accompanied by more aggressive growth, metastatic spread, and loss of iodide uptake ability, making the tumor resistant to the traditional therapeutic modalities and radioiodine [5]. Knowledge of genetic alterations occurring in thyroid cancer has rapidly expanded in the past decade. This improved knowledge has provided new insights into thyroid cancer etiology and has offered novel diagnostic tools and prognostic markers that enable improved and personalized management of patients with thyroid nodules [6].

TC is the most common malignancy of the endocrine system. It accounts for approximately 2% of all newly diagnosed cancer cases and majority of endocrine cancer related deaths each year [7, 8]. An estimated 12.66 million people were diagnosed with cancer across the world in 2008, and 7.56 million people died from the disease. This equates to around 188 cases for every 100,000 people (using the crude rate). Among the 20 most commonly diagnosed cancers worldwide, thyroid cancer figures on 17th (2% of all cancers) number (2008 estimates) [9]. There were 213,179 new thyroid cancer cases and 163,000 cases among females worldwide by the year 2008 [10]. Its prevalence continues to rise; in 2008, it became the sixth most diagnosed cancer among women in United States Around 56,460 cases (men – 13,250, women – 43,210) and 1780 deaths (men – 780, women – 1000) from thyroid cancer occurred in 2012 [11]. The data indicated that there were 60,220 new cases in 2013, accounting for 3.6% of all new cancer cases. There were 1850 thyroid cancer-related deaths in 2013, accounting for 0.3% of all cancer deaths. There are currently ~534,973 TC patients in USA. The reasons for increased incidence are unclear, with potential explanations including increased screening, more widespread diagnostic testing of asymptomatic thyroid nodules, changing demographics, and environmental risk factor. TC accounts for approximately 10% of malignancies diagnosed in persons aged 15–29 years. Follicular cancers include papillary thyroid cancer (PTC, 80%), follicular thyroid cancer (FTC, up to 11%), Hürthle cell cancer (3%), and anaplastic thyroid cancer (ATC, 2%). Medullary thyroid cancer (MTC) accounts for about 4% of thyroid cancers [12]. As expected from the size of Asia's population, the majority of cancer cases occurred there. Between 1984 and 1993, over 5614 thyroid cancer cases were recorded in India which included 2007 males and 3617 females and the age standardized rate (ASR) in 1993 was $1.0/\text{year}/10^5$ and $1.9/\text{year}/10^5$ for males and females, respectively [13]. The age-adjusted incidence rates of thyroid cancer per 100,000 are about 1 for males and 1.8 for females as per the Mumbai Cancer Registry, which covered a population of 9.81 million subjects. The commonest cancer type was papillary, followed by follicular cancer. TC is the 8th most common cancer in the valley of Kashmir and 7th most common cancer among women of Kashmir valley. Among all types of cancers in the Kashmir valley, the frequency of TC has increased from 2.3% in 1995 to 5.4% in 2010, keeping overall frequency of 3.2% [14].

2. Classification of thyroid tumors

The classification of thyroid tumors is given by the World Health Organization (WHO) and Armed Forces Institute of Pathology (AFIP) with slight difference [15]. According to AFIP, priority is given to the cell of origin and incorporating, in each cell type, special tumor types and subtypes designated as "variants". Classification scheme adopted by the Armed Forces Institute of Pathology (AFIP) is depicted in **Figure 2**.

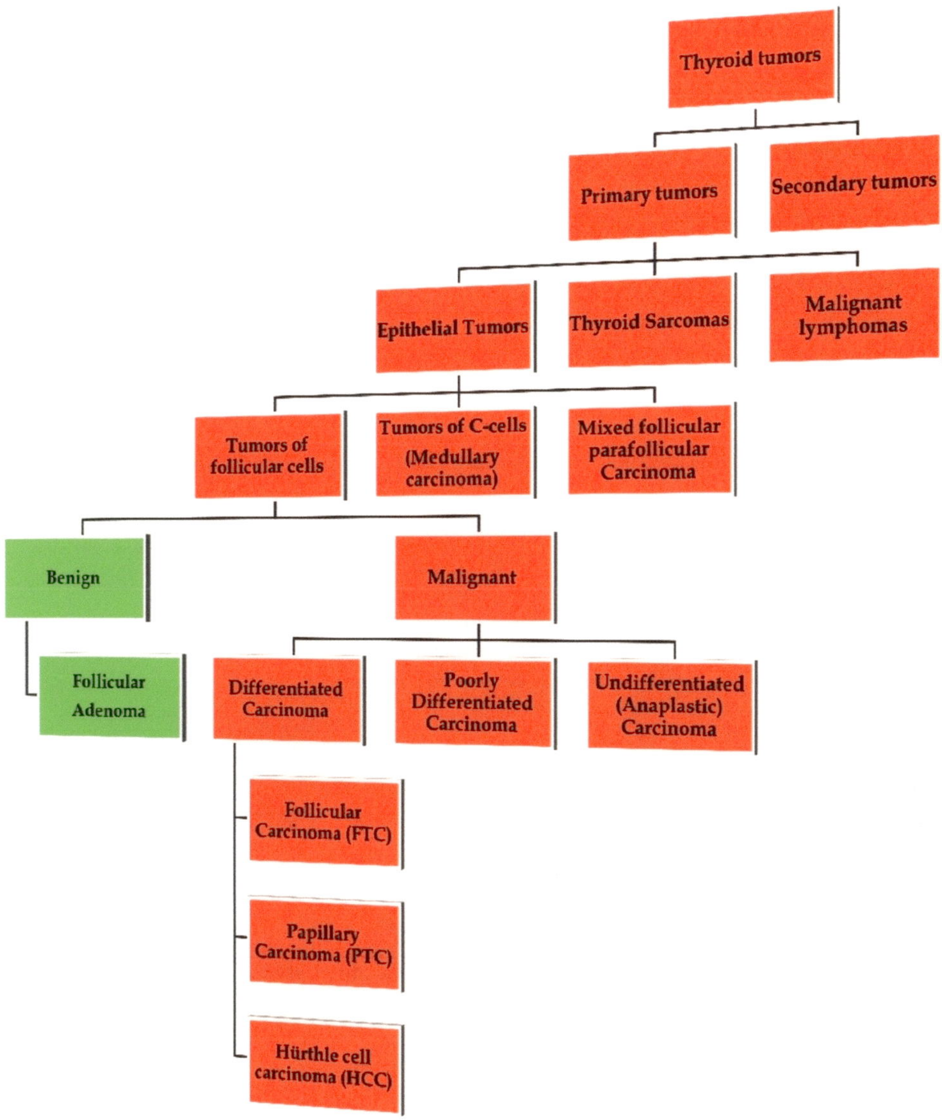

Figure 2. Classification of thyroid tumors as per Armed Forces Institute of Pathology (AFIP).

3. Staging of thyroid carcinoma

There are different stages of TC as designated by the American Joint Committee on Cancer (AJCC) [15]. The SEER modified 7th edition AJCC staging is given in **Tables 1** and **2**.

Primary tumor (T)	
TX	Primary tumor cannot be assessed
T0	No evidence of primary tumor is found
T1	Tumor size ≤ 2 cm in greatest dimension and is limited to the thyroid
T1a	Tumor ≤ 1 cm, limited to the thyroid
T1b	Tumor > 1 cm but ≤ 2 cm in greatest dimension, limited to the thyroid
T2	Tumor size > 2 cm but ≤ 4 cm, limited to the thyroid
T3	Tumor size > 4 cm, limited to the thyroid or any tumor with minimal extrathyroidal extension (e.g., extension to sternothyroid muscle or perithyroid soft tissues)
T4a	Moderately advanced disease; tumor of any size extending beyond the thyroid capsule to invade subcutaneous soft tissues, larynx, trachea, esophagus, or recurrent laryngeal nerve
T4b	Very advanced disease; tumor invades prevertebral fascia or encases carotid artery or mediastinal vessel
All anaplastic carcinomas are considered stage IV:	
T4a	Intrathyroidal anaplastic carcinoma
T4b	Anaplastic carcinoma with gross extrathyroid extension
Regional lymph nodes (N)	
Regional lymph nodes are the central compartment, lateral cervical, and upper mediastinal lymph nodes:	
NX	Regional nodes cannot be assessed
N0	No regional lymph node metastasis
N1	Regional lymph node metastasis
N1a	Metastases to level VI (pretracheal, paratracheal, and prelaryngeal/Delphian lymph nodes)
N1b	Metastases to unilateral, bilateral, or contralateral cervical (levels I, II, III, IV, or V) or retropharyngeal or superior mediastinal lymph nodes (level VII)
Distant metastasis (M)	
M0	No distant metastasis is found
M1	Distant metastasis is present

Table 1. TNM classification for thyroid cancer (SEER modified 7th edition AJCC staging).

Stage grouping			
Separate stage groupings are recommended for papillary or follicular (differentiated), medullary, and anaplastic (undifferentiated) carcinoma			
Papillary and follicular thyroid cancer (age < 45y):			
Stage	**T**	**N**	**M**
I	Any T	Any N	M0
II	Any T	Any N	M1
Papillary and follicular; differentiated (age ≥ 45y):			
Stage	**T**	**N**	**M**
I	T1	N0	M0
II	T2	N0	M0

http://dx.doi.org/10.5772/63740

Stage grouping			
Separate stage groupings are recommended for papillary or follicular (differentiated), medullary, and anaplastic (undifferentiated) carcinoma			
III	T3	N0	M0
IVA	T1-3	N1a	M0
	T4a	N1b	M0
IVB	T4b	Any N	M0
IVC	Any T	Any N	M1
Anaplastic carcinoma (all anaplastic carcinomas are considered stage IV):			
Stage	**T**	**N**	**M**
IVA	T4a	Any N	M0
IVB	T4b	Any N	M0
IVC	Any T	Any N	M1
Medullary carcinoma (all age groups):			
Stage	**T**	**N**	**M**
I	T1	N0	M0
II	T2, T3	N0	M0
III	T1–T3	N1a	M0
IVA	T4a	N0	M0
	T4a	N1a	M0
	T1	N1b	M0
	T2	N1b	M0
	T3	N1b	M0
	T4a	N1b	M0
	T4a	N0, N1b	M0
	T1-T4a	N1b	M0
IVB	T4b	Any N	M0
IVC	Any T	Any N	M1

Table 2. Stage grouping of thyroid cancer (SEER modified 7th edition AJCC staging).

4. Risk factors of thyroid cancer

4.1. Gender and age

Females exhibit a better prognosis than men. TC is 2–4 times more frequent in women. It is rare in patients aged <16 years, presenting an annual incidence of 0.02–0.3/100.000 [16, 17]. Its incidence increases with ageing, and the average age at diagnosis is 45–50 years.

4.2. Ethnic differences

TC incidence has a geographic and ethnic variability. The incidence of TC in areas such as Iceland, Hawaii, the Philippines, Japan, and Israel is higher than in North America, Canada, and US. In US, the TC is more frequent in Caucasian descent subjects. All these findings suggest that such differences may be attributable to both environmental (e.g., dietary habits) and genetic factors [18].

4.3. Previous exposure to ionizing radiation

Previous exposure to ionizing radiation for external irradiation of the neck increases the incidence of thyroid nodules, either benign or malignant. Palpable nodules are detected in 20–30% of people exposed to radiation and in pediatric patients undergoing radiation therapy for oncological and hematological malignancies such as lymphoma or leukemia [19, 20].

4.4. Age at the time of irradiation

Irradiation is no longer an increased risk after 15–20 years of age. In children exposed to doses of 1 Gy, the excess risk for TC is equal to 7.7 [21]. Several studies have shown an increased risk of TC in children aged between 5 months and 10 years after the Chernobyl nuclear disaster [22].

4.5. Previous history of benign thyroid disease (BTD)

People with benign thyroid conditions like an enlarged thyroid (goiter), thyroid nodules (adenomas), and inflammation of the thyroid (thyroiditis) are more likely to develop thyroid cancer. Approximately 1 in 5 thyroid cancers (20%) occur in people who have had a BTD in the past [23].

4.6. Contribution of iodine in the food

In areas of sufficient iodine intake, PTC is more prevalent (80% of TCs), whereas in iodine-deficient areas, FTCs and ATCs are 2–3 times more frequently reported as compared to areas with adequate iodine intake [24].

4.7. Body mass index

High body mass index (BMI) has been shown as a risk factor for TC according to several case-control studies. There is a fivefold risk in obese men and 2 times in obese women. In postmenopausal women, weight gain of >14% positively correlates with the onset of TC [25].

4.8. Hormonal factors

According to the period of life in which thyroid cancer occurs, the female:male incidence ratio is different. In women of child bearing age, this ratio is about 4:1 and 1.5:1 in older, prepuberal, and menopause individuals [26]. TSH regulates the growth and function of the thyroid gland [27]. Growth of some thyroid cancers is dependent on TSH secretion and suppression of TSH release by administration of thyroxin is often an effective treatment for thyroid carcinomas. The thyroxine-binding globulin level in normal females is 10–20% higher than in males and in pregnancy, a 50% increase in the level of thyroxine-binding globulin results in a similar magnitude increase in TSH level [28]. It therefore appears likely that TSH levels of non pregnant normal females will be elevated above the level in males at some point in the menstrual cycle although not necessarily throughout the cycle. An elevated risk was also reported in women who used estrogens for gynecological problems. In some studies, higher levels of estrogen receptors (ERs) were found in neoplastic than in normal thyroid tissues [29]. The ligand-bound dimer ER can interact with an estrogen-responsive element, resulting in transcriptional activation of the target gene [30]. 17 β-estradiol stimulates cell cycle progression early in G1 phase by induction of cyclin D1 gene expression. In different cell lines, the induction of cell growth was found to correlate with increased expression of cyclin D1 protein levels [31].

4.9. Smoking status

Although relatively little is known about the etiology of thyroid cancer beyond its association with radiation exposure and some previous thyroid disorders [32], data are slowly accumulating as to the protective effect of cigarette smoking on this disease. Thyroid cancer has been negatively associated with cigarette smoking in a number of studies, possibly consistent with the greater occurrence of the disease in women than in men [33]. There are at least five distinct proposed mechanisms for the effect of tobacco smoke on thyroid function. The *first* one relates to a smoking-related reduction in TSH secretion, as it has long been hypothesized that elevated levels of TSH may increase the risk of thyroid cancer. The lower body weight among smokers compared to nonsmokers is a *second* proposed explanation, as increased body weight was associated with a slightly increased thyroid cancer risk in the above-mentioned pooled analysis. A *third* possible biological pathway lies in the potential anti-estrogenic effect of cigarette smoke; a role for estrogen in the etiology of thyroid cancer is hypothesized because of the higher incidence of this cancer in females relative to males [34]. The *fourth* is higher levels of thyroxine-binding globulin and testosterone among smokers compared to nonsmokers and the *fifth* is the higher levels of thyrotoxins in tobacco smoke in heavy smokers compared to light and moderate smokers [35].

4.10. Oxidative stress

Oxidative stress (OS) is a state of excessive free radicals and reactive metabolites. In essence, OS represents an imbalance between the production of oxidants and their elimination by anti oxidative systems in the body. Many studies have linked OS to thyroid cancer by showing its association with abnormally regulated oxidative or antioxidative molecules [36].

5. Molecular biology of thyroid cancer

Thyroid tumors represent an appropriate model for the study of epithelial neoplastic transformation. The roles of somatic mutations, gene rearrangement (s), and level of gene expression in carcinogenesis are now well established. The application of molecular techniques to thyroid tumors has focused particular attention on the role of point mutations activating (or inhibiting) the genes for the TSH receptor (*TSHR*), *RAS*, *BRAF*, *Gsp*, *P53*, etc, specific rearrangements of the oncogenes *RET* and *TRK* and alterations in the pattern of expression of the oncogene *BRAF*, *MET*, etc [37]. The theory of sequential progression of well-differentiated thyroid carcinoma to poorly differentiated and undifferentiated thyroid carcinoma is because of genetic imbalances [38]. **Figure 3** depicts the model of multi-step carcinogenesis of thyroid neoplasms.

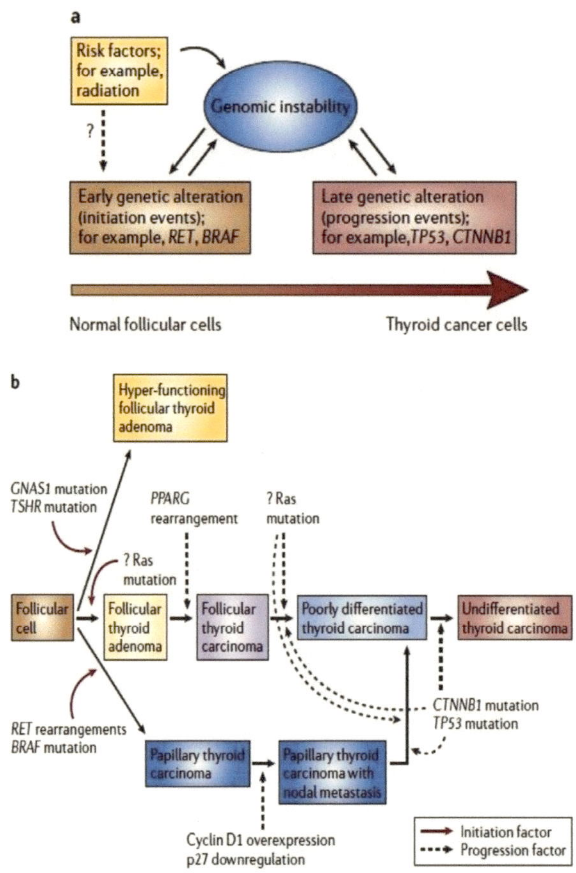

Figure 3. Model of multi-step carcinogenesis of thyroid neoplasms. The proposed model of thyroid carcinogenesis is based on general concepts and specific pathways. (a) Risk factors, such as exposure to radiation, induce genomic instability through direct and indirect mechanisms, resulting in early genetic alterations. (b) Scheme of step-wise dedifferentiation of follicular cell-derived thyroid cancer along with genetic alterations.

Biomarkers, also known as *molecular markers, biological markers*, or *tumor markers* have become useful not only for detecting thyroid cancer early, but also for detecting recurrent and persistent disease and for predicting the effectiveness of surgical removal, radioiodine ablation, and chemotherapy since the past 40 years, and they include genetic mutations and molecular changes. Nowadays, high-throughput genomic and proteomic assays are being used to identify a multitude of biomarker signature for each tumor type at any given stage [39, 40]. These biomarkers are discussed in detail as under.

5.1. Serum-based biomarkers

Serum biomarkers represent the first generation of thyroid biomarkers. Ideally, a serum biomarker is one that is highly sensitive and specific, can establish diagnostic certainty and can be easily measured.

5.1.1. Calcitonin

Para follicular C cells secrete calcitonin, which is a serum-based marker for MTC [41]. Overall, calcitonin is more sensitive for documenting recurrent tumor but CEA levels are better predictors of tumor aggressiveness. *RET* mutations have replaced calcitonin to a greater because it is more sensitive and specific [42].

5.1.2. Thyroglobulin

Tg is a valuable serum marker for detecting recurrent or persistent well-differentiated thyroid cancer of follicular cell origin, as there should be no Tg present after a total thyroidectomy unless residual thyroid tissue is present. More recently, molecular studies using reverse transcriptase-polymerase chain reaction (RT-PCR) have been used to measure tissue-tumor-specific messenger RNA levels of Tg in the circulation [43].

5.2. Mutation-based biomarkers

Genetic alterations in thyroid tumors can be divided into two categories: *inheritable (germline) mutations and sporadic (somatic) mutations*. Investigations into the inheritable and sporadic mutations in thyroid cancer have proceeded in parallel with one another. The single known inheritable gene mutation associated with thyroid cancer is a point mutation in the *RET* proto-oncogene that causes medullary thyroid cancer [44]. The first sporadic mutation identified in thyroid cancer was described in 1987 and involved a genetic defect in the *RAS* protein family [45] followed by somatic *RET/PTC* translocations in 1990 and *P53/NTRK1* mutations in 1992. In the year 2000, *PAX8/PPARgamma* translocations were found in follicular thyroid cancers [46] followed by the discovery of *BRAF* mutations, first in melanoma, then in PTC in 2003 [47]. The mutation-based biomarkers are discussed below in detail.

5.2.1. Chromosomal rearrangements

RET/PTC is a chromosomal rearrangement found in PTC. These chimeric genes contain the portion of *RET* encoding intact tyrosine kinase domain fused to an active promoter of another gene that drives the expression and ligand-independent dimerization of the *RET/PTC* protein, leading tumorigenesis in thyroid cells [48]. *RET/PTC1* and *RET/PTC3* are the most common rearrangement types in which *RET* is fused to either *CCDC6* (also known as H4) or *NCOA4* (also known as *ELE1* or *RFG*), respectively [49]. Both of these rearrangement types are paracentric, intrachromosomal inversions. *RET/PTC2* and nine more recently discovered types of *RET/PTC* rearrangements are all interchromosomal rearrangements formed by *RET* fusion to genes located on different chromosomes [50]. *RET/PTC* rearrangement occurs in 10–20% of PTC. Thyroid adenomas and other benign nodules and nonneoplastic thyroid lesions have 10–45% of *RET/PTC* rearrangements [51]. Chromosomal rearrangements involving another receptor tyrosine kinase gene, *NTRK1* have been reported to occur in up to 10–15% of PTC in some series of patients although the prevalence of this rearrangement in papillary carcinomas from many geographical areas is probably <2–5% [52]. *PAX8/PPARγ* rearrangement leads to the fusion between a portion of the paired-box gene 8 gene (*PAX8)* and peroxisome proliferator-activated receptor gamma gene (*PPARγ*). The fusion oncoprotein contributes to malignant transformation by targeting several cellular pathways. The *PPARγ* rearrangements are found in follicular thyroid adenomas (0–31%) and follicular thyroid carcinomas (25–63%) [53].

5.2.2. RET point mutations (familial medullary thyroid cancer)

The *RET* gene encodes the *RET* receptor expressed in neuroendocrine and neural cells. The nucleotide sequence of the *RET* gene was determined and in 1989 and was mapped to chromosome 10q11.2 [54, 55]. In 1993, the specific germline mutations of the *RET* gene were found to develop MTC [56]. Point mutations of the *RET* gene that causes MTC result in a gain of function of the *RET* receptor. The hereditary *RET* point mutations are the most specific biomarkers in clinical use today for diagnosing patients who will develop MTC. No other currently used thyroid cancer biomarker is as sensitive or specific.

5.2.3. RAS mutations

The beginning of *RAS* research can be traced back to 1964 when Jennifer Harvey observed that a preparation of a murine leukemia virus, taken from a leukemic rat, induced sarcomas in newborn rodents [57]. The nucleotide sequences of the v-h-ras and v-k-ras oncogenes were not published until the autumn of 1982, a time when the excitement in the *RAS* field was shifting towards the recently isolated human oncogenes. By 1983, a new human transforming gene was identified and found to be a third member of the *RAS* gene family. This gene was designated *NRAS* [58]

5.2.3.1. RAS signaling

RAS proteins are signal switch molecules that regulate cell fates by coupling receptor activation to downstream effector pathways that control diverse cellular responses including proliferation, differentiation, and survival [59]. Human cancers frequently express mutant RAS proteins, termed 'oncogenic RAS'. RAS proteins are GDP/GTP binding proteins that functions as a molecular switches to mediate downstream signaling from a variety of extracellular stimuli. The RAS proteins are activated when the protein binds GTP and be-

http://dx.doi.org/10.5772/63740

comes inactive upon GTP hydrolysis to GDP by RAS proteins. The action of RAS proteins is regulated by several guanine-nucleotide exchange factor (GNEFs) and GTPase-activating proteins (GAPS). RAS proteins regulate cellular responses to many extracellular stimuli, including soluble growth factors. GTP-bound RAS can interact productively with more than 20 effectors, including Raf, phosphatidylinositol 3-kinase (PI3K) and Ral guanine nucleotide-dissociation stimulator (RALGDS), to regulate various cellular responses including proliferation, survival, and differentiation [60]. RAS–GTP also binds the catalytic subunit of type I PI3Ks causing translocation of PI3K to the plasma membrane and subsequent activation. PI3K phosphorylates phosphatidyl inositol-4,5-bisphosphate (PIP2) to generate phosphatidylinositol-3,4, 5-triphosphate, which activates downstream kinases such as Akt [61] (**Figure 4**).

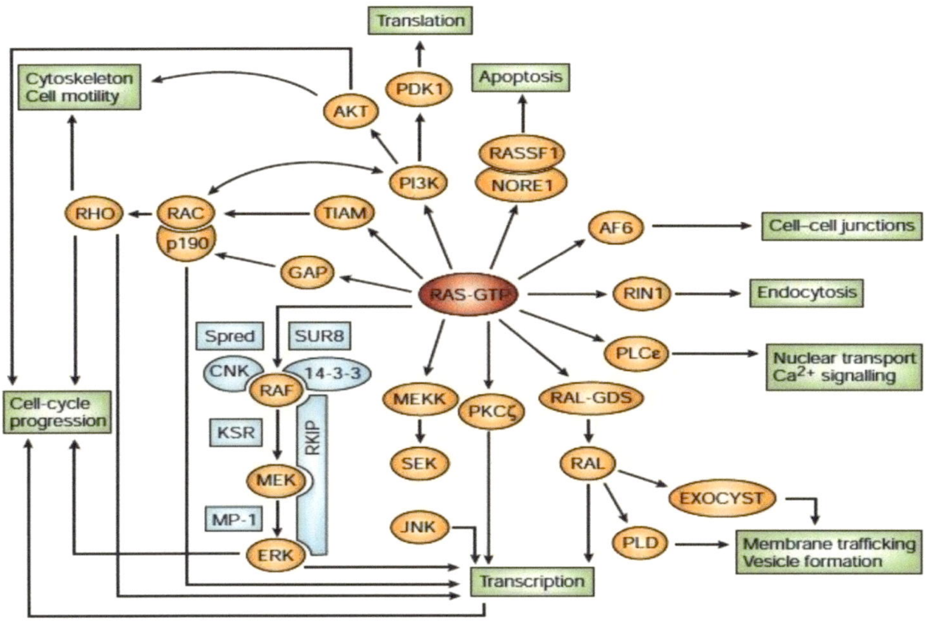

Figure 4. Overview of known RAS effectors and their corresponding biological responses. Active RAS-GTP induces a wide variety of cellular processes, such as transcription, translation, cell-cycle progression, apoptosis or cell survival, through direct interaction with various effectors. GAP proteins also interact with RAS-GTP and might also act as effectors. Modulators of some of these pathways are also indicated. The blue boxes represent adaptor complexes.

5.2.3.2. Oncogenic RAS mutations and abnormal signaling

Somatic missense *RAS* mutations found in cancer cells involve amino acid substitutions at positions 12, 13, and 61 impairing the intrinsic GTPase activity and conferring resistance to GAPs, thereby causing active, GTP-bound conformation to accumulate [62]. Glutamine 61 is essential for GTP hydrolysis, and substituting any amino acid at this position except glutamic acid blocks hydrolysis. Replacing glycine 12 of *RAS* with any other amino acid except proline also biochemically activates RAS. Substituting proline for glycine 12 renders RAS resistant to

GAPs but has increased intrinsic GTP hydrolysis. Consistent with this idea, the transforming potential of HRAS proteins with different codon 61 substitutions is inversely related to intrinsic GTPase activities [63]. Oncogenic RAS proteins deregulate downstream effector pathways to confer the abnormal functional properties of cancer cells: deregulated cell growth, survival, and differentiation.

5.2.3.3. Role of oncogenic RAS gene in thyroid cancer

Activating *RAS* mutations occur in ~30% of human cancers. Activated oncogenes of the *RAS* family have been identified in a wide range of solid and hematological malignancies. Mutations that cause activation of the *RAS* proto-oncogene have been well defined, and several groups have studied the occurrence of different mutations in thyroid neoplasia. The *RAS* mutations generally occur in up to 20–50% of thyroid neoplasms. However, the prevalence of mutations in specific histological classes varies widely. In papillary carcinomas, *RAS* mutations are relatively infrequent, as they occur in 10–20% of tumors. In FTC, *RAS* mutations are found in 40–50% of tumors and may also correlate with tumor dedifferentiation and less favorable prognosis [64]. RAS mutations are found in 20–40% of poorly differentiated and anaplastic carcinomas, 20–40% of benign follicular adenomas [65]. *RAS* mutations may predispose well-differentiated cancers to de differentiation and anaplastic transformation. Because *RAS* mutations are found in the entire spectrum of thyroid cancers, and with increasing frequency as tumors become more undifferentiated, *RAS* mutations have been suggested to be a biomarker for a more aggressive form of thyroid cancer [64]. In Thyroid cancer, *NRAS* codon 61 and *HRAS* codon 61 mutations are most common.

5.2.4. BRAF mutations

Point mutations, small in-frame deletions/insertions, and/or chromosomal rearrangement are the events by which BRAF can be activated. The most common BRAF activation is due to a point mutation involving substitution of thymine by adenine at nucleotide position 1799, resulting in a valine-to-glutamate replacement at residue 600 [66]. This *BRAF* V600E mutation constitutes 98–99% of all *BRAF* mutations found in thyroid cancer. Lys601Glu point mutation and small, in-frame insertions or deletions and *AKAP9/BRAF* rearrangement are other alterations in *BRAF* [67]. The *BRAF* V600E mutation is found in 40–45% PTCs. The mutation also occurs in 20–40% of poorly differentiated thyroid carcinomas and 30–40% of ATCs [68].

ARAF, BRAF, and *CRAF* are three *RAF* paralogs. These are downstream molecules of the membrane-bound RAS [69]. RAS stimulates RAF activation, which in turn activates MEK and ERK. ERK regulates cell proliferation, differentiation, senescence, and apoptosis. This pathway is hyper-activated in 30% of cancers with activating mutations in *RAS* occurring in approximately 15–30% of cancers, and recent data have shown that *BRAF* is mutated in about 7% of cancers [70], identifying it as another important oncogene on this pathway. The *BRAF* gene is located on the long (q) arm of chromosome 7 at position 34. More precisely, the *BRAF* gene is located from base pair 140,433,811 to base pair 140,624,563 on chromosome 7.

5.2.4.1. BRAF mutations from A to Z

BRAF mutations are found in 27–70% of malignant melanomas, 36–53% of PTC, 5–22% of colorectal cancers, and <30% of serous ovarian cancer, but they also occur at a low frequency of 1–3% in a wide variety of other cancers [70, 71]. There are more than 40 mutations identified in the *BRAF* gene so far, among which *BRAF* V600E mutation accounts for more than 90% [72, 73]. A few other activated *BRAF* mutants are only rarely found in thyroid cancer, such as the *BRAF* K601E, *AKAP9-BRAF* [74], *BRAF* V599ins [75], K601del, and a recently characterized novel *BRAF* mutant, V600D, FGLAT 601–605ins, resulting from an insertion of 18 nucleotides at nucleotide T1799 of the *BRAF* gene [76].

5.2.4.2. BRAF mutation in thyroid cancer

Although there are lots of alterations in *BRAF* gene in thyroid cancer, the most important mutation found in TC is *BRAF* V600E. This mutation is exclusive to PTC and PTC-derived ATC (44% and 24%, respectively), as it does not occur in any other type of TC.

5.2.4.2.1. Association of BRAF mutation with high-risk clinicopathological characteristics of PTC

Many studies have investigated the relationship of *BRAF* mutation with clinicopathological characteristics of PTC. Although the results are not entirely consistent, most of the studies from various ethnic and geographical backgrounds demonstrate a significant association of BRAF mutation with one or more conventional high-risk clinicopathological characteristics of PTC [77]. Among the various clinicopathological risk factors, extrathyroidal invasion, lymph node metastasis, and advanced clinicopathological stages III and IV most reliably predict thyroid cancer progression, recurrence, aggressiveness, and ultimately, higher morbidity and mortality [78]. Interestingly, among the various clinicopathological characteristics of PTC, many studies have found that *BRAF* mutation is also most commonly associated with these three risk predictors. This suggests that *BRAF* mutation may play a role in promoting the progression of PTC to ATC. Thus, BRAF mutation is a driving force behind the aggressive pathological characteristics of PTC and predicts a poorer prognosis for patients with PTC

5.2.4.2.2. Association of BRAF mutation with recurrence of PTC and loss of radioiodine avidity in recurrent tumors

Many studies have investigated the predictive value of the *BRAF* mutation for PTC recurrence and have shown the association of *BRAF* mutation in the primary PTC with loss of radioiodine avidity in the recurrent tumors [79].

5.2.4.2.3. Molecular bases for BRAF mutation-promoted invasiveness and progression of PTC

The oncogenic strength of *BRAF* mutation and the molecular events coupled to them in the cell cause genetic instability [80]. *BRAF* mutation has a close association with aberrant methylation of several important tumor suppressor genes in PTC including tissue inhibitor of matrix metalloproteinase-3 (*TIMP3*), death-associated protein kinase (*DAPK*), *SLC5A8*, and retinoic acid receptor 2 (*RAR2*) [81] which can further promote invasiveness and progression of PTC. Interestingly, a recent study demonstrated overexpression of VEGF in association with *BRAF* mutation in PTC [82]. Therefore, adding to the mutation-induced progression and invasiveness of PTC, the authors also showed that *BRAF* V600E promoted activation of the nuclear transcription factor NF kappaB-coupled signaling, which in turn promoted matrigel invasion of thyroid cancer cells. The efficacy of radioiodine treatment for thyroid cancer depends on the integrity of the iodide-metabolizing system of the thyroid cell [83]. Interestingly, *BRAF* mutation was found to be associated with decreased expression of thyroperoxidase (TPO) [84], Na^+/I^- symporter (NIS) [85], Tg [86], and pendrin [87] in primary or recurrent PTC tumors. Conditional expression of *BRAF* V600E in rat thyroid cell lines led to silencing of all these thyroid-specific iodide metabolizing genes [88]. Methylation was shown to be a mechanism mediating the silencing of some of these thyroid genes.

5.2.4.2.4. Testing of BRAF mutation as new dimension to risk stratification and clinical management of PTC

BRAF mutation may represent a novel and useful prognostic molecular marker for PTC. Like several conventional clinicopathological factors, particularly extrathyroidal invasion, lymph node metastasis, and diseases stages III and IV. *BRAF* mutation similarly has a high predictive value for PTC recurrence [85]. This novel prognostic factor may assist in deciding how aggressive the initial treatment of the patient should be and in deciding how vigilantly and aggressively patients should be managed after the initial treatment. PTC patients with *BRAF* mutation may need to be more closely monitored by a more liberal battery of diagnostic tests, such as more aggressive use of imaging methods.

5.2.5. P53 inactivation

P53 is known as *"policeman of the genome"* [89]. Alterations in the *P53* tumor suppressor gene by inactivating point mutations, usually involving exons 5–8, or by deletion result in progressive genome destabilization, additional mutations, and propagation of malignant clones. Among thyroid tumors, *P53* mutations are generally restricted to poorly differentiated thyroid cancer (PDTC) and ATC. Point mutations of *P53* occur in approximately 60% of ATC and in 25% of PDTC [90]. Because of their high incidence in undifferentiated thyroid cancer, the presence of *P53* mutations may be predictive of a highly aggressive thyroid cancer.

5.3. DNA mutation panels

Mutations of the *RET/RAS/BRAF/MAPK* pathway gladiators are responsible for more than 70% of PTCs and 80% of FTCs, but the sensitivity and specificity of these mutations are too low to be clinically relevant. But, because almost 70–80% of thyroid cancers should have at least one of these mutations, a panel of all the mutations may be able to improve the diagnostic accuracy of thyroid tumor FNA cytology. Signatures from gene expression profiles will eventually be used to construct new DNA mutation panels for FNA-based diagnosis of thyroid nodules [91].

5.4. Epigenetic biomarkers

Currently, epigenetic refers to the study of heritable changes in gene expression that occurs without any alteration in the primary DNA sequence [92]. Epigenetic information that fulfills the requirement of heritability can be classified into three distinct types: *DNA methylation, histone modifications*, and *noncoding RNAs*. In thyroid cancer, DNA methylation, histone modifications, and microRNA silencing have all been studied, but there is minimal data on nucleosome positioning.

Aberrant methylation, or hypermethylation, of tumor suppressor genes has been identified in many human tumors including thyroid tumors [93]. Hypermethylation of multiple genes has been identified in association with the PIK3/AKT pathway in FTC and of the MAPK pathway in PTC. Hypermethylation has also been identified in benign thyroid tumors, though to a lesser extent than in thyroid carcinomas. A close association between *BRAF* mutation and aberrant methylation of several tumor-suppressor genes in PTC has been reported [81]. Aberrant methylation also involves thyroid-specific genes such as the *NIS*, the promoter of the TSH receptor, the genes for the putative thyroid follicular cell apical iodide transport (*pendrin* and *SCL5A8*) [93]. Suppression of these thyroid iodide-metabolizing molecules results in the loss of cancer cells ability to concentrate iodine, rendering tumors insensitive to radioiodine therapy.

5.4.1. TSHR function and signaling

TSH is the main regulator of thyroid gland growth and development. Binding of TSH to TSHR stimulates thyroid epithelial cell proliferation and regulates the expression of differentiation markers such as Tg, TPO, and the NIS, necessary for the synthesis of thyroid hormones. Two G protein-dependent pathways are activated by TSHR: (i) Gαs-adenylate-cAMP activates protein kinase A (PKA)—phosphorylates the transcription factor CREB, thereby increasing its transcriptional activity and (ii) Gαq-phospholipase C–releasing inositoltriphosphate (IP3) and diacylglycerol (DAG)—activates protein kinase C, which promotes proliferation via the *RAF/MEK/ERK* pathway. Complex cross-talk occurs between these pathways and other signaling pathways including the PI3/Akt, PKC/NFkB, and JAK/STAT pathways [94, 95].

5.4.2. TSHR alterations related to thyroid cancer

Excesses or defaults in TSHR activity may play a role in thyroid disease and cancer. Both can be achieved by a number of mechanisms including mutations in critical domains, improper epigenetic marking of the gene, or incorrect transcriptional regulation.

5.4.3. Altered levels of TSHR expression

Quantitative analysis of promoter hypermethylation in thyroid cancer has involved *RASSF1A, TSHR, RARβ2, DAPK, S100, p16, CDH1, CALCA, TIMP3, TGF-β*, and *GSTpi* [81]. The *TSHR* gene promoter is frequently hypermethylated in thyroid carcinoma, with preferential methylation in undifferentiated carcinoma. In contrast, *TSHR* gene promoter is unmethylated in the normal thyroid and in benign tumors (thyroid adenoma). TSHR stimulates several key steps in thyrocyte concentration of iodine, including uptake by NIS and oxidation before incorporation into Tg by thyroid peroxidase [96]. Promoter hypermethylation resulting in decreased expression of *TSHR* and *NIS* may result in a decreased ability to concentrate iodine, rendering ablative doses of 131I ineffective. Promoter hypermethylation of *TSHR* is reported in 34–59% of patients with PTC [97]. NIS expression and iodide uptake requires functional TSHR. Low or absent TSHR expression correlates with worse prognosis in thyroid carcinomas [98].

5.4.4. BRAF mutational status and silencing of TSHR gene

It is thought that the loss of responsiveness to 131I is because of the loss of function of iodine-metabolizing proteins, such as NIS and TSHR. Tumor cells harboring *BRAF* V600E mutation have decreased NIS and TSHR gene expression compared with similar cells without the mutation. Several recent in vitro and in vivo mouse studies have demonstrated that BRAF inhibition with small-molecule MAPK pathway inhibitors restores the expression of iodine-metabolizing proteins and increases susceptibility to radioiodine ablation [99]. *BRAF* mutations are associated with decreased expression of mRNAs for the NIS and the TSH receptors that are considered markers of thyroid differentiation [100] (**Figure 5**).

The molecular mechanism involved in this V600E *BRAF*-induced silencing of thyroid genes is also unclear. Liu et al. showed the restorability of the expression of several key thyroid iodide-metabolizing genes by suppressing BRAF/MEK/MAP kinase pathway in thyroid cells expressing the V600E *BRAF* mutant. Using TSHR gene as a model, they showed that the effect

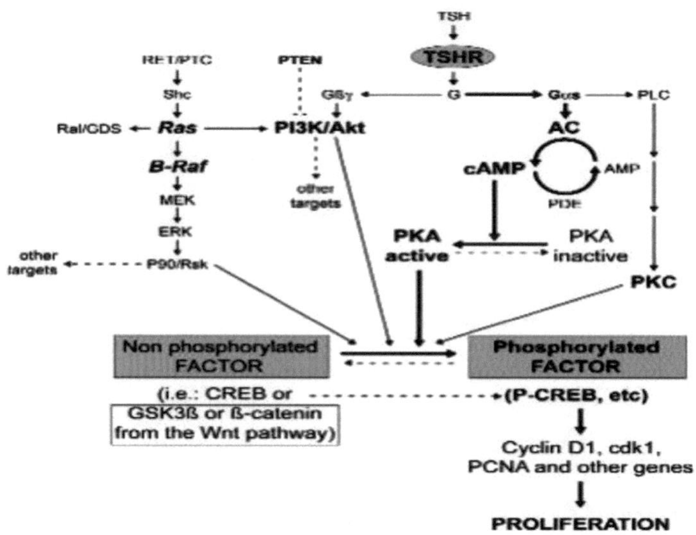

Figure 5. Classical TSHR signaling pathway and the framing network in thyrocyte proliferation. The bold arrows represent the classical TSHR signaling pathway towards proliferation. Normal arrows integrate cross talking molecules from other signaling pathways. Dashed lines represent other targets that may or may not be related to this pathway. Commonly altered molecules in thyroid cancer that may alter the integrity of the signaling network are enclosed in a square. Examples of integration between the classical TSHR/PKA and the MAPK/ERK, PI3K/Akt and Wnt/β-catenin pathways are provided.

of the *BRAF/MEK/MAP* kinase pathway on thyroid gene expression occurred through alteration of gene promoter activity, which may involve methylation [101].

5.5. Genomics

It includes the mapping and sequencing of the genome, as well as the analysis of the information gained from mapping and sequencing in the context of their biological significance and biomedical application. cDNA microarrays, oligonucleotide arrays, and serial analysis of gene expression (SAGE) are the various gene expression profiling technologies currently in use [102] which allow the study and comparison of the expression of thousands of genes simultaneously in varying conditions and will someday lead to the development of DNA signatures unique to each patient leading to patient specific treatment. In 2001, the first gene expression profile in thyroid cancer was done [103].

5.6. Proteomics

Proteomics is defined as the study of protein structure and function. The term was first introduced as an analogy to "genomics", but in this case referring to the entire protein spectrum [104]. Several immunohistochemical markers representing different components of the cell, such as the membrane, the cytoplasm, or the nucleus, have been studied in thyroid neoplasms [105]. The proteomic information also takes into account post-translational changes that are not detected at the mRNA level, as well as protein expression. The advantage of proteomics is the ability to detect biomarkers leaked into circulation from the patient's serum or plasma. Proteomics combines multidimensional separation systems based on mass spectrometry analysis and protein chip technology to detect complex mixture of proteins and peptides from either tissue or serum with high sensitivity and specificity [106]. The first study that established a proteomic profile of benign and malignant human thyroid tissue was reported in 2002 [107].

5.6.1. BRAF protein overexpression in thyroid cancer

The BRAF copy number gain, which results from either numerical changes of chromosome 7 or gene amplification, occurs in a significant portion of benign and malignant follicular thyroid tumors, including those of conventional and oncocytic types. This abnormality is associated with overexpression of BRAF protein and did not coincide with the presence of other mutations leading to activation of the MAPK pathway, suggesting that BRAF copy number gain may represent another mechanism of BRAF activation in thyroid tumors. It has been known for a long time that clonal numerical changes of chromosome 7 are common in benign and malignant thyroid tumors, and most of them are chromosome gains, particularly trisomy 7 [108]. Although gains of chromosome 7 lead to the increase in copy number of many genes located on this chromosome, data suggest that BRAF may represent an important target for the selection and clonal progression. The numerical changes of BRAF include gains of one to three extra copies of the gene and result in the modest overexpression (near to double) of the protein. This increased protein expression leads to additional stimulation of the MAPK pathway, although significantly lower as compared to more than 400-fold increase of BRAF kinase activity imposed by V600E point mutation [109]. A study by Kondo et al. revealed focal expression of wild-type BRAF in nonneoplastic thyroids and diffuse expression in benign adenomas and well-differentiated carcinomas regardless of their *BRAF* gene mutational status. Increased expression of wild-type *BRAF* may play important roles in the proliferation of transformed follicular cells [1].

6. Molecular analysis of *BRAF* and *RAS* genes

The study was aimed and designed to analyze the mutations, if any, in the coding exons (1 and 2) of RAS gene family (*NRAS, HRAS* and *KRAS*) and exon 15 of *BRAF* gene along with the analysis of BRAF protein expression and to establish the correlation of *RAS* and *BRAF* gene mutation and BRAF expression with clinicopathological variables of thyroid cancer patients. A total of 60 consecutive thyroid tumors and their adjacent normal tissues surgically resected either by total thyroidectomy/hemi-thyroidectomy or lobectomy over a period of 3 years were included in the study for sequence analysis of *RAS* gene family (*HRAS, NRAS*, and *KRAS*) and *BRAF* gene. By histopathological conformation, all the resected samples were established as thyroid cancer. Majority of the patients had attended the hospital with a clinical presentation of a lump or nodule. In this study, 80% (48 of 60) of cases were females and 20% (12 of 60) were males with a male: female ratio of 1:4. The cases in the age group of <45 were 60% (36 of 60) and exceeded than ≥45 years which were 40% (24 of 60). Only 10% (6 of 60) of patients were smokers who were all males and 90% (46 of 60) were nonsmokers. Benign thyroid diseases were found in 80% (48 of 60) patients. Tumor samples were histologically confirmed as differentiated thyroid carcinomas [PTC—70% (42 of 60) and FTC—13.4% (8 of 60), respectively] except few cases of MTC—6.6% (04 of 60) and Hürthle cell cancer—10% (6 of 60). Well-differentiated cancer grade was present in 95% (57 of 60) thyroid cancer patients. The clinicoepidemiological and pathological characteristics of these patients are listed in **Table 3**.

DNA isolated from the samples (tumor tissues and corresponding normal tissues) (**Figure 6**) was subjected to PCR to amplify the hot spot coding exon 15 of *BRAF* gene. Besides these, six other coding exons of *RAS* family of genes were amplified (1 and 2 exons of *HRAS, NRAS* and *KRAS*). The representative pictures of each exon of both the genes are given in **Figure 7**. After PCR amplification, the PCR products were subjected to DNA sequence analysis.

To identify the sequence variations, the electrophoregram obtained after sequencing of the PCR products was compared manually with the reference sequence of the *BRAF* and *RAS* genes deposited in the NCBI gene bank database. In addition, the electrophoregrams of both the genes were compared with the corresponding reference sequence of *BRAF* and *RAS* gene by aligning in "Cluster X software" to find somatic aberrations like insertions, deletions, or substitutions.

Variable	Parameter	Cases (n = 60)	
		n	% n
Sex	Female	48	80
	Male	12	20
Age, years	<45	36	60
	≥45	24	40
Dwelling	Rural	51	85
	Urban	09	15
Smoking status	Nonsmoker	54	90
	Smoker	06	10
Benign thyroid disease	Yes	48	80
	No	12	20
TSH levels	Elevated	25	41.6
	Normal	35	58.4
Histological types	Papillary	42	70
	Follicular	08	13.4
	Others	10	16.6
Grade	Well differentiated	57	95
	Poorly differentiated	03	05
Stage, <45 years	Stage I	34	56.6
	Stage II	02	3.4
Stage, ≥45 years	Stages I and II	15	25
	Stage III and above	09	15
Lymph node metastasis	Yes	15	25
	No	45	75
Vascular/capsular invasion	Yes	26	43
	No	34	67

TSH = Thyroid-stimulating hormone, n = Number.

Table 3. Clinicoepidemiological and clinicopathological variables of thyroid cancer patients used for mutational analysis in our center (SKIMS, India).

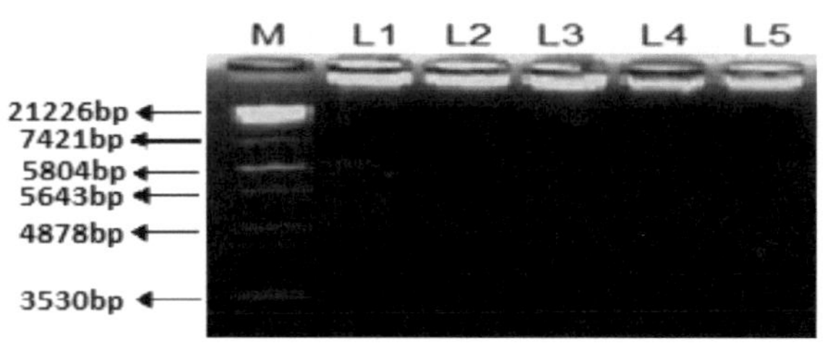

Figure 6. 1% Agarose gel electrophoresis of DNA isolated from blood, tumor tissue, and adjacent normal tissue of thyroid cancer patient. Lane M consists of lambda DNA-EcoRI digest. Lanes 1–3: DNA derived from thyroid tumor tissue. Lane 4: DNA derived from adjacent normal tissue. Lane 5: DNA derived from blood of thyroid cancer patient.

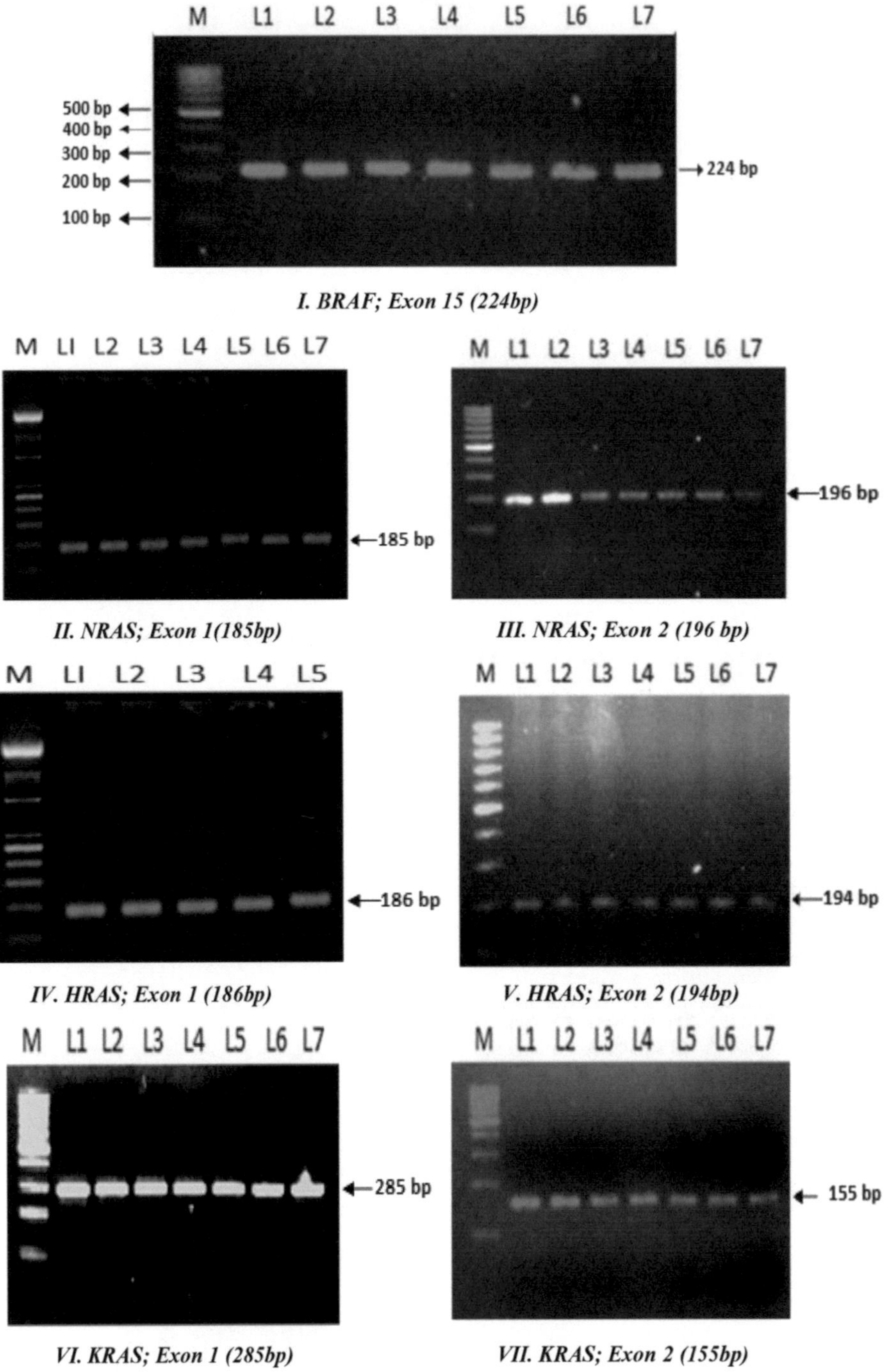

Figure 7. PCR amplification of different exons of BRAF and RAS genes. Lane M: molecular size marker 100 bp. Lanes 1–5, 6 and 7: amplified product from DNA of patient samples.

6.1. Mutational spectrum of BRAF gene

Total mutations of *BRAF* in this study were found to be 25% (15 of 60). All of them were transversions (T > A) at nucleotide position 1799 in exon 15. This mutation affects codon 600 of *BRAF* gene. This V600E mutation was further confirmed by reverse sequence of the same samples (**Figures 8** and **9**). The matched constitutional DNA contained the wild-type sequence in every case, demonstrating the somatic nature of these mutations in thyroid cancer.

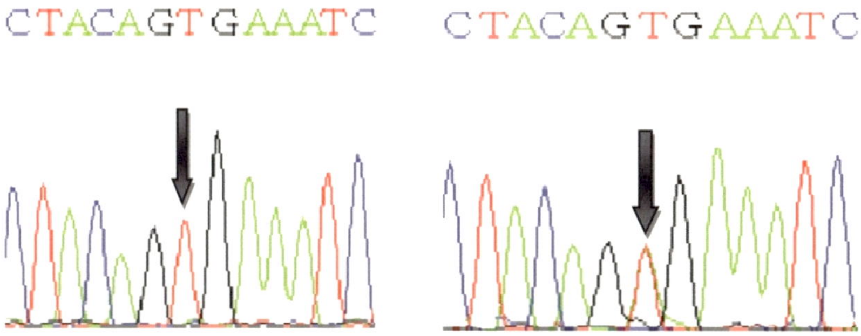

Figure 8. Partial electropherograms (forward) of the adjacent normal (left) and mutants (right) in exon 15 of the BRAF gene codon 600 (TGA→CGA).

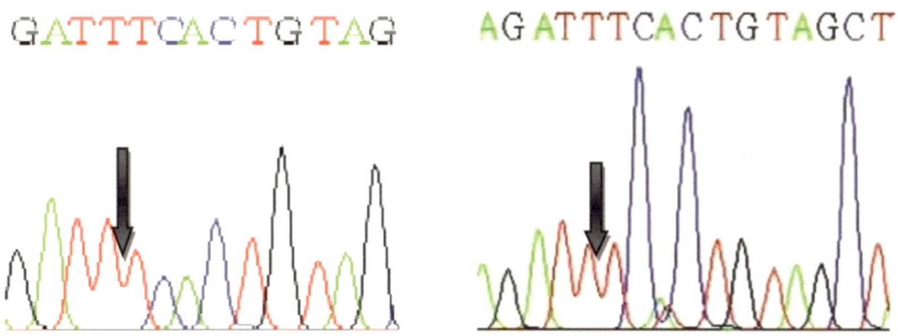

Figure 9. Partial electropherograms (reverse) of the adjacent normal (left) and mutants (right) in exon 15 of the BRAF gene codon 600 (TGA→CGA).

Among 25% (15/60) mutations of *BRAF* gene found in this study, 40% (10 of 25) of cases having elevated TSH levels were harboring mutation compared to 14.2% (05 of 35) cases having normal TSH levels and this difference showed a strong statistical significance ($P < 0.05$) (**Table 4**). Among the various histological types of thyroid cancer, mutations were restricted only to PTC. So, 35.7% (15 of 42) of PTC patients were having mutation in codon 600 of *BRAF* gene compared to follicular and other types of thyroid cancer which did not contain any mutation and this difference in mutation frequency between different histological types of tumors was statistically significant ($P < 0.05$). All the mutations were found in well-differentiated thyroid carcinomas (26.3% – 15 of 57) when compared to poorly differentiated thyroid carcinomas ($P < 0.05$). In thyroid cancer patients having <45 years of age, 23.5% (8 of 34) of patients with stage I disease had mutation compared to 100% (02 of 02) in stage II patients. Similarly, thyroid cancer patients having ≥45 years of age, 33.3% (05 of 15) of patients with stage I disease have mutation compared to stage II patients who were free from mutation ($P < 0.05$). In this study, 34.6% (9 of 26) patients having vascular and capsular invasion were having mutation compared to only 17.6% (06 of 34) of mutation positive patients free from invasion ($P < 0.05$). No significant association of this mutation was found in this report with any other clinicoepidemiological characteristics of thyroid cancer patients (**Table 4**) [110].

Characteristics	Cases (n = 60)		Mutants n = 15 (25%)		Wild type n = 45 (75%)		P-Value
	n	% n	n	% n	n	% n	
Sex							
Female	48	80	12	25	36	75	>0.05
Male	12	20	03	25	09	75	
Age, years							
<45	36	60	10	27.7	26	72.3	>0.05
≥45	24	40	05	20.8	19	79.2	
Dwelling							
Rural	51	85	13	25.4	38	74.6	>0.05
Urban	09	15	02	22.2	07	77.8	
Smoking status							
Nonsmoker	54	90	13	24.1	41	75.9	>0.05
Smoker	06	10	02	33.3	04	66.7	
Benign thyroid disease							
Yes	48	80	13	27.1	35	72.9	>0.05
No	12	20	02	16.7	10	83.3	
TSH levels							
Elevated	25	41.6	10	40	15	60	**<0.05**
Normal	35	58.4	05	14.2	30	85.8	
Histological types							
Papillary	42	70	15	35.7	27	64.3	**<0.05**
Follicular	08	13.4	00	00	08	100	
Others	10	16.6	00	00	10	100	
Grade							
Well differentiated	57	95	15	26.3	42	73.7	**<0.05**
Poorly differentiated	03	05	00	00	03	100	

Characteristics	Cases (n = 60)		Mutants n = 15 (25%)		Wild type n = 45 (75%)		P-Value
	n	% n	n	% n	n	% n	
Stage, <45 years							
Stage I	34	56.6	08	23.5	26	76.5	**<0.05**
Stage II	02	3.4	02	100	00	00	
Stage, ≥45 years							
Stages I and II	15	25	05	33.3	10	66.7	**<0.05**
Stage III and above	09	15	00	00	09	100	
Lymph node metastasis							
Yes	15	25	07	46.6	08	53.4	**<0.05**
No	45	75	08	17.7	37	82.3	
Vascular/capsular invasion							
Yes	26	43	09	34.6	17	65.4	>0.05
No	34	67	06	17.6	28	82.4	

TSH = Thyroid-stimulating hormone, n = number.

Table 4. Clinicoepidemiological and clinicopathological variables of thyroid cancer patients versus the mutant phenotypes of the BRAF gene.

The substitution of the negatively charged glutamic acid for an uncharged valine at position 600 may mimic the normal physiological phosphorylation of T599 and S602 resulting in a constitutively activated BRAF kinase [71] and stimulating BRAF activity up to 700-fold [111]. Studies along with an updated meta-analysis continue to show a strong relationship of *BRAF* mutation with aggressive clinicopathological characteristics of PTC [112, 113]. In conclusion, our study shows that the *BRAF* mutations characterize the aggressive pathway of thyroid tumorigenesis.

6.2. Mutational spectrum of RAS genes

Exons 1 and 2 each of *NRAS, HRAS*, and *KRAS* genes were screened for mutations in 60 tissue samples of thyroid cancer cases. Total six exons of *RAS* gene family were screened for mutations especially in codons 12, 13, and 61. No mutations were observed in any of the six exons studied, particularly in codons 12, 13, and 61 (**Figure 10**). Studies on a variety of tumors have demonstrated some "hot spots" in *RAS* gene family that are susceptible to point mutations. Many studies have detected different types of *RAS* mutations in human thyroid tumors [114, 115], but *RAS* gene family members have not been screened for mutation in the same sample series in thyroid tumors in Kashmiri patients. Activating *RAS* mutations have been reported to occur in ~30% of human cancers [116]. Our study was limited to screening of two hot spot exons of each *RAS* family of genes but in contrast to most of the studies showed no activating mutations in the thyroid tumors [117, 118]. Furthermore, many studies have

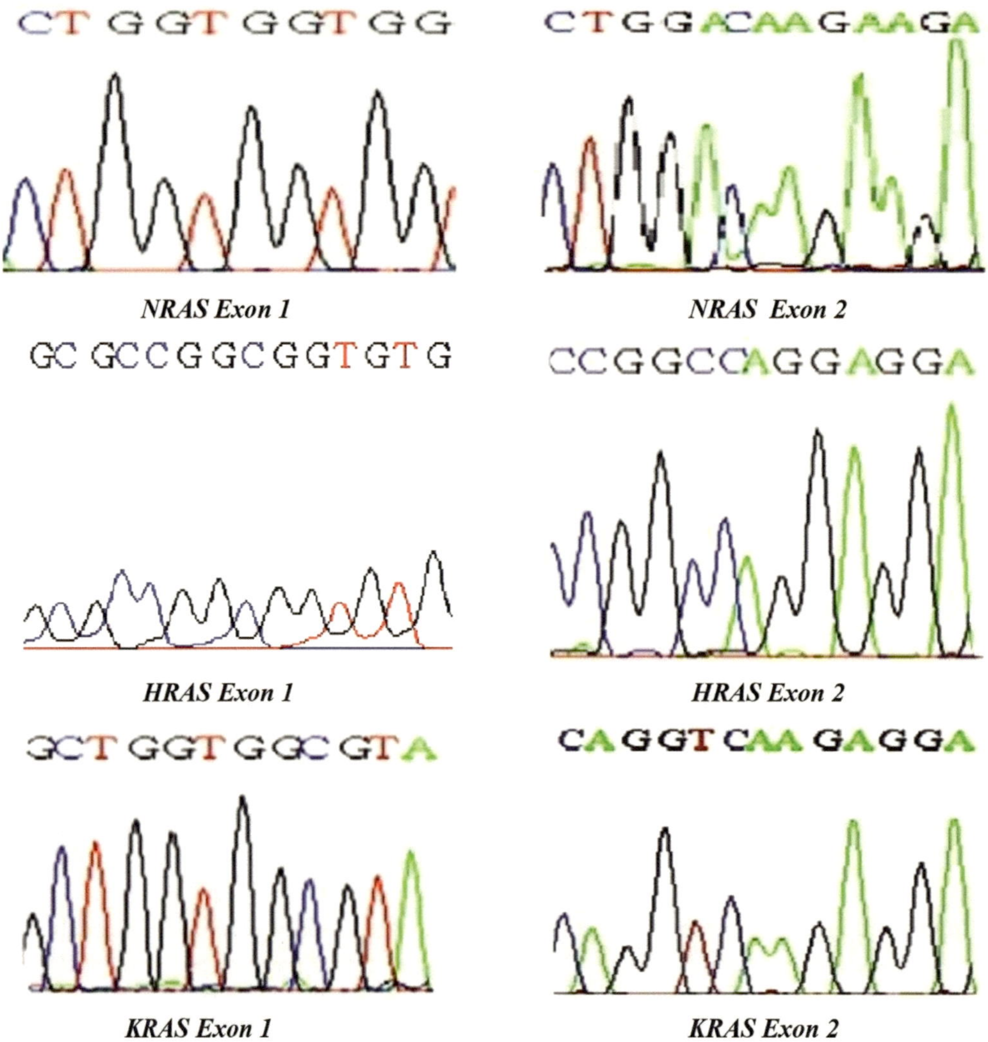

Figure 10. Partial electropherograms (forward) of exons 1 and 2 of the NRAS, HRAS, and KRAS genes.

reported mutual exclusiveness of *BRAF, RAS* as well as *RET/PTC* rearrangements in papillary thyroid cancers [1, 119]. As PTC is more prevalent in our region *BRAF* mutations predominate; hence, *RAS* mutations were not found in our study due to their mutual exclusiveness. In conclusion, it is evident from our study that although thyroid cancer is highly prevalent in this region, the mutational events for *RAS* genes do not seem to be involved in the thyroid carcinogenesis.

6.3. Polymorphic study of HRAS T81C SNP

DNA sequencing of *HRAS* exon 1 showed frequent T to C substitution in codon 27 of exon 1 at cDNA position 81, which is located in a wobble base position (**Figure 11**). The substitution

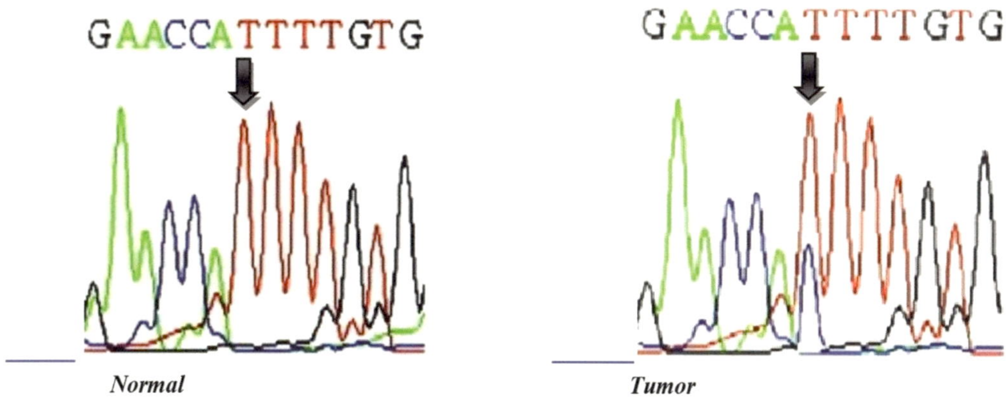

Figure 11. Partial electropherograms (forward) of the adjacent normal (left) and mutants (right) in exon 1 of the HRAS gene codon 27 (CAT→CAC).

(T81C) in codon 27 was found in 16 of 60 (26.6%) tumor tissue samples. *HRAS* 81 T > C substitution was found in 12 of 42 (28.5%) PTC tissues and 04 of 08 (50%) FTC tissues. *HRAS* T81C was frequently observed and was considered to be an informative SNP. Since this polymorphism has been reported only once in thyroid cancer; further, evaluation was imperative, to elucidate the conformity of the results in the backdrop of different ethnic backgrounds; thus, we conducted a case-control polymorphic study of *HRAS* T81C to assess the role of this SNP in thyroid cancer in Kashmiri population (North India). A total of 140 peripheral blood samples from confirmed thyroid cancer patients were collected from the department of Nuclear Medicine, SKIMS over a period of two years. Also 170 blood samples were collected from control subjects who were not having any sort of malignancy from the same hospital and belonging to the same geographical area, ethnic background for polymorphic analysis of *HRAS* T81C SNP. The cases included 19% (26 of 140) males and 81% (114 of 140) female patients (1:4.4), and the controls consisted of 82.4% (140 of 170) males and 17.6% (30 of 170) females. Of the total number of cases, 89% (124 of 140) were nonsmokers and 11% (16 of 140) were smokers. The subjects were considered nonsmokers only if until the day of sample collection they had not consumed tobacco and subjects were considered smokers if they are smoking presently or had quit smoking since last 6 months or less before sample collection. Only 29% (40 of 140) patients were above 45 years of age, and 71% (100 of 140) patients were below 45 years of age. **Table 5** shows demographic information and other parameter of cases and controls. The representative pictures of the amplicons and the RFLP are shown in **Figure 12**. The distribution of *HRAS* T81C allele frequency, its genotypes in cases and controls are shown in **Tables 6** and **7**. Due to the very low frequency of the 'CC' genotype and an increased risk associated with TC and CC genotypes, TC + CC was compared against TT. Frequencies of TT, TC, and CC genotypes among cases were 41.4%, 38.6%, and 20%, while in controls 84.1%, 11.7%, and 4.2%, respectively, with odds ratio (OR) of 7.4; 95% confidence interval (CI) = 4.3–12.7. The cases had a higher frequency of the rare allele (TC + CC) (58.6%) than the controls (15.9%), and this pattern of distribution of rare alleles among two groups showed statistical significance (P < 0.05). This finding shows an increased risk with TC + CC combination of genotypes against TT genotype. The frequency of mutant C allele was 39.3% in cases and 10% in controls. This observation showed a highly statistical significance of rare allele (C) between cases and controls (P < 0.05) with an O.R (95% C.I) of 5.8 (3.7–8.7). When classified further into groups, our study interestingly found higher percentage of rare allele (TC + CC) in FTC (82%, 18 of 22) compared to PTC (54%, 64 of 118) (P < 0.05). Association of variant allele with other clinicopathological characteristics is given in **Table 7**. While age, dwelling, gender, smoking status, and genotype (TC + CC) were associated with thyroid cancer in odds adjusted univariate analysis, the same parameters were associated with this disease in multivariate logistic regression analysis [120].

Characteristics	Cases n = 140 (%)	Controls n = 170 (%)	χ^2-Value	P-Value
Age group				
<45	100 (71)	60 (35)	40.14	**<0.05**
≥45	40 (29)	110 (65)		
Sex				
Female	114 (81)	30 (17.6)	125.56	**<0.05**
Male	26 (19)	140 (82.4)		
Dwelling				
Rural	112 (80)	50 (29.4)	78.75	**<0.05**
Urban	28 (20)	120 (70.6)		
Smoking				
Never	124 (89)	50(29.4)	109.12	**<0.05**
Ever	16 (11)	120 (70.6)		
Benign thyroid disease				
Yes	84 (60)			
No	56 (40)			
TSH levels				
Elevated	100 (71)			
Normal	40 (29)			
Histological types				
Papillary	118 (84)			
Follicular	22 (16)			
Tumor grade				
WD	134 (96)			
PD	06 (04)			
Stage, <45 years				
Stage I	94 (67)			
Stage II	06 (4.3)			

Characteristics	Cases n = 140 (%)	Controls n = 170 (%)	χ^2-Value	P-Value
Stage, ≥45 years				
Stages I and II	36 (25.7)			
Stage III and above	04 (03)			
Vascular/capsular invasion				
Yes	68 (48.5)			
No	72 (51.5)			
Lymph node metastasis				
Yes	52 (37)			
No	88 (63)			

TSH = thyroid-stimulating hormone, WD = well-differentiated thyroid cancer, PD = poorly differentiated thyroid cancer.

Table 5. Frequency distribution analysis of selected demographic and risk factors in thyroid cancer cases and controls taken for HRAS T81C polymorphic study.

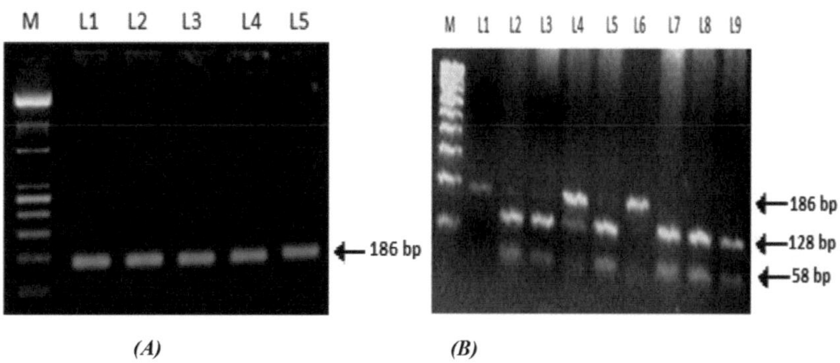

Figure 12. (A) PCR-amplified product of HRAS exon 1 (186 bp). (B): fragment digestion of PCR product by DraIII. TT allele (186 bp) shown in lanes 1 and 6; the TC heterozygous (186 bp, 128 bp and 58 bp) in lane 4; and homozygous CC variant (128 bp and 58 bp) in well 2, 3, 5, 7–9; M = 100 bp ladder.

	Cases n = 140 (%)	Controls n = 170 (%)	OR (95% CI)	P-Value
Genotype				
TT	58 (41.4)	143 (84.1)	6.6 (3.6–12.0)	**<0.05**
TC	54 (38.6)	20 (11.7)	9.8 (4.0–23.6)	**<0.05**
CC	28 (20)	07 (4.2)		
Allele type				
T	170 (60.7)	306 (90)	5.8 (3.7–8.7)	**<0.05**
C	110 (39.3)	34 (10)		

Table 6. Distribution of HRAS T81C genotypes and its allele frequency in cases and controls.

	Cases n (%)	TT	TC + CC	Controls n (%)	TT	TC + CC	OR (95% CI)	Adjusted OR (95% CI)	P-value
Overall genotype	n = 140	58	82	n = 170	143	27	7.4 (4.3–12.7)	7.4 (4.3–12.7)	**<0.05**
Age group									
<45	100 (71)	40	60	60 (35)	49	11	6.7 (3–14.4)	3.9(1.7–9.2)	**<0.05**
≥45	40 (29)	18	22	110 (65)	94	16	7.1 (3.1–15.6)	6.9(2.6–17.7)	**<0.05**
Sex									
Female	114 (81)	50	64	30 (17.6)	26	04	8.3 (2.6–25.3)	7.6(2.0–28.8)	**<0.05**
Male	26 (19)	08	18	140 (82.4)	117	23	11.4(4.3–29.2)	11.5(3.6–36.9)	**<0.05**
Dwelling									
Rural	112 (80)	40	72	50 (29.4)	34	16	3.8 (1.8–7.7)	3.7(1.5–9.1)	**<0.05**
Urban	28 (20)	18	10	120 (70.6)	109	11	5.5 (2.0–14.8)	5.2(1.4–9.1)	**<0.05**
Smoking									
Never	124 (89)	48	76	50(29.4)	33	17	03(1.5–5.9)	3.1(1.3–7.4)	**<0.05**
Ever	16 (11)	10	06	120 (70.6)	110	10	6.6 (1.98–21.7)	7.2(1.2–42.0)	**<0.05**
Benign thyroid disease									
Yes	84 (60)	34	50				1.1 (0.5–2.42)		>0.05
No	56 (40)	24	32						
TSH levels									
Elevated	100 (71)	44	56				0.7 (0.3–1.6)		>0.05
Normal	40 (29)	14	26						
Histological types									
Papillary	118 (84)	54	64				0.26 (0.06–1.0)		**<0.05**
Follicular	22 (16)	04	18						
Tumor									
Grade	134 (96)	56	78				0.7 (0.05–8.6)		>0.05
WD	06 (04)	02	04						
PD									
Stage, < 5 years									
Stage I	94 (67)	38	56				0.7 (0.06–8.7)		>0.05
Stage II	06 (4.3)	02	04						
Stage, ≥45 years									
Stages I and II	36 (25.7)	16	20				1.25(0.15–9.8)		>0.05
Stages III and above	04 (3)	02	02						
Vascular/capsular invasion									
Yes	68 (48.5)	32	36				0.63 (0.32–1.2)		>0.05
No	72 (51.5)	26	46						
Lymph node metastasis									
Yes	52 (37)	22	30				0.9 (0.39–2)		>0.05
No	88 (63)	36	52						

TSH = thyroid-stimulating hormone, WD = well-differentiated thyroid cancer, PD = poorly differentiated thyroid cancer.

Table 7. Association between HRAS T81C phenotypes and clinicopathologic characteristics of thyroid cancer patients.

In thyroid cases, however, we found higher frequency of variant genotypes as compared to other studies conducted on various cancers [121]. Our study revealed a sevenfold increased risk of thyroid cancer in carriers of the variant genotype (TC + CC) in cases. Therefore, our report reveals a significant risk for thyroid cancer, both either when stratified with C allele or in combination of the variant genotypes TC + CC compared with the TT genotype. Consistent with the tissue specificity hypothesis and various studies that had confirmed that the *HRAS* gene plays a more important role in bladder cancer acquired amino acid mutations in the hotspot codons 12, 13, and 61, which prolong the GTP-bound activated state of the *HRAS* product [122]. This polymorphism does not lead to the alteration of RAS protein structure, and it affects the cancer susceptibility possibly through linkage disequilibrium with other potential functional variants of *HRAS*. One of the linkage candidates is a region of variable tandem repeats about 1 kb downstream exon 4, with a possible transcriptional enhancer activity [123]. Another associated polymorphic site is hexanucleotide repeat located about 80 bp upstream of the 5′-end of exon 1 [124]. Yet another report has shown that *HRAS* T81C might be serving as a marker of other polymorphisms in intron D2 of *HRAS* that would act as regulators of IDX inclusion [125]. In conclusion, *HRAS* T81C SNP has been found to moderately increase thyroid cancer risk with variant alleles implicated more in follicular thyroid tumors.

6.4. Analysis of protein expression of BRAF

In this part of study, a total of 60 previously analyzed TC and their adjacent normal tissues were further analyzed for BRAF protein expression. **Table 3** depicts the clinicopathological characteristics of the studied subjects. **Figure 13** shows the representative picture of the extracted proteins run on SDS PAGE. Out of 60 cases of thyroid cancer, 90% (54 of 60) showed overexpression of BRAF protein (**Figure 14**) and the rest 10% (6 of 60) of the cases showed normal protein (BRAF) expression. Overexpression of BRAF protein in males was observed to be 84% (10 of 12) and in females as 91.6% (44 of 48). Among nonsmokers 96.3% (52 of 54) showed overexpression compared to smokers who showed only 33.4% (2 of 6) overexpression in BRAF protein and the difference is statistically significant ($P > 0.05$). BRAF protein overexpression was found to be in 97.7% (41 of 42) of PTC, 75% (6 of 8) of FTC, and 70% (07 of 10) of medullary/

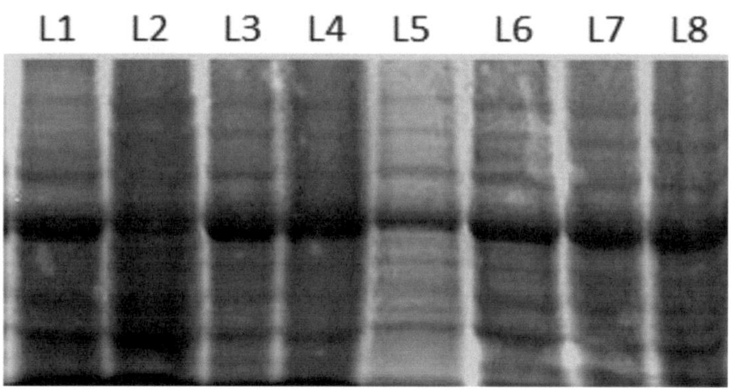

Figure 13. Representative gel picture of 10% SDS-PAGE. In each case 24 μl sample (20μl of the crude protein extract + 4 μl sample buffer) from tumor tissue and adjacent normal was loaded.

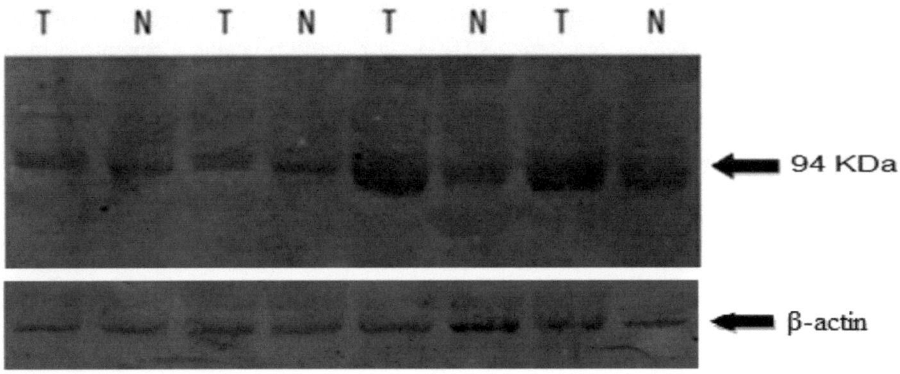

Figure 14. Western blot analysis of BRAF protein in thyroid tumor and adjacent normal tissues. Representative immunoblot showing the expression of BRAF protein in thyroid tumor tissue as compared to their adjacent normals. Extracts from samples were separately run for β-actin protein expression as loading control. Lanes T: protein extracted from tumor tissue. Lanes N: protein extracted from normal tissues. Membrane was probed with a polyclonal antibody specific for BRAF protein.

Hürthle cell carcinomas with a statistically significant association ($P > 0.05$). When we compared *BRAF* gene mutational status with BRAF protein expression, 86.7% (13 of 15) of *BRAF* mutation positive patients were having overexpression of BRAF protein, whereas 91.2% (41 of 45) of patients having wild-type *BRAF* status were having overexpressed BRAF protein ($P > 0.05$). No significant association of BRAF overexpression with any other clinicopathological characteristics was found (**Table 8**) [110].

		Normal expression n (%)	Over expression n (%)	OR (95% CI)	P-Value
Clinico pathological variables	**Overall cases n = 60 (%)**	**06 (10%)**	**54 (90%)**	–	–
Sex					
Female	48 (80%)	04 (8.4%)	44 (91.6%)	Reference	>0.05
Male	12 (20%)	02 (16%)	10 (84%)	2.2 (0.35–13.6)	
Age, years					
<45	36 (60%)	02 (5.5%)	34 (94.5%)	Reference	>0.05
≥45	24 (40%)	04 (16%)	20 (84%)	3.4 (0.54–20)	
Dwelling					
Rural	51 (85%)	04 (7.8%)	47 (92.2%)	Reference	>0.05
Urban	09 (15%)	02 (22.2%)	07 (77.8%)	3.3 (0.5–21.4)	
Smoking status					
Nonsmoker	54 (90%)	02 (3.7%)	52 (96.3%)	Reference	**<0.05**

		Normal expression n (%)	Over expression n (%)	OR (95% CI)	P-Value
Smoker	06 (10%)	04 (66.6%)	02 (33.4%)	52 (5.2–468)	
Benign thyroid disease					
Yes	48 (80%)	04 (8.3%)	44 (91.7%)	Reference	>0.05
No	12 (20%)	02 (16.6%)	10 (83.4%)	2.2 (0.35–13.7)	
TSH levels					
Elevated	25 (41.6%)	02 (8%)	23 (92%)	Reference	>0.05
Normal	35 (58.4%)	04 (11.5%)	31 (88.5%)	1.5 (0.24–8.9)	
Histological types					
Papillary	42 (70%)	01 (2.3%)	41 (97.7%)	Reference	**<0.05**
Follicular	08 (13.4%)	02 (25%)	06 (75%)	13.6 (1–174)	
Others	10 (16.6%)	03 (30%)	07 (70%)	17.5 (1.6–192)	
Tumor grade					
WD	57 (95%)	05 (8.7%)	52 (91.3%)	Reference	>0.05
PD	03 (05%)	01 (33.3%)	02 (66.7%)	5.2 (0.36–67.6)	
Stage, <45 years					
Stage I	34 (56.6%)	03 (8.8%)	31 (91.2%)	Reference	>0.05
Stage II	02 (3.4%)	01 (50%)	01 (50%)	10.3 (0.4–208)	
Stage, ≥45 years					
Stages I and II	15 (21.6%)	01 (6.6%)	14 (93.4%)	Reference	>0.05
Stages III and above	09 (15%)	01 (11.1%)	08 (88.9%)	1.75 (0.08–31.8)	
Lymph node metastasis					
Yes	15 (25%)	02 (13.3%)	13 (86.7%)	Reference	>0.05
No	45 (75%)	04 (8.8%)	41 (91.2%)	0.63 (0.10–3.8)	
Vascular/capsular invasion					
Yes	26 (43%)	03 (11.5%)	23 (88.5%)	Reference	>0.05
No	34 (67%)	03 (8.8%)	31 (91.2%)	0.75 (0.13–4.1)	
BRAF V600E Mutation					
Positive	15 (25%)	02 (13.3%)	13 (86.7%)	Reference	>0.05
Negative	45 (75%)	04 (8.8%)	41 (91.2%)	0.63 (0.4- 1.0)	

TSH = Thyroid-stimulating hormone, WD = well-differentiated thyroid cancer, PD = poorly differentiated thyroid cancer.

Table 8. Association of clinicopathological and clinicoepidemiological characteristic with BRAF protein overexpression.

As an important positive regulator of the MAP kinase signaling pathway, BRAF protein forms a multiprotein complex with MEK (downstream regulatory molecule), hence keeping MAP kinase pathways always on. Therefore, by positive regulation of the MAP kinase signaling pathway, BRAF can accelerate the proliferation of tumor cells. As we could not identify a distinct association between BRAF expression and BRAF mutation in thyroid tumors in accordance with other studies, possibly there might be another potential mechanism of BRAF activation other than mutational events. BRAF copy number gain in thyroid tumors has recently been studied by fluorescence in situ hybridization (FISH) where trisomy, tetrasomy for chromosome 7 was the most common alteration in tumors [108]. Although gains of chromosome 7 lead to the increase in copy number of many genes located on this chromosome, our data suggest that *BRAF* gene may represent an important target for the selection and clonal progression. Furthermore, *BRAF* copy number is directly proportional to amount of BRAF protein [1]. Therefore, it is tempting to speculate that weak stimulation of the MAPK pathway may participate in thyroid carcinogenesis.

7. Analysis of promoter methylation of *TSHR* gene

This study was aimed and designed to analyze the promoter hypermethylation of *TSHR* gene by methylation-specific PCR (MS-PCR) and to correlate it with clinicopathological characteristics of thyroid cancer patients and *BRAF* mutation. For this study, sixty (60) thyroid cancer tissues and their corresponding normal tissues were analyzed. The clinicopathological characteristics of the studied subjects are given in **Table 3**. In case when promoter region was highly methylated (both alleles) only the methylated band was detected and when promoter was partially methylated both methylated and unmethylated bands were detected. The representative picture of promoter hypermethylation of *TSHR* gene by methylation-specific PCR (MSP) is given in **Figure 15**.

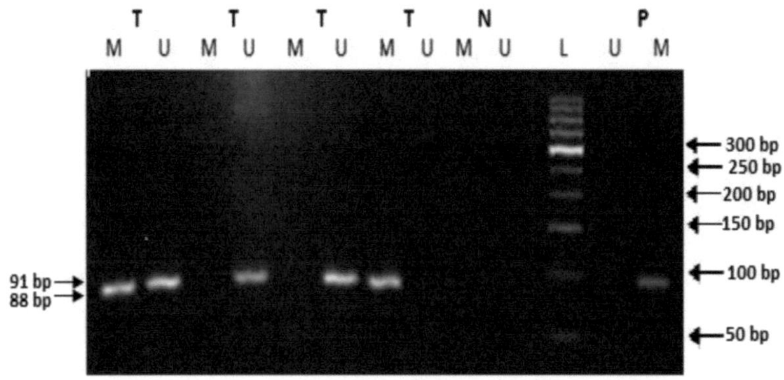

Figure 15. Representative picture of promoter hypermethylation of TSHR gene by MSP (4% agarose). L: 50 bp DNA marker. U (91 bp) indicates presence of unmethylated TSHR. M (88 bp) indicates presence of methylated TSHR. P and N indicate positive and negative controls, respectively. Distilled water was used as negative control in place of DNA.

http://dx.doi.org/10.5772/63740

Variable	Cases n = 60 (%)	*TSHR* methylation (n = 60)		OR (95% CI)	P-Value
		Positive n = 15 (25%)	Negative n = 45 (75%)		
Gender					
Female	48 (80)	12 (25)	36 (75)	Reference	>0.05
Male	12 (20)	03 (25)	09 (75)	1 (0.23–4.3)	
Age					
<45	36 (60)	10 (27.7)	26 (72.3)	Reference	>0.05
≥45	24 (40)	05 (20.8)	19 (79.2)	1.5 (0.45–5.1)	
Dwelling					
Rural	51 (85)	13 (25.5)	38 (74.5)	Reference	>0.05
Urban	09 (15)	2 (22.2)	07 (77.8)	1.2 (0.21–6.5)	
Smoking status					
Nonsmoker	54 (90)	13 (24)	41 (76)	Reference	>0.05
Smoker	06 (10)	02 (33.3)	04 (66.7)	0.63 (0.1–3.8)	
Benign thyroid disease					
Yes	48 (80)	13 (27)	35 (73)	Reference	>0.05
No	12 (20)	02 (16.6)	09 (83.4)	1.7 (0.32–8.8)	
TSH levels					
Elevated	25 (41.6)	10 (40)	15(60)	Reference	**<0.05**
Normal	35 (58.4)	5 (14.2)	30(85.8)	4 (1.1–13.8)	
Histological types					
Papillary	42 (70)	12 (28.5)	30 (71.5)	Reference	>0.05
Follicular	08 (13.4)	02 (25)	06 (75)	1.2 (0.2–6.8)	
Others	10 (16.6)	01 (10)	09 (90)	3.6 (0.4–31.3)	
Grade					
WD	57 (95)	14 (24.5)	43 (75.5)	Reference	>0.05
PD	03 (05)	01 (33.3)	02 (66.7)	0.65 (0.05–7.6)	
Stage, <45 years					
Stage I	34 (56.6)	09 (26.4)	25 (73.6)	Reference	>0.05
Stage II	02 (3.4)	01 (50)	01 (50)	0.36 (0.01–6.3)	
Stage, ≥ 45 years					
Stages I and II	15 (25)	04 (26.6)	11 (73.4)	Reference	>0.05
Stages III and above	09 (15)	01 (11.1)	08 (88.9)	2.9 (0.26–31)	
Lymph node metastasis					
Yes	15 (25)	06 (40)	09 (60)	Reference	>0.05
No	45 (75)	09 (20)	36 (80)	2.7 (0.75–9.4)	
Vascular/capsular invasion					
Yes	26 (43)	06 (23)	20 (77)	Reference	>0.05
No	34 (67)	09 (26.4)	25 (73.6)	0.83 (0.25–2.6)	

TSH = thyroid-stimulating hormone, WD, PD = well and poorly differentiated thyroid cancer.

Table 9. Association of TSHR promoter methylation with different variables of thyroid cancer patients.

The promoter region of *TSHR* gene was found to be methylated in 25% (15 of 60) of the thyroid cancer patients studied. The promoter methylation was found to be 27.7% (10 of 36) in patients <45 years of age compared to 20.8% (5 of 24) in patients ≥45 years of age. When methylation was compared with smoking status of patients, 33.3% (2 of 6) of smokers had methylated promoter region than 24% (13 of 54) of nonsmokers but the association was statistically insignificant ($P > 0.05$). When patients were grouped according to histological types, 28.5% (12 of 42) of PTC patients and 25% (2 of 8) of FTC patients had methylated promoter region, also 10% (01 of 10) of patients having other types of thyroid cancers were having methylation in promoter region ($P > 0.05$). Patients having elevated TSH levels showed strong association with methylation (OR = 4.0, $P = 0.02$) than patients having normal TSH levels. Association of *TSHR* promoter methylation with other clinicopathological characteristics is given in **Table 9** [126].

TSHR stimulates thyroid epithelial cell proliferation and several key steps in thyrocyte concentration of iodine, including uptake by *NIS* and oxidation before incorporation into Tg by thyroid peroxidase. Excesses or defaults in *TSHR* activity may play a role in thyroid disease and cancer. Aberrant methylation of the *TSHR* gene leads to loss of *TSHR* gene expression [96]. Promoter hypermethylation resulting in decreased expression of *TSHR* and *NIS* may result in a decreased ability to concentrate iodine, rendering ablative doses of 131I ineffective [97]. To summarize, our results showed a higher frequency of *TSHR* gene methylation in thyroid tumors and demonstrated it as a molecular pathway underlying the silencing of this gene. Moreover, the ability to achieve restoration of gene expression by nonnucleoside demethylating agents (such as procainamide) and nucleoside-analogue demethylating agents (such as azacitidine and decitabine) [96] suggests that DNA demethylating agents could be used to improve the efficiency of TSH promoted radioiodine therapy in epithelial thyroid cancers, particularly in those that have lost the response to TSH manipulation.

7.1. Association of TSHR promoter methylation with BRAF mutation spectrum

Now that we found *BRAF* and *TSHR* gene hypermethylation are highly implicated in thyroid tumors, we explored their association in the same group of patients. For this part of study, 60 thyroid cancer tissues and their corresponding normal tissues were analyzed. These were the same patients, wherein mutational analysis of *BRAF* gene and hyper methylation of *TSHR* was carried out. Here, we compared the *BRAF* mutations with *TSHR* promoter methylation. Out of 60 patients, *TSHR* methylation was found in 25% (15 of 60) patients and *BRAF* was found in 25% (15 of 60) patients. Out of 15 patients wherein mutations of *BRAF* gene were found, *TSHR* promoter was methylated in 73.3% (11 of 15) patients (**Table 10**). The presence of methylation in *TSHR* gene was found to be significantly associated with the *BRAF* mutation positive status ($P < 0.05$). Similarly, out of 45 patients, wherein mutations of *BRAF* gene were absent, *TSHR* promoter was methylated in only 8.8% (4 of 45) patients and rest of 91.2% (41 of 45) patients showed absence of *TSHR* promoter methylation (**Table 10**). Among the thyroid cancer patients studied, *TSHR* promoter methylation was significantly greater in patients with *BRAF* mutated (73.3%) than those with wild-type *BRAF* (8.8%) [126].

BRAF mutation	No. of cases (n = 60)	*TSHR* methylation (n = 60)		P-Value
		Positive n = 15 (25%)	Negative n = 45 (75%)	
Present	15	11(73.3%)	04(26.7%)	0.005
Absent	45	04(8.8%)	41(91.2%)	

Table 10. Association of BRAF mutation with TSHR promoter methylation.

Several recent *in vitro* and *in vivo* mouse studies have demonstrated that *BRAF* inhibition with small-molecule MAPK pathway inhibitors restores the expression of iodine-metabolizing proteins and increases susceptibility to radioactive iodine (RAI) [99, 127]. Our finding is an addition to the link of promoter methylation of *TSHR* gene with V600E *BRAF* and also represents an interesting further step from previous studies showing promoter methylation as a mechanism in silencing of this gene in thyroid cancer [96]. Our results also conclude that *TSHR* methylation is significantly associated with *BRAF* mutation spectrum. These diagnostic and therapeutic implications of *TSHR* gene methylation and its link with *BRAF* mutation in thyroid tumor clearly deserve further clinical investigation in other ethnic populations as well as our population of Kashmir and because of very few studies done, our results need to be further verified in larger cohort of patients to confirm the link between *BRAF* mutations and *TSHR* promoter methylation.

8. Conclusion

In conclusion, thyroid tumors represent an appropriate model for the study of epithelial neoplastic transformation. Thyroid cancers accumulate a number of alterations at the genomic level, and it has been proposed that genomic instability has a crucial role in the progression of thyroid neoplasms. Recent advances have improved our understanding of its pathogenesis; these include the identification of genetic alterations in *RET, RAS,* and *BRAF* that activate a common effector pathway involving the MAP kinase signaling cascade. Several thyroid-specific protein molecules play a key role in iodide-metabolizing process, including thyroid-stimulating hormone receptor (*TSHR*), sodium iodide symporter (*NIS*), *Tg, TPO,* and the thyroid gene transcription factors TTF-1 and Pax-8. Loss of expression of the genes for these molecules is common in aggressive thyroid cancer and is a sufficient cause for the loss of radioiodine avidity and failure of radioiodine therapy in this cancer.

Although TC is one of the least deadly forms of cancer, research in the field has remained on the cutting edge of science and technology, but better diagnostic tests and predictors of tumor aggressiveness are necessary. Nowadays, novel treatments are being designed based on our enhanced understanding of this disease process. The use of sophisticated genetic tools is generating a wealth of information for the better management of patients with TC.

Our study shows that the *BRAF* mutations as well its protein overexpression characterize the aggressive pathway of thyroid tumorigenesis. The high implication of this gene can thus be exploited for diagnosis and follow-up of thyroid cancer patients. On the other hand, *RAS* genes do not seem to be involved in the thyroid carcinogenesis in our series of patients with thyroid tumors with an exception of a germ line alteration in *HRAS* T81C SNP that moderately increase thyroid cancer risk. Moreover, the ability to achieve restoration of gene expression of thyroid iodide metabolizing genes by demethylating agents (such as azacitidine and decitabine) suggests that DNA demethylating agents could be used to improve the efficiency of radioiodine therapy in epithelial thyroid cancers. We found higher frequency of *TSHR* gene methylation in thyroid tumors, an event underlying the silencing of this gene supporting the above hypothesis about the role of *TSHR* hypermethylation in aggressive thyroid tumors. *BRAF* mutation is associated with silencing of various thyroid iodide-metabolizing genes including *TSHR* and loss of radioiodine avidity, and this is supported by our results that conclude with *TSHR* methylation being significantly associated with *BRAF* mutation spectrum. These diagnostic and therapeutic implications of *TSHR* gene methylation and its link with *BRAF* mutation in thyroid tumor clearly deserve further clinical investigation in other ethnic populations as well as our population of Kashmir.

Because of very few studies done on thyroid cancer from this region and relatively lesser sample size of our study the results need to be further verified in larger cohort of patients to confirm the link between various molecular assaults and thyroid carcinogenesis.

Author details

Syed Mudassar[1*], Mosin S. Khan[1], Shariq R. Masoodi[2], Khursheed A. Wani[3], Mahboob Ul Hussain[4] and Khurshid I. Andrabi[4]

*Address all correspondence to: syed.mudassar@skims.ac.in; mosinskims@gmail.com

1 Department of Clinical Biochemistry, Sher-I-Kashmir Institute of Medical Sciences, Soura, Srinagar, Kashmir, India

2 Department of Endocrinology, Sher-I-Kashmir Institute of Medical Sciences, Soura, Srinagar, Kashmir, India

3 Department of General Surgery, Sher-I-Kashmir Institute of Medical Sciences, Soura, Srinagar, Kashmir, India

4 Department of Biotechnology, University of Kashmir, Srinagar, Kashmir, India

References

[1] Tetsuo K, Tadao N, Shin-ichi M, et al. Enhanced B-Raf protein expression is independent of V600E mutant status in thyroid carcinomas. Human Pathol. 2007; 38: 1810–1818.

[2] Corner J, Bailey C (Eds.). Cancer Nursing Care in Context. Oxford: Blackwell Publishing; 2001.

[3] Yarbro C, Frogge M, Goodman M. Cancer Nursing: Principles and Practice. 6th ed. Boston: Jones and Bartlett Publishers; 2005.

[4] Mazzaferri EL, Massoll N. Management of papillary and follicular (differentiated) thyroid cancer: new paradigms using recombinant human thyrotropin. Endocr Relat Cancer. 2002; 9: 227–247.

[5] Alessandro A, Clodoveo F, et al. New targeted molecular therapies for dedifferentiated thyroid cancer. J Oncol. 2010; 2010: 1–6.

[6] Nikiforov Y, Gnep DR. Pediatric thyroid cancer after the Chernobyl disaster: pathomorphologic study of 84 cases (1991–1992) from the Republic of Belarus. Cancer. 19947; 4: 748–766.

[7] Sarlis NJ, Benvenga S. Molecular signaling in thyroid cancer. Cancer Treat Res. 2004; 122: 237–264.

[8] Sarlis NJ. Expression patterns of cellular growth-controlling genes in non-medullary thyroid cancer: basic aspects. Rev Endocr Metab Disord. 2000; 1: 183–196.

[9] A Cancer Stats Cancer Worldwide. International Agency for Research in Cancer (World Health Organization). Cancer Research UK; 2011.

[10] Jemal DV, Freddie Bray, Melissa M, et al. Global cancer statistics. CA Cancer J Clin. 2011; 61: 69–90.

[11] Howlader N, Noone AM, Krapcho M, Neyman N, et al. SEER Cancer Statistics Review, 1975–2009 (Vintage 2009 Populations). National Cancer Institute. Bethesda; 2012.

[12] Rebecca LB, Jonas A, Ezra EW. Thyroid cancer: burden of illness and management of disease. Journal of Cancer. 2011; 2: 193–199.

[13] Rao DN. Epidemiological Observations of Thyroid Cancer. Thyroid Cancer—An Indian Perspective. Radiation Medicine Centre, Bhabha Atomic Research Centre and Tata Memorial Hospital; 2000.

[14] Arshad AP, Mushtaq AS. Burden of cancers in the valley of Kashmir: 5 year epidemiological study reveals a different scenario. Tumor Biol. 2012; 33: 1629–1637.

[15] Hedinger C, Williams E, Sobin L. Histological typing of thyroid tumors. In: World Health Organization International Histological Classification of Tumors. Berlin: Springer Verlag; 1988.

[16] Franceschi S, Boyle P, Maisonneuve P, et al. The epidemiology of thyroid carcinoma. Crit Rev Oncog. 1993; 4: 25–52.

[17] Landis SH, Murray T, Bolden S, Wingo PA. Cancer statistics. CA Cancer J Clin. 1998; 48: 329–337.

[18] Parkin DM, Whelan SL, Ferlay J, Powell J, Teppo L. Cancer Incidence in Five Continents. In: IARC Scientific Publication no. 155. vol. 8. France: IARC Press; 2003.

[19] Hanson GA, Komorowski RA, Cerletty JM, Wilson SD. Thyroid gland morphology in young adults: normal subjects versus those with prior low-dose neck irradiation in childhood. Surgery. 1983; 94: 984–988.

[20] Pui CH, Cheng C, Leung W, et al. Extended follow up of long-term survivors of childhood acute lymphoblastic leukemia. N Engl J Med. 2003; 349: 640–649.

[21] Ron E, Lubin JH, Shore RE, et al. Thyroid cancer after exposure to external radiation: a pooled analysis of seven studies. Radiat Res. 1995; 141: 259–277.

[22] Leenhardt L, Aurengo A. Post-chernobyl thyroid carcinoma in children, Best Pract Res. Clin Endocrinol Metabol. 2000; 14: 667–677.

[23] Farbota LM, Calandra DB, Lawrence AM, Paloyan E. Thyroid carcinoma in Graves' disease. Surgery 1985; 98: 1148–1153.

[24] Belfiore A, Rosa GL, Porta GA, et al. Cancer risk in patients with cold thyroid nodules: relevance of iodine intake, sex, age, and multinodularity. Am J Med. 1992; 93: 363–369.

[25] Suzuki T, Matsuo K, Hasegawa Y, et al. Anthropometric factors at age 20 years and risk of thyroid cancer. Cancer Causes Control. 2008; 19: 1233–1242.

[26] Franceschi S, Preston-Martin S, Dal ML, et al. A pooled analysis of case-control studies of thyroid cancer. IV. Benign thyroid diseases. Cancer Causes Control. 1999; 10: 583–595.

[27] Ingbar SH, Woeber KA. The thyroid gland. In: Williams RH, editor. Textbook of Endocrinology. Philadelphia: WB Saunders Co; 1974. pp. 95–232.

[28] Malkasian GD, Mayberry WE. Serum total and free thyroxine and thyrotropin in normal and pregnant women, neonates, and women receiving progestogens. Am J Obstet Gynecol. 1970; 108: 1234–1238.

[29] Yane K, Kitahori Y, Konishi N, et al. Expression of the estrogen receptor in human thyroid neoplasms. Cancer Lett. 1994; 84: 59–66.

[30] Auricchio F, Migliaccio A, Castoria G, et al. Protein tyrosine phosphorylation and estradiol action. Ann NY Acad Sci. 1996; 784: 149–172.

[31] Diana M, Beatrice S, et al. Estrogen promotes growth of human thyroid tumor cells by different molecular mechanisms. J Clin Endocrinol Metabol. 2001; 86: 120–129.

[32] Ron E. Thyroid cancer. In: Schottenfeld D, Fraumeni JF, editors. Cancer Epidemidology and Prevention. 2nd ed. New York: Oxford University Press; 1996. pp. 1000–1021.

[33] Kreiger N, Parkes R. Cigarette smoking and the risk of thyroid cancer. Eur J Cancer. 2000; 36: 1969–1973.

[34] Mack WJ, Preston M, et al. A pooled analysis of case–control studies of thyroid cancer: cigarette smoking and consumption of alcohol, coffee, and tea. Cancer Causes Control. 2003; 14: 773–785.

[35] Konstantinos T, Faidon C. Endocrine effects of tobacco smoking. Clin Endocrinol. 2004; 61: 664–674.

[36] Lassoued S, Mseddi M, Mnif F, Abid M, Guermazi F, Masmoudi H, El Feki A, Attia H. A comparative study of the oxidative profile in Graves' disease, Hashimoto's thyroiditis, and papillary thyroid cancer. Biol Trace Element Res. 2010; 138: 107–115.

[37] Horacio GS. Genetic alterations in human epithelial thyroid tumours. Clin Endocrinol. 1998; 48: 531–546.

[38] Tetsuo K, Tadao N, Shin-ichi M, et al. Enhanced B-Raf protein expression is independent of V600E mutant status in thyroid carcinomas. Human Pathol. 2007; 38: 1810–1818.

[39] Milhaud G, Calmette C, Taboulet J et al. Hypersecretion of calcitonin in neoplastic conditions. Lancet. 1974; 1: 462–463.

[40] Srinivas PR, Kramer BS, et al. Trends in biomarker research for cancer detection. Lancet Oncol. 2001; 2: 698–704.

[41] Holyoke ED, Block GE, Jensen E, et al. Biologic markers in cancer diagnosis and treatment. Curr Probl Cancer. 1981; 6: 1–68.

[42] Eng C. RET proto-oncogene in the development of human cancer. J Clin Oncol. 1999; 17: 380–93.

[43] Wong J, Lu Z, Doery J, Fuller P. Lessons from a review of thyroglobulin assays in the management of thyroid cancer. Int Med J. 2008; 38: 441–444.

[44] Mulligan LM, Kwok JB, Healey CS, et al. Germ-line mutations of the RET proto-oncogene in multiple endocrine neoplasia type 2A. Nature. 1993; 363: 458–460.

[45] Knyazev PG, Fedorov SN, et al. Molecular-genetic analysis of myc and c-Ha-ras proto-oncogene alterations in human carcinoma. Haematol Blood Transfus. 1987; 31: 469–473.

[46] Kroll TG, Sarraf P, Pecciarini L, Chen CJ, Mueller E, et al. PAX8-PPAR gamma1 fusion oncogene in human thyroid carcinoma. Science. 2000; 289: 1357–1360.

[47] Kimura ET, Nikiforova MN, et al. High prevalence of BRAF mutations in thyroid cancer: genetic evidence for constitutive activation of the RET/PTC–RAS–BRAF signaling pathway in papillary thyroid carcinoma. Cancer Res. 2003; 63: 1454–1457.

[48] Jhiang SM, et al. Targeted expression of the RET/PTC1 oncogene induces papillary thyroid carcinomas. Endocrinology. 1996; 137: 375–378.

[49] Santoro M, et al. Molecular characterization of RET/PTC3: a novel rearranged version of the RET proto-oncogene in a human thyroid papillary carcinoma. Oncogene. 1994; 9: 509–516.

[50] Klugbauer S, Rabes HM. The transcription coactivator HTIF1 and a related protein are fused to the RET receptor tyrosine kinase in childhood papillary thyroid carcinomas. Oncogene. 1999; 18: 4388–4393.

[51] Wirtschafter A, et al. Expression of the RET/PTC fusion gene as a marker for papillary carcinoma in Hashimoto's thyroiditis. Laryngoscope. 1997; 107: 95–100.

[52] Nikiforov YE, Nikiforova MN. Molecular genetics and diagnosis of thyroid cancer. Nat Rev Endocrinol. 2011; 7: 569–580.

[53] Marques AR, Espadinha C, Catarino AL, et al. Expression of PAX8-PPAR gamma 1 rearrangements in both follicular thyroid carcinomas and adenomas. J Clin Endocrinol Metab. 2002; 87: 3947–3952.

[54] Ishizaka Y, Itoh F, Tahira T, et al. Human RET proto-oncogene mapped to chromosome 10q11.2. Oncogene 1989; 4: 1519–1521.

[55] Yamamoto M, Miki T, et al. Tight linkage of the ret proto-oncogene with the multiple endocrine neoplasia type 2A locus. Jpn J Clin Oncol. 1991; 21: 149–152.

[56] Donis-Keller H, Dou S, et al. Mutations in the RET proto-oncogene are associated with MEN 2A and FMTC. Hum Mol Genet. 1993; 2: 851–856.

[57] Harvey JJ. An unidentified virus which causes the rapid production of tumors in mice. Nature. 1964; 204: 1104–1105.

[58] Shimizu K, Goldfarb M, Perucho M, Wigler M. Isolation and preliminary characterization of the transforming gene of a human neuroblastoma cell line. Proc Natl Acad Sci USA. 1983; 80: 383–387.

[59] Vetter IR, Wittinghofer A. The guanine nucleotide binding switch in three dimensions. Science. 2001; 294: 1299–1304.

[60] Mitin N, Rossman KL, Der CJ. Signaling interplay in Ras superfamily function. Curr Biol. 2005; 15: 563–574.

[61] Bader A, Kang S, Zhao L, Vogt P. Oncogenic PI3K deregulates transcription and translation. Nat Rev Cancer. 2005; 5: 921–929.

[62] Trahey M, McCormick FA. Cytoplasmic protein stimulates normal N-ras p21 GTPase, but does not affect oncogenic mutants. Science. 1987; 238: 542–545.

[63] Donovan S, Shannon K M, Bollag G. GTPase activating proteins: critical regulators of intracellular signaling. BBA Rev Cancer. 2003; 1602: 23–45.

[64] Garcia-Rostan G, Zhao H, Camp R, et al. RAS mutations are associated with aggressive tumor phenotypes and poor prognosis in thyroid cancer. J Clin Oncol 2003; 21: 3226–3235.

[65] Motoi N, et al. Role of RAS mutation in the progression of thyroid carcinoma of follicular epithelial origin. Pathol Res Pract 2000; 196: 1–7.

[66] Cohen Y, Xing M, Mambo E, et al. BRAF mutation in papillary thyroidcarcinoma. J Natl Cancer Inst. 2003. 95: 625–627.

[67] Trovisco V, Vieira de Castro I, Soares P, et al. BRAF mutations are associated with some histological types of papillary thyroid carcinoma. J Pathol. 2004; 202: 247–251.

[68] Xing M. BRAF mutation in thyroid cancer. Endocr Relat Cancer. 2005; 12: 245–262.

[69] Robinson MJ, Cobb MH. Mitogen-activated protein kinase pathways. Curr Opin Cell Biol. 1997; 9: 180–186.

[70] Davies H, Bignell GR, Cox C, et al. Mutations of the BRAF gene in human cancer. Nature. 2002; 417: 949–954.

[71] Nikiforova MN, Kimura ET, Gandhi M, et al. BRAF mutations in thyroid tumors are restricted to papillary carcinomas and anaplastic or poorly differentiated carcinomas arising from papillary carcinomas. J Clin Endocrinol Metab. 2003; 88: 5399–5404.

[72] Wan PT, Garnett MJ, Roe SM, et al. Mechanism of activation of the RAF-ERK signaling pathway by oncogenic mutations of B-RAF. Cell. 2004; 116: 855–867.

[73] Garnett MJ, Marais R. Guilty as charged: BRAF is a human oncogene. Cancer Cell. 2004; 6: 313–319.

[74] Ciampi R, Knauf JA, Kerler R, et al. Oncogenic AKAP9–BRAF fusion is a novel mechanism of MAPK pathway activation in thyroid cancer. J Clin Invest. 2005; 115: 94–101.

[75] Moretti S, Macchiarulo A, De Falco V, Avenia N, Barbi F, Carta C, et al. Biochemical and molecular characterization of the novel BRAF (V599Ins) mutation detected in a classic papillary thyroid carcinoma. Oncogene 2006; 25: 4235–4240.

[76] Hou P, Liu D, Xing M. Functional characterization of the T1799–1801del and A1799–1816ins BRAF mutations in papillary thyroid cancer. Cell Cycle. 2007; 6: 377–379.

[77] Rodolico V, Cabibi D, Pizzolanti G, et al. BRAF (V600E) mutation and p27(kip1) expression in papillary carcinomas of the thyroid 1 cm and their paired lymph node metastases. Cancer. 2007; 110: 1218–1226.

[78] Sherman SI, Angelos P, Ball DW, Beenken SW, et al. Thyroid carcinoma. J Natl Compr Canc Netw. 2005; 3: 404–457.

[79] Xing M, Westra WH, et al. BRAF mutation predicts a poorer clinical prognosis for papillary thyroid cancer. J Clin Endocrinol Metab. 2005; 90: 6373–6379.

[80] Mitsutake N, Knauf JA, Mitsutake S, et al. Conditional BRAF V600E expression induces DNA synthesis, apoptosis, dedifferentiation, and chromosomal instability in thyroid PCCL3 cells. Cancer Res. 2005; 65: 2465–2473.

[81] Hoque MO, Rosenbaum E, Westra WH, et al. Quantitative assessment of promoter methylation profiles in thyroid neoplasms. J Clin Endocrinol Metab. 2005; 90: 4011–4018.

[82] Jo YS, Li S, Song JH, Kwon KH, et al. Influence of the BRAF V600E mutation on expression of vascular endothelial growth factor in papillary thyroid cancer. J Clin Endocrinol Metab. 2006; 91: 3667–3670.

[83] Nilsson M. Iodide handling by the thyroid epithelial cell. Exp Clin Endocrinol Diabetes. 2001; 109: 13–17.

[84] Giordano TJ, Kuick R, Thomas DG, Misek DE, et al. Molecular classification of papillary thyroid carcinoma: distinct BRAF, RAS, and RET/PTC mutation-specific gene expression profiles discovered by DNA microarray analysis. Oncogene. 2005; 24: 6646–6656.

[85] Riesco-Eizaguirre G, Gutierrez-Martinez P, et al. The oncogene BRAF V600E is associated with a high risk of recurrence and less differentiated papillary thyroid carcinoma due to the impairment of Na/I targeting to the membrane. Endocr Relat Cancer. 2006; 13: 257–269.

[86] Durante C, Puxeddu E, Ferretti E, et al. BRAF mutations in papillary thyroid carcinomas inhibit genes involved in iodine metabolism. J Clin Endocrinol Metab. 2007; 92: 2840–47.

[87] Mian C, Barollo S, Pennelli G, Pavan N, Rugge M, et al. Molecular characteristics in papillary thyroid cancers (PTCs) with no (131) I uptake. Clin Endocrinol. 2008; 68:108–16.

[88] Liu D, Hu S, Hou P, Jiang D, Condouris S, Xing M. Suppression of BRAF/MEK/MAP kinase pathway restores expression of iodide-metabolizing genes in thyroid cells expressing the V600E BRAF mutant. Clin Cancer Res. 2007; 13: 1341–1349.

[89] Farid NR, Shi Y, Zou M. Molecular basis of thyroid cancer. Endocr Rev. 1994; 15: 202–232.

[90] Dobashi Y, Sugimura H, Sakamoto A, et al. Stepwise participation of p53 gene mutation during dedifferentiation of human thyroid carcinomas. Diagn Mol Pathol. 1994; 3: 9–14.

[91] Nikiforov YE, Steward DL, et al. Molecular testing for mutations in improving the fine-needle aspiration diagnosis of thyroid nodules. J Clin Endocrinol Metab. 2009; 94: 2092–2098.

[92] Sharma S, Kelly TK, Jones PA. Epigenetics in cancer. Carcinogenesis. 2010; 31: 27–36.

[93] Xing M. Gene methylation in thyroid tumorigenesis. Endocrinology. 2007; 148: 948–953.

[94] Alvarez-Nuñez F, Bussaglia E, et al. Thyroid Neoplasia Study Group PTEN promoter methylation in sporadic thyroid carcinomas. Thyroid 2006; 16: 17–23.

[95] Latif R, Morshed SA, Zaidi M, Davies TF. The thyroid stimulating hormone receptor: impact of thyroid-stimulating hormone and thyroid-stimulating hormone receptor antibodies on multimerization, cleavage, and signaling. Endocrinol Metab Clin North Am. 2009; 38: 319–41.

[96] Xing M, Usadel H, Cohen Y, et al. Methylation of the thyroid-stimulating hormone receptor gene in epithelial thyroid tumors: a marker of malignancy and a cause of gene silencing. Cancer Res. 2003; 63: 2316–2321.

[97] Smith JA, Fan CY, Zou C, Bodenner D, Kokoska MS. Methylation status of genes in papillary thyroid carcinoma. Arch Otolaryngol. 2007; 133: 1006–1011.

[98] Mirebeau-Prunier D, Guyetant S, Rodien P, Franc B, Baris O, Rohmer V, et al. Decreased expression of thyrotropin receptor gene suggests a high-risk subgroup for oncocytic adenoma. Eur J Endocrinol. 2004; 150: 269–76.

[99] David AK, Daniel B, et al. Thyroid stimulating hormone increases iodine uptake by thyroid cancer cells during BRAF silencing. J Surg Res. 2012; 111: E1–9.

[100] Maria GC, Nicoletta F, Giuseppe B. Epigenetics modifications and therapeutic prospects in human thyroid cancer. Front Endocrinol. 2012; 3: 1–8.

[101] Dingxie L, Shuiying H, et al. Suppression of BRAF/MEK/MAP kinase pathway restores expression of iodide-metabolizing genes in thyroid cells expressing the V600E BRAF mutant. Clin Cancer Res. 2007; 13: 1341–1349.

[102] Mandruzzato S. Technological platforms for microarray gene expression profiling. Adv Exp Med Biol. 2007; 593: 12–18.

[103] Huang Y, Prasad M, Lemon WJ, et al. Gene expression in papillary thyroid carcinoma reveals highly consistent profiles. Proc Natl Acad Sci. 2001; 98: 15044–15049.

[104] Wilkins MR, Pasquali C, et al. From proteins to proteomes: large scale protein identification by two-dimensional electrophoresis and amino acid analysis. Nat Biotechnol. 1996; 14: 61–65.

[105] Fischer S, Asa SL. Application of immune histochemistry to thyroid neoplasms. Arch Pathol Lab Med. 2008; 132: 359–372.

[106] Wang JX, Yu JK, Wang L, et al. Application of serum protein fingerprint in diagnosis of papillary thyroid carcinoma. Proteomics. 2006; 6: 5344–5349.

[107] Srisomsap C, Subhasitanont P, et al. Detection of cathepsin B up-regulation in neoplastic thyroid tissues by proteomic analysis. Proteomics. 2002; 2: 706–712.

[108] Belge G, Roque L, Soares J, et al. Cytogenetic investigations of 340 thyroid hyperplasias and adenomas revealing correlations between cytogenetic findings and histology. Cancer Genet Cytogenet. 1998; 101: 42–48.

[109] Ciampi R, Zhu Z, Yuri EN. BRAF copy number gains in thyroid tumors detected by fluorescence in situ hybridization. Endocr Pathol. 2005; 16: 99–106.

[110] Mosin S Khan, Arshad A Pandith, Niyaz Azad, Mahboob Ul Hussain, Shariq R Masoodi, Khursheed A Wani, Khurshid I Andrabi and Syed Mudassar. Impact of molecular alterations of BRAF in the pathogenesis of thyroid cancer. Mutagenesis 2014; 29: 131–137.

[111] Emma R, Cantwell-Dorris, John J, Orla MS. BRAF V600E: Implications for carcinogenesis and molecular therapy. Mol Cancer Ther. 2011; 10: 385–394.

[112] Elisei R, Ugolini C, Viola D, et al. BRAF V600E mutation and outcome of patients with papillary thyroid carcinoma: a 15-year median follow-up study. J Clin Endocrinol Metab. 2008; 93: 3943–9.

[113] Xinying L, Asim B, Abdel M, Emad K. BRAF mutation in papillary thyroid carcinoma. Int J Clin Exp Med. 2012; 5: 310–315.

[114] Esapa CT, Johnson SJ, Kendall-Taylor P, et al. Prevalence of Ras mutations in thyroid neoplasia. Clinical Endocrinol (Oxf). 1999; 50: 529–35.

[115] Basolo F, Pisaturo F, et al. N-ras mutation in poorly differentiated thyroid carcinomas: correlation with bone metastases and inverse correlation to thyroglobulin expression. Thyroid. 2000; 10: 19–23.

[116] Lemoine NR, Mayall ES, Wyllie FS, et al. Activated RAS oncogenes in human thyroid cancers. Cancer Res. 1998; 48: 4459–63.

[117] Karga H, Lee JK, Vickery AL, et al. Ras oncogene mutations inbenign and malignant thyroid neoplasms. J Clin Endocrinol Metab. 1991; 73: 832–6.

[118] Said S, Schlumberger M, Suarez HG. Oncogenes and antioncogenesin human epithelial thyroid tumors. J Endocrinol Investig. 1994; 17: 371–9.

[119] Nikiforova MN, Nikiforov YE. Molecular diagnostics and predictors in thyroid cancer. Thyroid. 2009; 19: 1351–61.

[120] Mosin S Khan, Arshad A Pandith, Mahboob Ul Hussain, Mohammad Iqbal, Nighat P Khan, Khurshid A Wani, Shariq R Masoodi, Syed Mudassar. Lack of mutational events of RAS genes in sporadic thyroidcancer but high risk associated with HRAS T81C singlenucleotide polymorphism (case–control study). Tumor Biol. 2013; 34: 521–529.

[121] Ivkovic TC, Loncar B, Spaventi R, et al. Association of H-ras polymorphisms and susceptibility to sporadic colon cancer. Int J Oncol. 2009; 35: 1169–73.

[122] Lowy DR, Willumsen BM. Function and regulation of ras. Annu Rev Biochem. 1993; 62: 851–91.

[123] Trepicchio WL, Krontiris TG. Members of the rel/NF-B family of transcriptional regulatory proteins bind the HRAS1 minisatellite DNA sequence. Nucleic Acids Res. 1992; 20: 2427–34.

[124] Kotsinas A, Gorgoulis VG, Zacharatos P, et al. Additional characterization of a hexanucleotide polymorphic site in the first intron of human HRAS gene: comparative study of its alterations in non small cell lung carcinomas and sporadic invasive breast carcinomas. Cancer Genet Cytogenet. 2001; 126: 147–54.

[125] Castro P, Soares P, Gusma L, Seruca R, Sobrinho M. H-RAS 81 polymorphism is significantly associated with aneuploidy in follicular tumors of the thyroid. Oncogene. 2006; 25: 4620–4627.

[126] Mosin S Khan, Arshad A Pandith, Shariq R Masoodi, Khursheed A Wani, Mahboob Ul Hussain, Syed Mudassar. Epigenetic silencing of TSHR gene in thyroid cancer patients in relation to their BRAF V600E mutation status. Endocrine 2014; 47: 449–455.

[127] Nucera C, Nehs MA, Nagarkatti SS, et al. Targeting BRAF V600E with PLX4720 displays potent anti-migratory and anti-invasive activity in preclinical models of human thyroid cancer. Oncologist. 2001; 16: 296–305.

Chapter 3

Atypia of Undetermined Significance/Follicular Lesion of Undetermined Significance (AUS/FLUS): Interpretation and Algorithm for Follow-Up

Lei Zhang, Beverly Wang, Jianyu Rao and
Douglas Bell

Additional information is available at the end of the chapter

http://dx.doi.org/10.5772/64155

Abstract

The Bethesda System for Reporting Thyroid Cytology (TBSRTC) has proven to be an effective and robust thyroid fine needle aspiration (FNA) classification scheme to guide the clinical treatment of patients with thyroid nodules. However, a tendency of increasing diagnosis of atypia of undetermined significance/follicular lesion of undetermined significance (AUS/FLUS) is observed. This is commensurate with the incorporation of new molecular tests for classifying indeterminate thyroid nodules. Moreover, a sizable portion of AUS/FLUS is correlated with follicular variant papillary carcinoma (FVPTC). A suggestion of reclassifying noninvasive FVPTC (NI-FVPTC) or noninvasive follicular thyroid neoplasm with papillary-like nuclear features (NIFTP) as a neoplasm rather than a carcinoma would significantly change the risk of malignancy in AUS/FLUS category. We review the diagnostic criterion and subclassifying suggestions of AUS/FLUS, features indicating follicular variant neoplasm in AUS/FLUS category, and commercially available molecular tests for AUS/FLUS subgrouping. We propose a multidisciplinary approach to AUS/FLUS follow-up.

Keywords: atypia of undetermined significance/follicular lesion of undetermined significance (AUS/FLUS), diagnosis, risk of malignancy, follow-up

1. Introduction

Fine needle aspiration (FNA) is continuously and widely considered to be the most accurate method for the evaluation of a thyroid nodule [1, 2]. To address a significant variability in the reporting of cytological findings in thyroid FNA samples, a consensus recommendation known as the Bethesda System for Reporting Thyroid Cytology (TBSRTC) was provided in 2007. It includes six diagnostic categories, which are associated with varying risks of malignancy: I = nondiagnostic (ND), II = benign, III = atypia/follicular lesion of undetermined significance (AUS/FLUS), IV = follicular neoplasm/suspicious for a follicular neoplasm (FN/SFN), V = suspicious for malignancy, and VI = malignant [3]. This reporting system is compatible with that recommended by the British Thyroid Association [4] (**Table 1**). The BSRTC has proven to be an effective and robust thyroid FNA classification scheme to guide the clinical treatment of patients with thyroid nodules [5–9]; it is endorsed as a standard practice in reporting thyroid aspiration cytology by the 2015 American Thyroid Association (ATA) guidelines [2]. The Bethesda reporting system for thyroid FNA was used in 90% of practices in a recent survey [10].

Bethesda diagnostic category [3]		**British Thyroid Association [4]**		**Cancer Risk [3]**	**Management [3]**
I	Nondiagnostic or unsatisfactory	**Thy1**	Nondiagnostic	1–4%	Repeat FNA with U/S
II	Benign	**Thy2**	Nonneoplastic	1–3%	Follow-up clinically
III	Atypia of undetermined significance (AUS) or follicular lesion of undermined significance (FLUS)	**Thy3a**	Atypical features present	~5–15%*	Repeat FNA
IV	Follicular neoplasm (FN) or suspicious for a follicular neoplasm (SFN)	**Thy3f**	Follicular neoplasm suspected	20–30%*	Lobectomy
V	Suspicious for malignancy (SM)	**Thy4**	Suspicious of Malignancy	60–75%*	Lobectomy or total thyroidectomy
VI	Malignant	**Thy5**	Diagnostic of malignancy	97–99%	Total thyroidectomy

* Reclassifying non-invasive follicular variant papillary thyroid carcinoma (NI-FVPTC) as neoplasm, and renaming it as noninvasive follicular thyroid neoplasm with papillary-like nuclear features (NIFTP) would have most pronounced effect on the indeterminate categories: a decrease of cancer risk 5.2-17.6% in AUS/FLUS, 8-15.1% in SF/FN and 17.6-41.5% in suspicious for malignancy [22, 23] (see 3.3).

Table 1. Thyroid fine needle aspiration diagnostic category.

However, with implementation of BSRTC there is a tendency of increasing diagnosis of AUS/FLUS [6–12], and the risk of malignancy (ROM) associated with AUS/FLUS seems to be higher than estimated before [6–17]. These trends are commensurate with the incorporation of new molecular tests for classifying indeterminate thyroid nodules [16–20], and increased diagnosis of follicular variant papillary thyroid carcinoma (FVPTC) by surgical pathology [21]. Of note, a significant portion of AUS/FLUS has a histologic diagnosis of FVPTC [11, 12, 22]. If non-invasive FVPTC (NI-FVPTC) is considered as a neoplasm rather than a carcinoma, e.g.

noninvasive follicular thyroid neoplasm with papillary-like nuclear features (NIFTP) as recently suggested, the risk of malignancy for AUS/FLUS would further change [16, 22, 23].

Although "indeterminate" thyroid nodules include AUS/FLUS (III), FN/SF (IV), and suspicious for malignancy (V) categories, AUS/FLUS remains the most "*undetermined*" in terms of management. The recommendations for FN/SF (IV) and suspicious for malignancy (V) are lobectomy or total thyroidectomy [3] with 61.2 and 86.0% of them potentially referring to surgery in practice [22], while the suggestion for AUS/FLUS cases is repeated FNA biopsy [3]. The risk of malignancy for AUS/FLUS diagnosed postoperatively ranges from 5 to 48% [24–27]. The wide range has posed anxiety to patients and difficulty in reaching clinical decision.

Hürthle cells are oncocytic cells, present in normal thyroid (increase with age), goiter, Hashimoto thyroiditis, Graves disease, radiation, chemotherapy, adenoma and carcinoma [29]. A Hürthle cell carcinoma is diagnosed if morphologic features indicative of malignancy are obvious. Otherwise, it is categorized as SN/FSN if the nodule is composed exclusively of Hürthle cells. It is downgraded to AUS/FLUS in a background of Hashimoto thyroiditis [3, 28, 29]. Hürthle cell lesions are considered "non-predictable" or "with higher malignant risk" [30], despite the fact that the risk of malignancy diagnosed by FNA in Hürthle cell lesions is similar to non-Hürthle cell lesions by other studies [28, 31].

We would discuss the scenarios triggering AUS/FLUS diagnosis, characters helpful for subclassifying AUS/FLUS, cytological features of FVPTC, and Hürthle cell lesion. An algorithm with integrated approaches of clinical, radiologic, pathologic, and molecular findings will be proposed for indeterminate thyroid nodules.

2. AUS/FLUS interpretation

2.1. Diagnosis of exclusion and incorporation of biomarkers

The AUS/FLUS thyroid nodules represent those not clearly benign or malignant [3]. The cytologic findings are not convincingly benign, yet the degree of cellular or architectural atypia is not sufficient for an interpretation of SF/FN, suspicious for malignancy, or malignancy [28]. It is a diagnosis of exclusion (**Figure 1**).

> Case 1 (**Figure 2**): The aspiration of a 2.6 cm × 2.5 cm × 1.7-cm isthmus solid nodule is from a 46-year-old female. The smears are cellular with scant colloid, unlike a benign thyroid nodule. Nuclear enlargement and overlapping resembling SF/FN are present, but are focal. Rare microfollicles are identified in cell-block section. There are no papillary carcinoma features such as nuclear groove, pseudoinclusion, or papillae. This case was categorized cytologically as AUS (case courtesy of Dr. Jaklyn McClendon, Anaheim Health Medical Center, CA).

The specimen was forwarded for ThyGenX Thyroid Oncogene Panel and ThyraMIR Thyroid miRNA Classifier. ThyGenX™ Oncogene Panel detected one NRAS point mutation (Q61R). The ThyraMIR™ microRNA Classifier was negative. Thyroid nodules with AUS diagnosis and NRAS mutation are at increased risk for malignancy (42–65% compared to 7–37% in NRAS-negative AUS, p = 0.038) [32]. However, RAS mutation has limited value-predicting malignancy in the absence of BRAF mutation among thyroid nodules with AUS/FLUS cytology [33];

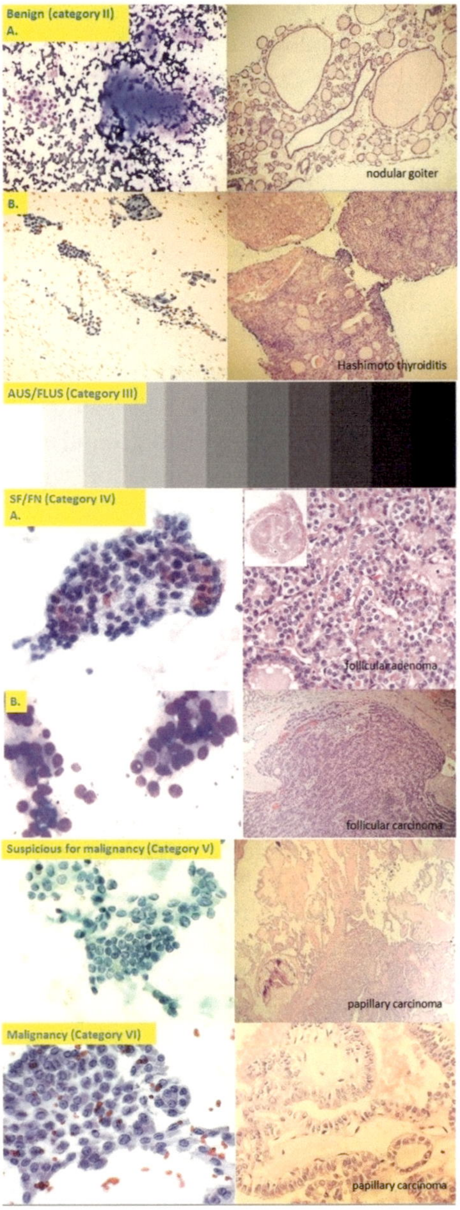

Figure 1. AUS/FLUS in the Bethesda Thyroid Diagnostic Category. The cytological interpretation is on the left, the corresponding histological diagnosis is on the right. Category I nondiagnostic or unsatisfactory is not illustrated. Category II is a group of benign lesions including nodular goiter with abundant colloid and honeycomb sheets of follicular cells (IIA), and Hashimoto thyroiditis characterized by follicular cells, Hürthle cells, lymphocytes and plasmacytes (IIB). Category IV indicates follicular lesions (SF/FN) featured by increased cellularity and microfollicles. Category V applies to aspirations with some but not all features of malignancy. Category VI includes lesions meeting diagnostic criteria of malignancy. AUS/FLUS: Atypia of undetermined significance/follicular lesion of undetermined significance SF/FN: suspicious for follicular neoplasm/follicular neoplasm.

RAS mutation has been detected in follicular adenoma (8–48%) and follicular carcinoma (0–52%) [34]. The probability of malignancy is reduced to 50:50 in combination with the mild atypia and negative ThyraMIR™ finding in this case.

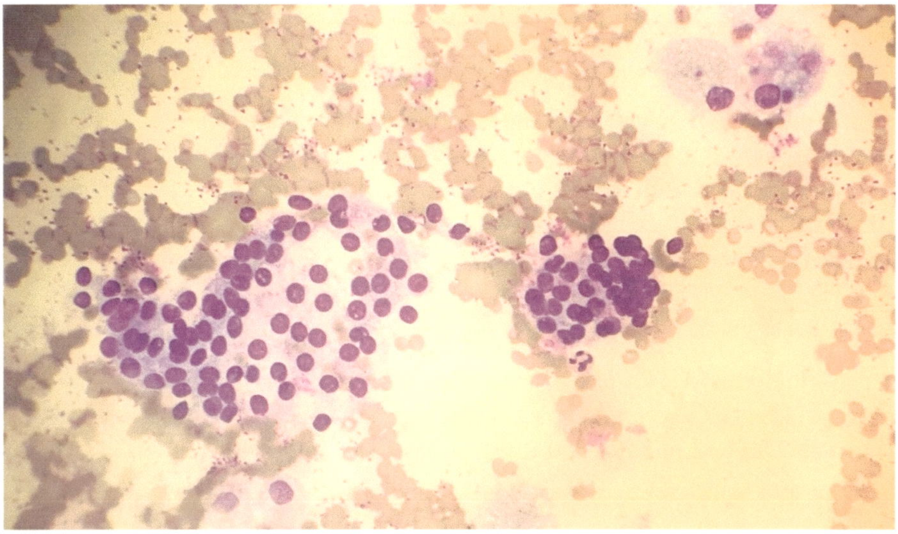

Figure 2. Atypia of undetermined significance. Focal crowded follicular cell clusters with scant colloid. (Case courtesy of Dr. Jaklyn McClendon, Anaheim Health Medical Center, CA.)

This case has also brought up a question of how ancillary studies would help subclassify AUS/FLUS. The various performances in molecular tests could be due to the nature of AUS/FLUS, which is a group of heterogeneous borderline lesions in transit from hyperplastic or adenomatoid nodule to adenoma, adenoma with atypia, and carcinoma. There is no single magic marker for subclassifying AUS/FLUS. Most tests use a panel of markers. New tests are emerging and extensive validation is required. Therefore, the 2015 American Thyroid Association (ATA) guidelines recommend ancillary studies but do not specify particular test(s) for AUS/FLUS follow-up [2].

2.2. Reproducibility of AUS/FLUS

2.2.1. Adequacy check

Recognizing that some of the equivocal FNA cases are the result of inadequate number of cells or poorly visualized cells, the Bethesda System for Reporting Thyroid Cytopathology (TBSRTC) has recommended adequacy evaluation with category I being nondiagnostic [3]. Blood diluted and obscured specimen may push the follicular cells into microfollicle-like structure, making the colloid imperceivable and masking the benign cytological details. A sparse preparation or interpretation hindered by sampling preparation artifact may not be justified for a category of AUS/FLUS [3, 35]. It is important not to place those cases in AUS/FLUS group for the reasons: although re-biopsy is the same immediate outcome for ND or AUS/FLUS, the risk of malignancy for two AUS/FLUS diagnoses is higher than that for one AUS/FLUS diagnosis [10, 36], and most cases with two AUS/FLUS diagnoses will go to surgery [36].

2.2.2. Correlation with clinical and ultrasound findings

Clinical findings such as spiculated margin, microcalcification, hypoechogenicity of ultrasonography, larger size of mass, male gender, and increased thyroid-stimulating hormone (TSH) level may be associated with increased risk of malignancy in AUS/FLUS diagnosis. On the other hand, cystic or complex nodules have a lower risk of malignancy [37–42]. Considering those features, a more definitive diagnosis could be reached [35].

2.2.3. Consensus diagnosis

Expert consultation and group consensus reviews have been reported to minimize the diagnosis of FLUS [43]. A second opinion has an overall diagnostic resolution rate of 42.5% for "indeterminate" thyroid nodules and 71.5% reclassification accuracy in AUS/FLUS category [44].

2.2.4. Quality assessment

The use of the individual diagnostic categories within BSRTC varied up to 12.7-fold. The ratio of "AUS/FLUS" (A) to "malignant" (M) diagnoses varied at a range of 0.5–4.9 with a median ratio of 2.0. Based on this, an A:M ratio of 1.0–3.0 is proposed for the proper use of AUS/FLUS diagnosis. AUS:M ratios of >3.0 are likely because of overdiagnosis of AUS or underdiagnosis of M. AUS:M ratios of <1.0 are mostly due to low AUS rates, at the likely expense of sensitivity [45]. Some study supports this quality measure, but disputes exist [46].

3. Cytology hints for subgrouping AUS/FLUS

3.1. Reactive change and benign cellular components mimicking atypia

3.1.1. Reactive atypia

Reactive atypia in thyroid are associated with cystic degeneration, thyroiditis (inflammation), physical or chemical trauma, radiation, and other nonspecific causes, in a very similar way to cervical cytology [28, 29]. They present as metaplastic Hürthle cells, squamous cells, degenerative/regenerative follicular cells, or proliferative fibroblasts. Cells can be alarmingly bizarre with nuclear grooves or nucleoli but never have high N:C ratio, crowded nuclei, papillae, or microfollicle [47].

Case 2 (**Figure 3**): The smear is prepared from a 4-cm left-neck complex lesion on a 65-year-old female. The significant finding is a cluster of hemosiderin-associated cells with large elongated or polygonal nuclei in contrast to a background of honeycomb-round follicular cells. Despite the presence of nuclear groove, no intranuclear pseudoinclusion or architectural disorder such as crowded nuclei or papillae is identified to further suggest malignancy. Concurrent Afirma gene expression classifier result is benign, and medullary thyroid cancer classifier is negative (Veracyte, Inc., San Francisco, CA).

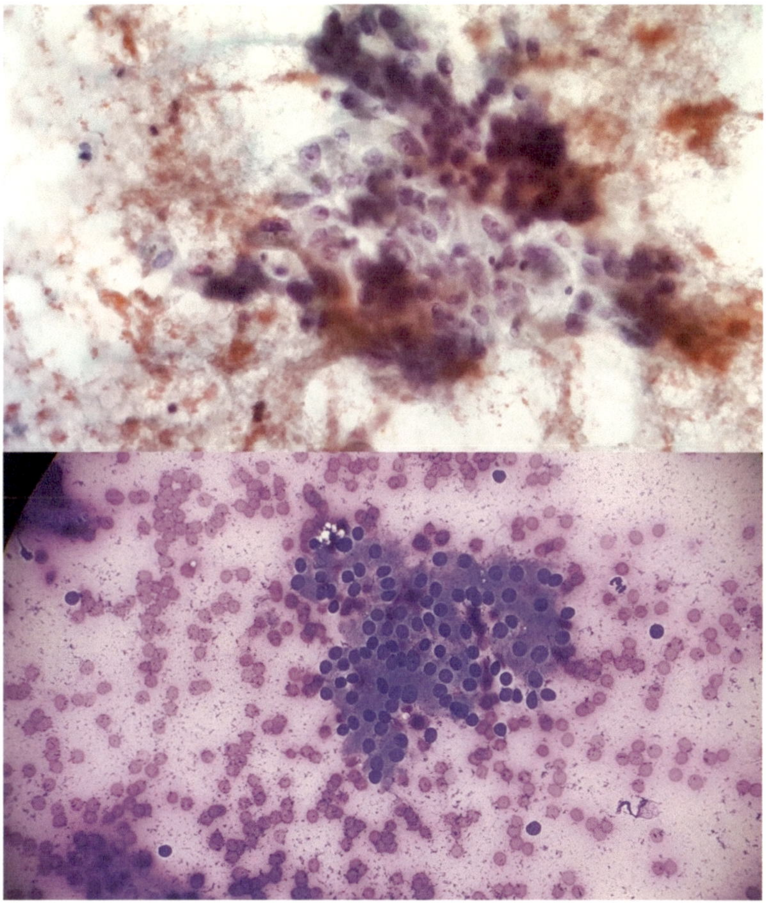

Figure 3. Atypical cells suggestive of benign cystic lining. The cells (upper) are larger compared to the rest of the follicular cells (lower), showing partially streaming appearance, irregular nuclear membrane and nuclear groove, pale chromatin, and small nucleoli. No nuclear overlapping or inclusion is present.

Atypical cystic lining cells need to be distinguished from cystic papillary carcinoma, which constitutes 10% of papillary carcinoma. The former does not have nuclear overlapping and inclusion [47].

Epithelioid cells in Hashimoto thyroiditis (**Figure 4**) or reparative fibroblasts can have atypical features such as large nuclei, taking an appearance of ugly ducklings among benign follicular cells. The low N:C ratio and non-clumping chromatin distinguish them from malignancy.

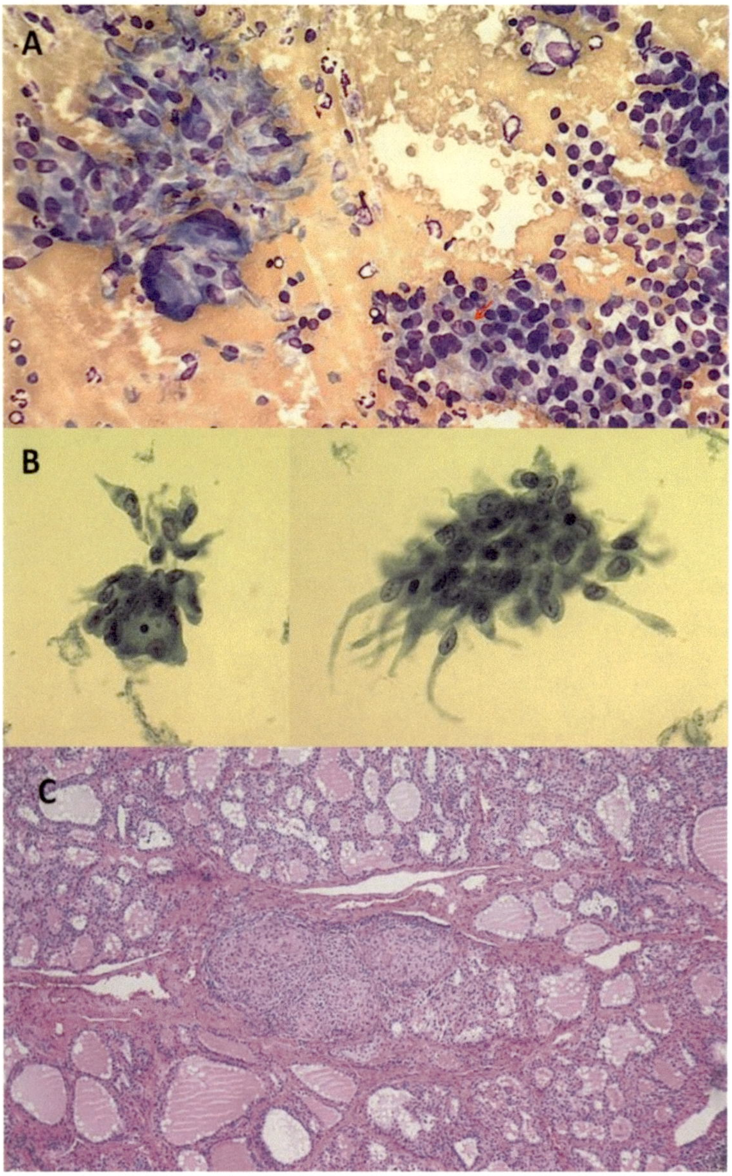

Figure 4. Granulomatous inflammation. (A) Epithelioid cells (left) in contrast to sheets of bland-appearing follicular cells mixed with several plasmacytes (arrow), Diff Quick stain. (B) Epithelioid cells in spindle-shaped and multinucleated form, Pap stain. (C) Resection shows Hashimoto thyroiditis with diffuse inflammation.

3.1.2. Perifollicular fibrosis

Perifollicular fibrosis refers to basement membrane-like material outlining follicles. Perifollicular fibrosis has been described in sporadic colloid nodule, adenomatoid hyperplasia, and in pediatric thyroid cancer following the Chernobyl disaster [24, 28, 48–50]. It is associated with benign or low-grade thyroid lesions. The incidence of perifollicular fibrosis seems to be higher in elderly people (>60) than in other age population (5–10 vs 2%) ([51] and unpublished data). In the elderly, it is often linked to a paucicellular aspiration with fibrosis.

Cases 3 and 4 (**Figure 5**): Perifollicular fibrosis is illustrated in two cases with Bethesda category of atypia and benign, respectively. The first case (A) is a 38-year-old male with a left thyroid nodule status post chemoradiation for Hodgkin disease. Surgical resection shows an atypical adenomatoid hyperplasia. The second case (B) is a 61-year-old female with a benign 1.3-cm complex thyroid nodule.

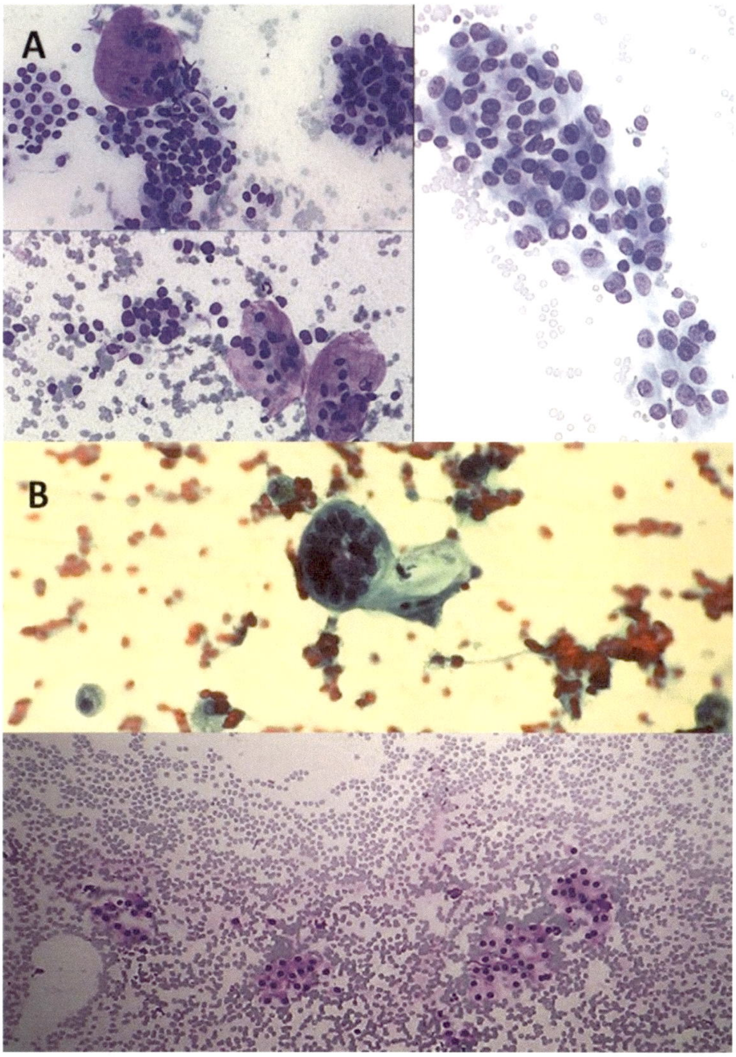

Figure 5. Perifollicular fibrosis (A) in a cellular specimen with atypical cells. Follicular cells are expelled off a balloon-like fibrous rind (perifollicular fibrosis, left, Diff Quick stain). The follicular cells are atypical with slightly larger, crowded nuclei and rare nuclear groove and inclusion (right, Pap stain). (B) In a benign thyroid nodule with sparser cells. A glassy hyaline rind is partially peeled off a follicle with hemosiderin macrophages (upper, Pap stain) and scattered benign follicular cells (lower, Diff-Quik stain) are seen in the background.

Perifollicular fibrosis was first described in post-Chernobyl nonneoplastic thyroid tissue [50]. The basement membrane-like structure surrounding follicles may inhibit tumor genesis and progression, although the mechanism underlying perifollicular fibrosis in radiation exposure might be different from that in natural aging.

3.1.3. Benign cellular components mimicking AUS/FLUS

Parathyroid gland is occasionally aspirated during thyroid nodule workup. In one molecular study for indeterminate thyroid nodules, three patients out of 441 who had a diagnosis of AUS/ FLUS were found to have parathyroid rather than thyroidal origin after biochemical study and surgery [19].

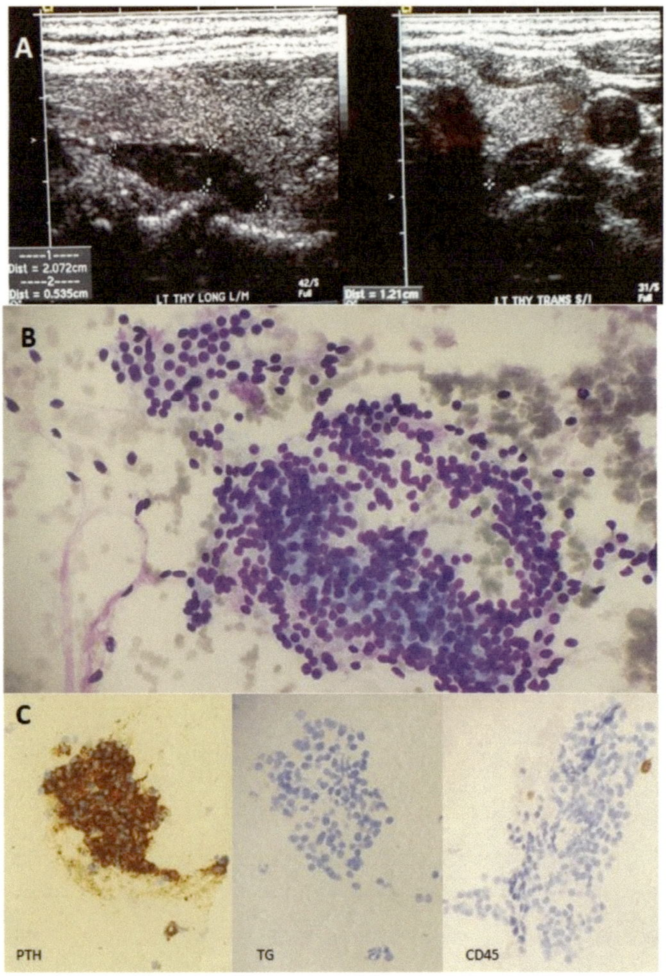

Figure 6. Parathyroid gland mimicking thyroid nodule. (A) An elongated nodule in the left posterior "thyroid" close to vessels. (B) Aggregates of structureless uniform cells with no colloid. (C) Immunohistochemistry performed on cell block confirmed parathyroid origin. PTH: parathyroid hormone; TG: thyroglobulin; CD45: white blood cell common antigen.

http://dx.doi.org/10.5772/64155

Case 5 (**Figure 6**): A 65-year-old female complained of "a lump in the throat." Ultrasonography identified a right isthmus movable 1.9-cm nodule and a left posterior 2-cm nodule. Image and cytological features of the left posterior nodule are shown in A and B. The monomorphic small cells are bland appearing with scant cytoplasm and no identifiable colloid. The immunohistochemistry (IHC) confirms parathyroid origin.

If IHC information is not available, this case may be mistaken for FLUS in the absence of colloid or benign thyroid nodule if colloid from adjacent thyroid is mixed up.

Ultimobranchial body or solid cell nest is a developmental remnant derived from fourth to fifth pharyngeal pouch, considered as a normal component of thyroid. It is found in about 60% of serially sectioned thyroid with a male predominance [52–54]. Incidental aspiration of them may lead to AUS diagnosis [55].

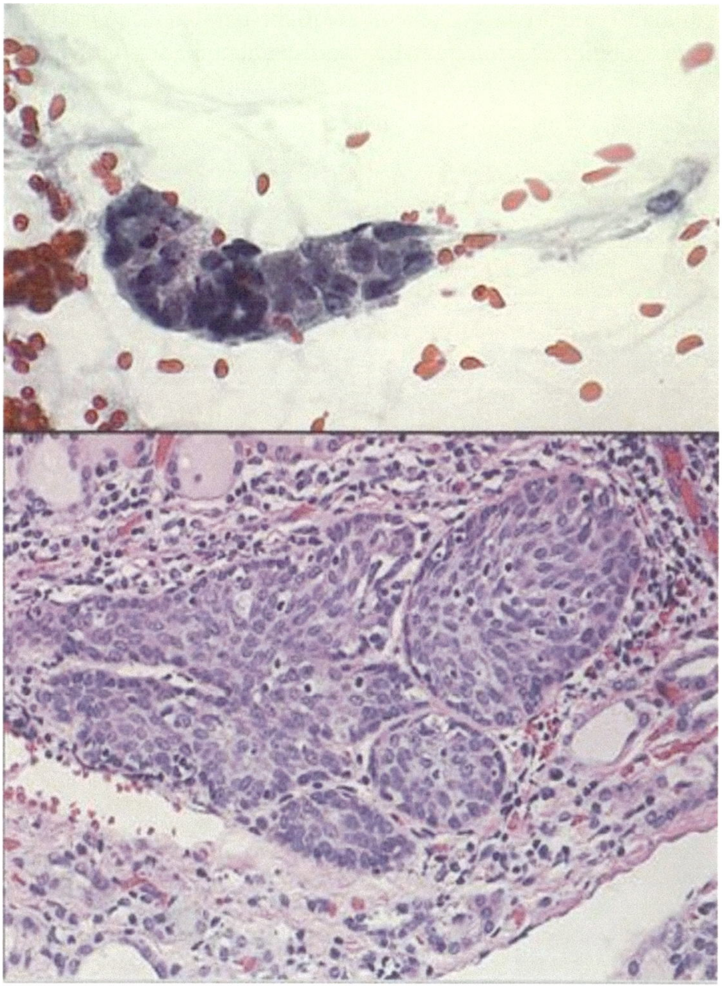

Figure 7. Ultimobranchial body. The aspiration shows cohesive polygonal cells. Histologic section shows a nest composed predominantly of similar polygonal or oval to spindle cells (main cells) mixed with a minor population of small cells with compact nuclei and clear cytoplasm.

Case 6 (**Figure 7**): The illustrated cell cluster is from a thyroid aspiration of a 46-year-old male. Cytological features distinguishing from malignancy include the absence of hyperchromatic nuclei or prominent nucleoli in tightly cohesive squamoid cells. Those cells are positive for Galectin-3, but negative for HMBE-1 [55].

3.2. Cytologic characters suggestive of malignancy

3.2.1. Nuclear atypia

It seems that nuclear atypia (a subgroup of AUS) is more predictive of malignancy than microfollicle (a subgroup of FLUS) [56]. Nuclear atypia suggestive of papillary carcinoma carry a higher risk of malignancy than AUS/FLUS interpretations made for other reasons, such as microfollicles, Hürthle cells, and suboptimal specimens [57]. This might be due to higher incidence of papillary carcinoma or follicular variant papillary carcinoma than follicular carcinoma, and incapability of cytology to distinguish adenoma from follicular carcinoma.

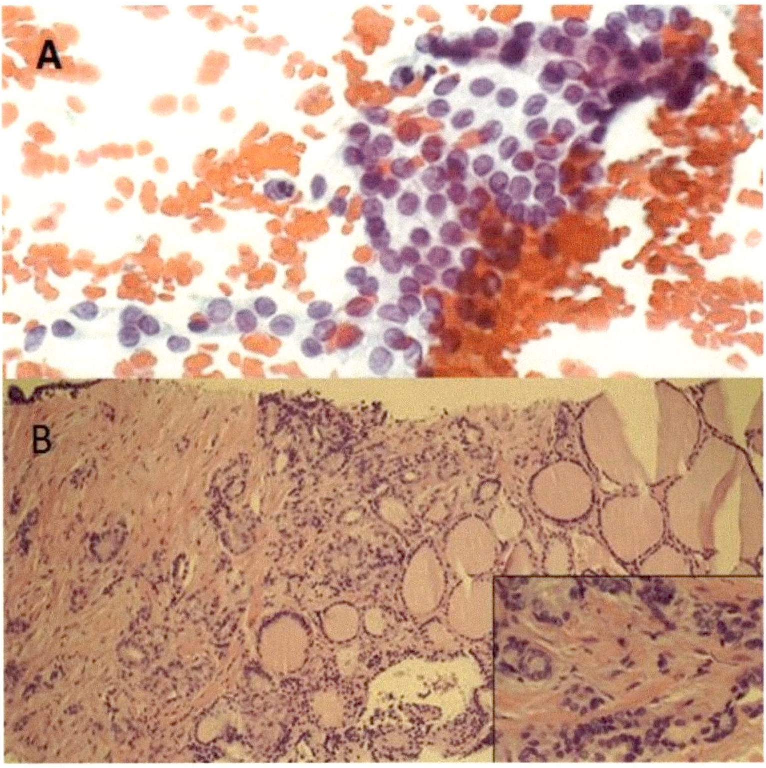

Figure 8. AUS upgraded to papillary carcinoma follicular pattern. (A) A combination of nuclear overlapping, groove, and pale chromatin indicates AUS, suspicious for malignancy. (B) A follow-up core biopsy confirmed papillary carcinoma follicular pattern with invasion.

Nuclear pseudoinclusion and papillae are diagnostic of papillary carcinoma. Other nuclear features such as enlarged nuclei, pale chromatin, nuclear groove, and crowded nuclei are more commonly seen in AUS/FLUS category. More prominence of these findings or a great of them should increase the suspicion of malignancy [57].

Case 7 (**Figure 8**): This is a case of AUS upgraded to malignancy in a 32-year-old female. The initial aspiration of a thyroid nodule demonstrates groups of follicular cells with various features of nuclear atypia including pale chromatin, nuclear groove, and nuclear overlapping. A core-needle biopsy (CNB) 1 month later confirmed papillary carcinoma of follicular pattern with invasion.

3.3. Follicular variant papillary thyroid carcinoma (FVPTC) and noninvasive follicular thyroid neoplasm with papillary-like nuclear features (NIFTP)

FVPTC is defined by histology as a tumor with PTC-type nuclei and follicular rather than papillary pattern (papillary architecture of <1%) [21]. Based on the presence or absence of invasion of capsule or parenchyma, it is subgrouped as invasive FVPTC (I-FVPTC) and noninvasive FVPTC. The NI-FVPTC is clinically indolent similar to adenoma [22, 58]. It is recently renamed as noninvasive follicular thyroid neoplasm with papillary-like nuclear features to avoid overtreatment [22, 23, 58]. The impact of reclassifying NI-FVPTC on the risk of malignancy would be most pronounced in the indeterminate categories: a decrease of ROM, 5.2–17.6%, in AUS/FLUS, 8–15.1% in SF/FN, and 17.6–41.5% in suspicious for malignancy [16, 22].

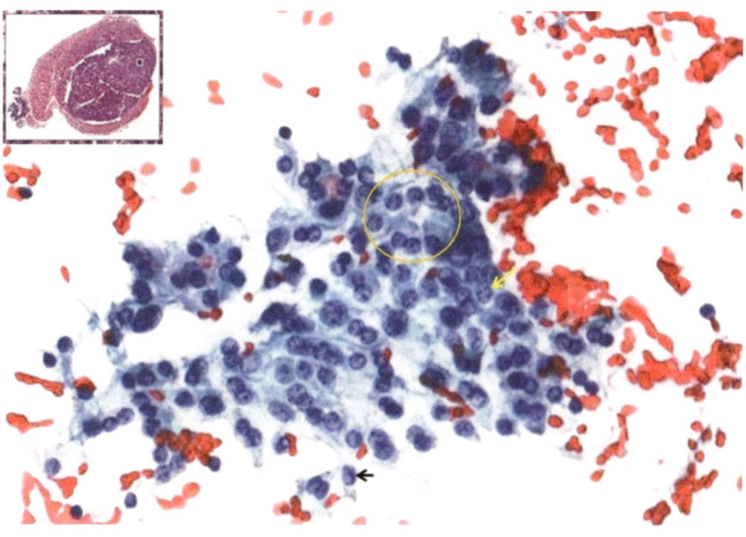

Figure 9. NIFNP/NI-FVPTC. NI-FVPTC characterized by pale nuclei with marginated chromatin (yellow arrow), nuclear groove (black arrow), and microfollicle (orange circle) in an encapsulated nodule (left-upper corner) without capsule or parenchyma invasion.

NIFTP or NI-FVPTC has a molecular file of RAS mutation and PAX8/PPARr translocation but lacking BRAF V600E mutation in keeping with follicular adenoma. I-FVPTC has an opposite molecular profile closer to classical papillary carcinoma than to follicular adenoma or NIFTP/NI-FVPTC (BRAFV600E > RAS mutations) [58].

Most NIFTP or NI-FVPTC are categorized as AUS/FLUS, SF/FN, or suspicious for malignancy in Bethesda system. The NIFTP/NI-FVPTC in AUS/FLUS category shows atypical PTC-type nuclear feature and microfollicles (**Figure 9**). However, I-FVPTC versus NIFTP/NI-FVPTC is a histologic diagnosis, not a cytology stratification. Whether the degree of nuclear atypia in FVPTC is predictive of invasion is unclear.

3.4. Hürthle cell lesion

Hürthle cell tumor of thyroid is a group of neoplasm with distinct biology, morphology, and natural history. However, it is not an independent entity in World Health Organization (WHO) category and therefore has been diagnosed as either benign adenoma, or papillary carcinoma or follicular carcinoma or poorly differentiated based on cytomorphology, architecture of papillae, follicle and solid/trabeculae, and evaluation of mitosis and necrosis [59]. Capsule invasion or vascular invasion is the criterion for malignancy, while pleomorphism by itself is not a feature of malignancy [28, 59]. Cytomorphological criteria have been shown to be helpful in distinguishing Hürthle cell neoplasm from Hürthle cell metaplasia (in nodular goiter or Hashimoto thyroiditis), but not Hürthle cell carcinoma from adenoma [60].

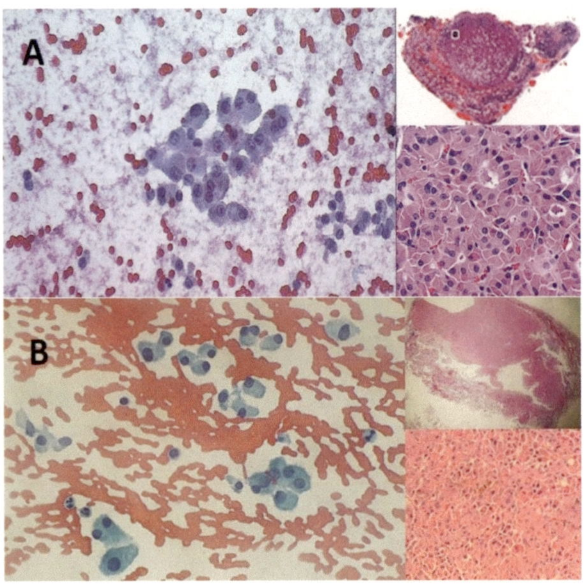

Figure 10. Hürthle cell lesion. (A) Predominant oncocytic cells on thyroid aspiration (left) and well-circumscribed nodule in the background of lymphocytic thyroiditis (Hashimoto disease) (right). (B) Loosely cohesive eosinophilic cells with binucleation on thyroid smears (left) and metastatic disease to the lung composed of the same cells (right) (case courtesy of Dr. Terry Welsh, Anaheim Health Medical Center, CA).

Lymphocytic thyroiditis is diagnosed based on a mixed cell population of lymphocytes, plasma cells, and follicular cells with Hürthle cell metaplasia. However, the differentiation of benign hyperplastic Hürthle cell nodule (or Hürthle cell adenoma) from Hürthle cell carcinoma can be very difficult based on cytology alone.

Case 8 (A and B) (**Figure 10**): A is a 56-year-old female presented with bilateral thyroid nodules. Surgical resection revealed hyperplastic oncocytic nodules in the background of lymphocytic thyroiditis. B is an 85-year-old female with one left thyroid nodule. Left lung wedge resection demonstrates metastatic lesion from thyroid (case courtesy of Dr. Terry Welsh, Anaheim Health Medical Center, CA). The smear preparations from A and B show similar oncocytic cells with the same cytological diagnosis of AUS/FLUS, Hürthle cell lesion.

After the lung lesion is diagnosed as thyroid metastasis (case B), a retrospective comparison of these two cytology cases was done. Hürthle cells in case B seem to be more loosely cohesive and have more binucleation. These architectural differences and cytological atypia are very subtle, requiring high grade of alert. Moreover, Hürthle cell metaplasia shows more pleomorphism than Hürthle cell carcinoma [27].

Retrospectively, the Hürthle cells in case A is positive for p27, but negative for HBME-1 and Galectin-3, in support of benign [54]. The triple immunostaining is not available for case B. The application of p27/HBME-1/Galectin-3 immunostaining in distinguishing benign Hürthle cell from Hürthle cell carcinoma needs to be studied.

A suspicious result from Afirma gene expression classifier does not increase the probability of malignancy in the Hürthle cell nodules. Patient should be counseled for the high possibility of unnecessary surgery based on suspicious interpretation of Afirma test for a Hürthle cell nodule [61, 62]. Molecular tests with both high sensitivity and specificity are needed for Hürthle cell nodules.

4. Algorithm for AUS/FLUS follow-up

4.1. Repeat FNA

Repeat FNA is the recommendation for AUS/FLUS in TBSRTC [3]. For an initial aspirate diagnosed as AUS/FLUS, repeat FNA is specifically endorsed by the American Thyroid Association as a suitable follow-up option, perhaps proving especially useful when limited cellularity contributes to the initial AUS/FLUS interpretation [2, 63].

For initial AUS/FLUS diagnosis, reclassification rate with repeat FNA is 56 and 69% [11, 64]. Most of the repeat FNA diagnoses are benign (69%, 47/74) [64]. The malignancy rate after surgery with or without repeat FNA for initial AUS/FLUS is 38.6 versus 15.6% [42, 65]. Repeat FNA helps the selection of patients with AUS/FLUS to triage to surgery, significantly reducing unnecessary surgery. Therefore, repeat FNA for nodules with AUS/FLUS on initial FNA is suggested.

Two consecutive AUS/FLUS diagnoses have higher malignancy risk of at least 31.0% than one AUS/FLUS diagnosis and a higher proportion of FVPTC [11, 36, 65]. Solid structure, increased nodular size (>2 cm), and irregular/microlobulated margins are found to be risk factors in two studies [42, 66] but not in the other [36]. Most cases with repeated AUS/FLUS will require surgery [11, 36, 42, 65].

For benign aspirates following initial AUS/FLUS, the malignancy risk is low (2 and 2.8%) so that clinical follow-up instead of surgical excision or continuous repeat FNA may be enough [64, 67], although one study has suggested a still higher risk of malignancy with one AUS/FLUS diagnosis compared to none [11]. The ultrasound features might be insignificant in predicting malignancy in this scenario [67].

A meta-analysis study has suggested that a core-needle biopsy has a higher conclusive rate than repeat FNA when the initial FNA produced inconclusive results [68]. This might be due to reduction in nondiagnostic category. Further prospective studies are necessary before follow-up CNB can be applied in daily practice.

4.2. Emerging molecular tests

Currently available commercial molecular tests for indeterminate (AUS/FLUS) thyroid nodules on fine needle aspiration have different strengths (**Table 2**). The Afirma gene expression classifier developed by Veracyte, Inc., is a "rule-out malignancy" test for the preoperative identification of benign thyroid nodules with indeterminate cytology. The Afirma test assesses gene expression from mRNA isolated from thyroid FNA samples by comparing the mRNA expression detected in a thyroid FNA against a panel of 167 molecular genes [17]. The other three later-developed assays test for 17 known thyroid cancer-related mutations and translocations [18], combined with miRNA, mRNA, and DNA mutation [19] or 14 thyroid cancer-related genes and 42 types of gene fusion related to thyroid cancer [20], aiming to increase diagnostic yields on positive-predictive value.

	Sensitivity (%)	Specificity (%)	Positive-predictive value (%)	Negative-predictive value (%)
Afirma gene expression classifier (Veracyte, Inc.) [17]	90	53	37.7	95
miRInform™ (Asuragen Inc.) [18]	63	99	94	88
Multi-Gene ThyroSeq Next-Generation Sequencing Assay (ThyroSeq®) [19]	90.9	92.1	76.9	97.2
ThyGenX and ThyraMIR™ [20]	94	80	68	97

Table 2. Commercial molecular tests for indeterminate (AUS/FLUS) thyroid nodules on fine needle aspiration.

The test performance may change when applied to individual clinics. One independent study has reported lower than previously reported negative- and positive-predictive value (75 compared to 95%, and 16 compared to 38%) for cytology diagnosis of AUS/FLUS and SN/FN combined [62]. One reason might be due to the lower malignancy rate for indeterminate thyroid nodules in the specialized academic center compared to the validation settings from Afirma (17 vs 24%). Adjusting the malignancy rate on Bethesda categories III and IV, another study from the same institution demonstrated still lower actual performance of Afirma™, miRInform™, and ThyroSeq™ v2 tests compared to published sensitivity and specificity [69]. Assessing the institutional performance of each test is necessary along with the prevalence of malignancy. This has called for attention that customization is needed for the application of the molecular tests.

4.3. Clinical cytological rescore prior to surgery

Diagnostic excision has been performed for high-risk thyroid nodules, and surgery is an indication for large goiter with symptoms. The synthesis of cytological interpretation, clinical factors including age, gender, nodular size, results of molecular testing, ultrasound findings, personal and family history, and the presence of additional nodules will impact the determination of the appropriate extent of initial surgical management [2, 42, 63, 70].

Quantitative methods are available to assemble clinical, ultrasonographic, and cytological findings into a scoring system to evaluate the malignant risk of thyroid nodules, especially in cases with indeterminate or repeated nondiagnostic FNA [70]. A similar scoring system integrating molecular test results would be desirable.

Acknowledgements

Cases are from the University of Chicago, Mercy Hospitals at Bakersfield, the University of California at Irvine, Anaheim Health Medical Center, and the University of California at Los Angeles. We thank Dr. McClendon and Dr. Welsh for the courtesy of cases and helpful discussion.

Author details

Lei Zhang[1*], Beverly Wang[2], Jianyu Rao[3] and Douglas Bell[4]

*Address all correspondence to: lei_248@hotmail.com

1 Anaheim Health Medical Center, California, United States

2 UC Irvine School of Medicine, UC Irvine Medical Center, California, United States

3 International Telepathology Dept. Pathology and Lab Med UCLA, David Geffen School of Medicine, California, United States

4 Biomedical Informatics Program, Department of Medicine, David Geffen School of Medicine at UCLA Program, California, United States

References

[1] Cooper DS, Doherty GM, Haugen BR, et al. Revised American Thyroid Association management guidelines for patients with thyroid nodules and differentiated thyroid cancer. Thyroid. 2009; 19: 1167–1214.

[2] Haugen BR, Alexander EK, Bible KC, et al. 2015 American thyroid association management guidelines for adult patients with thyroid nodules and differentiated thyroid cancer. Thyroid. 2016; 26(1): 1–133.

[3] Ali SZ, Cibas ES (editors). The Bethesda system for reporting thyroid cytopathology definitions, criteria and explanatory notes. ©Springer Science Business Media, LLC, New York Dordrecht Heidelberg London, 2010

[4] British Thyroid Association guidelines for the management of thyroid cancer. Clinical Endocrinology. 2014; 81(Suppl 1): 1–122.

[5] Bongiovanni M, Spitale A, Faquin WC, Mazzucchelli L, Baloch ZW. The Bethesda system for reporting thyroid cytopathology: a meta-analysis. Acta Cytopathology. 2012; 56: 333–339.

[6] Liu X, Medici M, Kwong N, et al. Bethesda categorization of thyroid nodule cytology and prediction of thyroid cancer types and prognosis. Thyroid. 2016; 26(2): 256–261.

[7] Hirsch D, Robenshtok E, Bachar G, et al. The implementation of the Bethesda system for reporting thyroid cytopathology improves malignancy detection despite lower rate of thyroidectomy in indeterminate nodules. World Journal of Surgery. 2015, 39(8): 1959–1965.

[8] Arul P, Akshatha C, Masilamani S. A study of malignancy rates in different diagnostic categories of the Bethesda system for reporting thyroid cytopathology: an institutional experience. Biomedical Journal. 2015; 38(6): 517–522.

[9] Bhasin TS, Mannan R, Manjari M, et al. Reproducibility of 'The Bethesda System for Reporting Thyroid Cytopathology': a multicenter study with review of the literature. Journal of Clinical and Diagnostic Research 2013; 7(6): 1051–14.

[10] Nassar A, Reynolds JP, Kerr SE, Jenkins SM, Lackore KA, Bernet V. Survey of cytopathologists and cytotechnologists for the clinical impact of the use of atypia or follicular lesion of undetermined significance. Cytojournal. 2015; 12: 14. doi: 10.4103/1742-6413.159246. eCollection

[11] Sullivan PS, Hirschowitz SL, Fung PC, et al. The impact of atypia/follicular lesion of undetermined significance and repeat fine-needle aspiration: 5 years before and after implementation of the Bethesda system. Cancer (Cancer Cytopathol). 2014; 122: 866–872.

[12] Fazeli R, VandenBussche CJ, Bishop BA, Ali SZ. Cytological diagnosis of follicular variant of papillary thyroid carcinoma before and after the Bethesda system for

reporting thyroid cytopathology. Acta Cytologica. 2016. Epub DOI 10.1007/s12022-009-9103-1

[13] Hyeon J, Ahn S, Shin JH, Oh YL. The prediction of malignant risk in the category "atypia of undetermined significance/follicular lesion of undetermined significance" of the Bethesda system for reporting thyroid cytopathology using subcategorization and BRAF mutation results. Cancer (Cancer Cytopathol). 2014; 122: 368–376.

[14] Straccia P, Rossi ED, Bizzarro T, et al. A meta-analytic review of the Bethesda system for reporting thyroid cytopathology: Has the rate of malignancy in indeterminate lesions been underestimated? Cancer (Cancer Cytopathol). 2015; 123: 713–722.

[15] Ho AS, Sarti EE, Jain KS, et al. Malignancy rate in thyroid nodules classified as Bethesda Category III (AUS/FLUS). Thyroid. 2014; 24(5): 832–839.

[16] Strickland KC, Howitt BE, Marqusee E, Alexander EK, Cibas ES, Krane JF, Barletta JA. The impact of noninvasive follicular variant of papillary thyroid carcinoma on rates of malignancy for fine-needle aspiration diagnostic categories. Thyroid. 2015; 25(9): 987–992.

[17] Alexander EK, Kennedy GC, Baloch ZW, et al. Preoperative diagnosis of benign thyroid nodules with indeterminate cytology. The New England Journal of Medicine. 2012; 367: 705–715.

[18] Beaudenon-Huibregtse S, Alexander EK, Guttler RB, Hershman JM, Babu V, Blevins TC, Moore P, Andruss B, Labourier E. Centralized molecular testing for oncogenic gene mutations complements the local cytopathologic diagnosis of thyroid nodules. Thyroid. 2014; 24: 1479–1487.

[19] Nikiforov YE, Carty SE, Chiosea SI, et al. Impact of the multi-gene ThyroSeq next-generation sequencing assay on cancer diagnosis in thyroid nodules with atypia of undetermined significance/follicular lesion of undetermined significance cytology. Thyroid. 2015; 25(11): 1217–1223.

[20] Labourier E, Shifrin A, Busseniers AE, et al. Molecular testing for miRNA, mRNA and DNA on fine-needle aspiration improves the preoperative diagnosis of thyroid nodules with indeterminate cytology. Journal of Clinical Endocrinology Metabolism. 2015; 100: 2743–2750.

[21] Rosai J. The encapsulated follicular variant of papillary thyroid carcinoma: back to the drawing board. Endocrinology Pathology. 2010; 21: 7–11.

[22] Faquin WC, Wong LQ, Afrogheh AH, et al. Impact of reclassifying noninvasive follicular variant of papillary thyroid carcinoma on the risk of malignancy in the Bethesda system for reporting thyroid cytopathology. Cancer Cytopathology. 2016; 124: 181–187.

[23] Nikiforov YE, Seethala RR, Tallini G, et al. Nomenclature revision for encapsulated follicular variant of papillary thyroid carcinoma A paradigm shift to reduce overtreat-

ment of indolent tumors. JAMA Oncology. 2016 Apr 14. doi: 10.1001/jamaoncol. 2016.0386. [Epub ahead of print]

[24] Yang J, Schnadig V, Logrono R, Wasserman PG. Fine needle aspiration of thyroid nodules: a study of 4703 patients with histologic and clinical correlations. Cancer. 2007; 111: 306–315.

[25] Wu HH-J, Rose C, Elsheikh TM. The Bethesda system for reporting thyroid cytopathology: an experience of 1,382 cases in a community practice setting with the implication for risk of neoplasm and risk of malignancy. Diagnostic Cytopathology. 2012 (2011); 40: 399–403.

[26] Jo VY, Stelow EB, Dustin SM, Hanley KZ. Malignancy risk for fine-needle aspiration of thyroid lesions according to the Bethesda system for reporting thyroid cytopathology. American Journal of Clinical Pathology. 2010; 134: 450–456.

[27] Theoharis CG, Schofield KM, Hammers L, Udelsman R, Chhieng DC. The Bethesda thyroid fine-needle aspiration classification system: year 1 at an academic institution. Thyroid. 2009;19:1215–1223.

[28] DeMay RM. Thyroid. In: *The Art & Science of Cytopathology*. 2nd ed. Chicago, IL: ASCP Press; 2012.

[29] Cibas ES, Ducatman BS. Cytology: diagnostic principles and clinical correlates. 4th ed. Edinburough: WB Saunders; 2014.

[30] Giorgadze T, Rossi ED, Fadda G, Gupta PK, Livolsi VA, Baloch Z. Does the fine-needle aspiration diagnosis of "Hurthle-cell neoplasm/follicular neoplasm with oncocytic features" denote increased risk of malignancy? Diagnostic Cytopathology. 2004; 31: 307–312.

[31] McKee S, Wu H, Wang XY, et al. Hurthle cell neoplasms diagnosed by fine needle aspiration are not associated with an increased risk of malignancy. Acta Cytologica. 2014; 58: 235–238.

[32] Jang EK, Kim WG, Kim EY, et al. Usefulness of NRAS codon 61 mutation analysis and core needle biopsy for the diagnosis of thyroid nodules previously diagnosed as atypia of undetermined significance. Endocrine. 2016; 52(2): 305–312.

[33] Yoon JH, Kwon HJ, Lee HS, et al. RAS mutations in AUS/FLUS cytology: does it have an additional role in BRAFV600E mutation-negative nodules? Medicine (Baltimore) 2015; 94(27): e1084. doi:10.1097/MD.0000000000001084

[34] Howell GM, Hodak SP, Yip L. RAS mutations in thyroid cancer. The Oncologist 2013; 18: 926–932.

[35] Henry M. The potential for overuse of atypical thyroid diagnoses. Cancer Cytopathology. 2012; 120(2): 108–110.

[36] Park VY, Kim EK, Kwak JY, et al. Malignancy risk and characteristics of thyroid nodules with two consecutive results of atypia of undetermined significance or follicular lesion of undetermined significance on cytology. European Radiology. 2015; 25: 2601–2607.

[37] Hong IK, Kim JH, Cho Yu, et al. Clinicopathological factors increased the risk of malignancy in thyroid nodules with atypical or follicular lesions of undetermined significance (AUS/FLUS) risk factor of malignancy in thyroid nodule with AUS/FLUS. Annals of Surgical Treatment and Research. 2016; 90(4): 201–206.

[38] Rosario PW. Thyroid nodules with atypia or follicular lesions of undetermined significance (Bethesda category III): importance of ultrasonography and cytological subcategory. Thyroid. 2014; 24(7): 1115–1120.

[39] Na DG, Baek JH, Sung JY, et al. Thyroid imaging reporting and data system risk stratification of thyroid nodules: categorization based on solidity and echogenicity. Thyroid. 2016; 26(4): 562–572.

[40] Yoon JH, Kwon HJ, Kim EK, et al. Subcategorization of atypia of undetermined significance/follicular lesion of undetermined significance (AUS/FLUS): a study applying thyroid imaging reporting and data system (TIRADS). Clinical Endocrinology (Oxford). 2015 Dec 7. doi: 10.1111/cen.12987. [Epub ahead of print].

[41] Barser H, Topaloglu O, Tam AA, et al. Higher TSH can be used as an additional risk factor in prediction of malignancy in euthyroid thyroid nodules evaluated by cytology based on Bethesda system. Endocrine. 2016, Mar 14 [Epub ahead of print].

[42] Kuru B, Atmaca A, Tarim IA, et al. Risk factors associated with malignancy and with triage to surgery in thyroid nodules classified as Bethesda category III (AUS/FLUS). European Journal of Surgical Oncology. 2016; 42: 87–93.

[43] Jing X, Knoepp SM, Roh MH, et al. Group consensus review minimizes the diagnosis of "Follicular lesions of undetermined significance" and improves cytohistologic concordance. Diagnostic Cytopathology. 2012; 40: 1037–1042.

[44] Gerhard R, Boemer SL. The value of second opinion in thyroid cytology: a review. Cancer Cytopathology. 2014, 122(8): 611–619.

[45] Krane JF, VanderLaan PA, Faquin WC, et al. The atypia of undetermined significance/follicular lesion of undetermined significance: malignant ratio: a proposed performance measure for reporting in the Bethesda system for thyroid cytopathology. Cancer Cytopathology. 2012; 120(2): 111–116.

[46] Fazeli R, Schneider EB, Ali SZ, Zeiger MA, Olson MT. Diagnostic frequency ratios are insufficient to measure laboratory precision with the Bethesda system for reporting thyroid cytopathology. Acta Cytologica. 2015; 59: 225–232.

[47] Faquin WC, Cibas ES, Renshaw AA. "Atypical" cells in fine-needle aspiration biopsy specimens of benign thyroid cysts. Cancer Cytopathology. 2005; 105: 71–79.

[48] Oertel YC, Oertel JE. Diagnosis of benign thyroid lesions: fine-needle aspiration and histopathologic correlation. Annals of Diagnostic Pathology. 1998; 2: 250–263.

[49] Sahoo M, Chintamani, Sekhri T, et al. Absence of microfollicular basement membrane: a new indicator in the diagnosis of follicular carcinoma thyroid. Diagnostic Cytopathology. 2008; 36: 519–522.

[50] Nikiforov Y, Gnepp DR. Pediatric thyroid cancer after the Chernobyl disaster. Cancer. 1994; 74: 748–766.

[51] Zhang L, DeMay RM. Prospective study of perifollicular fibrosis of thyroid: incidence, and diagnostic implication in cytopathology. American Society of Clinical Pathology 91st Meeting, 2013 Sep 19, Chicago, poster session 2.

[52] Harach HR. solid cell nests of the human thyroid in early stages of postnatal life. Systematic autopsy study. Acta Anatomica (Basel) 1986; 127(4): 262–264.

[53] Pianzola HM, Ottino A, Castelletto RH. Solid cell nests of the thyroid gland. Optic and immunohistochemical study at autopsies. Acta Anatomica (Basel). 1992; 143(1): 79–83.

[54] Moldavsky M, Szvalb S, Stayerman C. Solid cell nest in fine-needle aspiration of goiter. Diagnostic Cytopathology. 2002; 27(1): 66–67.

[55] Zhang L, Krausz T, DeMay RM. A pilot study of Galectin-3, HBME-1 and p27 triple immunostaining pattern for diagnosis of indeterminate thyroid nodules in cytology with correlation to histology. Applied Immunohistochemistry and Molecular Morphology 2015; 23(7): 481–490.

[56] Olson MT, Clark DP, Erozan YS, Ali SZ. Spectrum of risk of malignancy in subcategories of "atypia of undetermined significance". Acta Cytologica 2011; 55: 518–525.

[57] Nishino M, Wang HH. Should the thyroid AUS/FLUS category be further stratified by malignancy risk? Cancer Cytopathology. 2014; 122(7): 481–483.

[58] Xu B, Ghossein R. Encapsulated thyroid carcinoma of follicular cell origin. Endocrine Pathology. 2015; 26(3): 191–199.

[59] DeLellis R, Lloyd R, Heitz P, Eng C. Pathology and genetics of tumors of endocrine organs. World Health Organization Classification of Tumours. Lyon: IARC Press; 2004.

[60] Elliott DD, Pitman MB, Bloom L, et al. Fine-needle aspiration biopsy of Hurthle cell lesions of the thyroid gland: a cytomorphologic study of 139 cases with statistical analysis. Cancer. 2006; 108(2): 102–109.

[61] Brauner E, Holmes BJ, Krane JF, et al. Performance of the Afirma gene expression classifier in Hurthle cell thyroid nodules differs from other indeterminate thyroid nodules. Thyroid. 2015; 25(7): 789–796.

[62] McIver B, Castro MR, Morris JC, et al. An independent study of a gene expression classifier (Afirma) in the evaluation of cytologically indeterminate thyroid nodules. Clinical Endocrinology and Metabolism. 2014; 99: 4069–4077.

[63] Alexander EK, Faquin WC, Krane JF. Highlights for the cytology community from the 2015 American Thyroid Association clinical guidelines on the management of thyroid nodules and well-differentiated thyroid cancer. Cancer Cytopathology. 2015 Nov 30. doi: 10.1002/cncy.21662. [Epub ahead of print]

[64] Dincer N, Balci S, Yazgan A, et al. Follow-up of atypia and follicular lesions of undetermined significance in thyroid fine needle aspiration cytology. Cytopathology. 2013; 24: 385–390.

[65] Kuru B, Atmaca A, Kefeli M. Malignancy rate associated with Bethesda category III (AUS/FLUS) with and without repeat fine needle aspiration biopsy. Diagnostic Cytopathology. 2016, 44: 394–398.

[66] Yoo MR, Gweon HM, Park AY, et al. Repeat diagnoses of Bethesda category III thyroid nodules: what to do next? PLoS One. 2015; 10(6): e0130138. doi:10.1371/journal.pone.0130138

[67] Kim GR, Yoon JH, Kim EK, et al. Benign aspirates on follow-up FNA may be enough in patients with initial atypia of undetermined significance/follicular lesion of undetermined significance. International Journal of Endocrinology. 2014; 2014: Article ID 354612, 8 p. doi:10.1155/2014/354612

[68] Pyo JS, Sohn JH, Kang G. Core needle biopsy is a more conclusive follow-up method than repeat fine needle aspiration for thyroid nodules with initially inconclusive results: a systematic review and meta-analysis. Journal of Pathology and Translational Medicine. 2016 May;50(3):217–24. doi: 10.4132/jptm.2016.02.15. Epub 2016 Apr 14.

[69] Valderrabano P, Leon ME, Centeno BA, et al. Institutional prevalence of malignancy of indeterminate thyroid cytology is necessary but insufficient to accurately interpret molecular marker tests. European Journal of Endocrinology. 2016, 174(5): 621–629.

[70] Ianni F, Campanella P, Rota CA, et al. A meta-analysis-derived proposal for a clinical, ultrasonographic and cytological scoring system to evaluate thyroid nodules: the "CUT" score. Endocrine. 2016; 52: 313–321.

Chapter 4

Elastography: A New Ultrasound Technique in Nodular Thyroid Pathology

Dana Stoian, Timar Bogdan, Marius Craina,
Mihaela Craciunescu, Romulus Timar and
Adalbert Schiller

Additional information is available at the end of the chapter

http://dx.doi.org/10.5772/64374

Abstract

Elastography is a new technique for evaluating the stiffness of nodules. It is generally recognised that malignant thyroid lesions are harder than benign lesions. Different elastographic techniques are presented, with characteristics, advantages and limitations. Qualitative and semiquantitative methods are described. Comparison of the main existing techniques, static and dynamic elastographies, is presented in this chapter. Strain elastography seems to have a better diagnostic quality than shear wave elastography in the diagnosis of thyroid cancer disease. A positive elastogram, suggestive for malignancy is more useful in diagnosis than a positive grey-scale ultrasound evaluation. Elastography increases the specificity of grey scale ultrasound (US), it should be always integrated with its information and should be considered as a complement of conventional US.

Keywords: thyroid cancer, elastography, strain, shear wave, cutoff values

1. Introduction

Thyroid nodular disease is one of the most frequent endocrine pathologies in everyday practice. Epidemiologic studies have shown a prevalence of palpable thyroid nodules of 4–8% in iodine deficient areas [1], and up to 5% in women and 1% in men living in iodine sufficient areas [2]. The ultrasound (US) studies have revealed a much higher prevalence, up to 68% [3, 4]. The most important challenge in thyroid nodular disease is the correct identification of cancer cases, which occur in 7–15% of all thyroid nodules [5, 6].

The incidence of thyroid nodules has increased due to exposure to medical radiation, iodine intake, obesity and insulin resistance, genetics and inorganic phosphates [7, 8] with a 300% increase in the annual thyroid cancer rate [9].

Not only has the incidence of thyroid cancer significantly increased, but also there is an increase in demand for precise detection techniques, capable of dealing with small, incidentally discovered nodules: over 39% of all recently diagnosed thyroid cancers were below 1 cm [9]. High-resolution ultrasound evaluation is considered the most sensitive diagnostic modality for the detection and evaluation of thyroid nodules [10] being the first evaluation that is recommended in patients with suspect thyroid lesions.

There is a general consensus in all major guidelines [11–14] that fine needle ultrasound guided aspiration (FNAB) is the diagnostic of choice in order to establish the proper therapeutic option: refer to surgery or reevaluation. All guidelines recommend FNAB evaluation in cases of suspicious ultrasound characteristics, but these characteristics are not 100% superimposable: the American Thyroid Association (ATA) has stated that FNAB is the procedure of choice for the evaluation of thyroid nodules. FNAB should be performed in the presence of thyroid nodules >5 mm with suspicious US findings, hypoechoic solid nodules >1 cm, mixed cystic-solid nodules >1.5–2 cm with suspicious US findings, nodules with microcalcifications or abnormal cervical lymph nodes. The American Association of Clinical Endocrinology (AACE) recommends FNAB for hypoechoic solid nodules >1 cm, nodules with malignant US findings, regardless of size, and in patients with a special malignancy history. The Korean Guideline recommends FNAB in all suspicious nodules (taller than wide shape, irregular margins, marked hypoechoic texture, micro and macro-calcifications, speculated margins, extracapsular invasion) regardless of size and selective biopsy in probably benign nodules larger than 2 cm. The British Guidelines do not make any recommendation but suggest universal FNAB in cases with U3 (intermediate), U4 (suspicious) and U5 (malignant) nodules on ultrasound. Not only is it unclear which nodules should be referred to FNAB and which to follow up, but also there are a lot of data regarding the reluctance of the population to the FNAB procedure per se. FNAB results are not 100% accurate, with sensitivity and specificity up to 80% in very good centres [15]. They are considered a prediagnostic method and not a golden standard diagnostic method [16] due to the sensitivity achieved of 70 [17] to 85% [16] and also an application rate of 66% [17] use and accuracy of fine-needle aspiration cytology in histologically proven thyroid carcinoma according to an audit using a national anthology database [Cancer 2000; 90(6): 330–334]. The FNAB findings reported only 47 [17] to 55.3% [18] of proven cancers. The rate of false negative and false positive results of FNAB remains a challenge for this diagnostic method [16].

Elastography is a new method that evaluates the stiffness of the tissue since all thyroid nodules that are firm on palpation are suspicious for malignancy, which adds diagnostic value in respect of malignancy prediction [19, 20]. However, elastography is not widely used in clinical practice and not included in the major endocrine guidelines, but brings important information regarding the inelasticity of thyroid nodular lesions [21].

2. Elastography

Changes in tissue stiffness are present in cancerous disease, fibrotic changes or atherosclerosis. The vast majority of imaging techniques, such as computer tomography, magnetic resonance imaging and positron emission tomography, are focused on morphologic or functional characteristics; elastography assesses the stiffness of the tissue. Elastography is an application of the ultrasound technique, with specialised software that allows the measurement of different tissue stiffness [22].

The stiffness of the biological structures, viscous, anisotropic and non-linear is dependent on the degree of deformation. This deformation is obtained by external pressure, internal transversal deformation of tissue, induced by focused ultrasound beams called acoustic radiation force impulse (ARFI) excitation [23] or by inducing short duration focused acoustic beams, which generate shear waves that propagate transversally in the examined tissue.

These techniques bring qualitative information, imaging in colour maps with colour codes proportional to the tissue stiffness, or numerical evaluation of the stiffness, and are almost always a part of the ultrasound evaluation. The final diagnostic decision is a combination of conventional ultrasound and elastography [24]. There are important differences between manufactures, machines and techniques, and not all the results are comparable and therefore cannot be judged as a head-to-head comparison [25].

2.1. Elastography methods – strain elastography

Strain elastography requires an external palpation that induces a deformation of the subjacent tissue, parallel to the direction of the deformation force or endogenous stress such as vascular beam movements [26]. Repeated movements are registered. The stiff tissue moves less and shows lower deformation compared with the elastic tissue. The elastic images are added on the conventional 2B mode and displayed in a colour map from red (soft tissue) to blue (hard

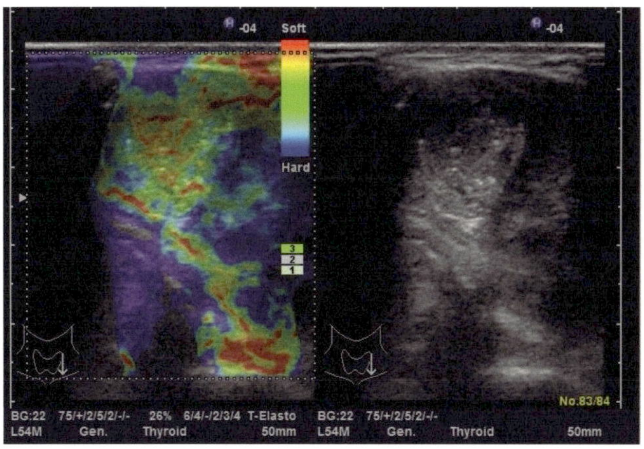

Figure 1. Hitachi device.Image on the left: strain elastography, red-green-blue colour map convention, soft nodule: green nodule. Image in the right: grey scale US: solid thyroid nodule, transversal section.

tissue). This qualitative evaluation is different in different manufacturers: in parallel with 2B images, superimposed to the grey scale images, at a refresh rate equal to that of grey scale = real-time elastography (RTE), offered by Hitachi Systems [27] or is displayed as a single image, representing the mean relative anelasticity strain over a time loop, predefined by the examiner, in the Toshiba machines.

Figures 1–3 show examples of solid thyroid nodules evaluated by strain elastography with different devices.

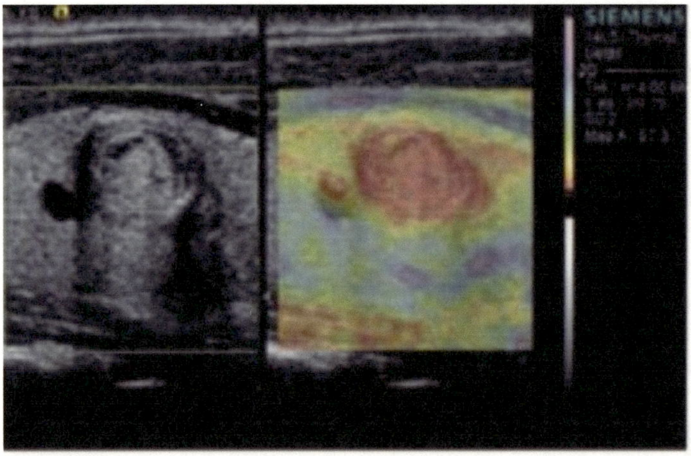

Figure 2. Siemens machine.Image on the left: grey scale US: solid thyroid nodule, longitudinal section. Image on the right: strain elastography, blue-green-red convention map: hard thyroid nodule: red colour.

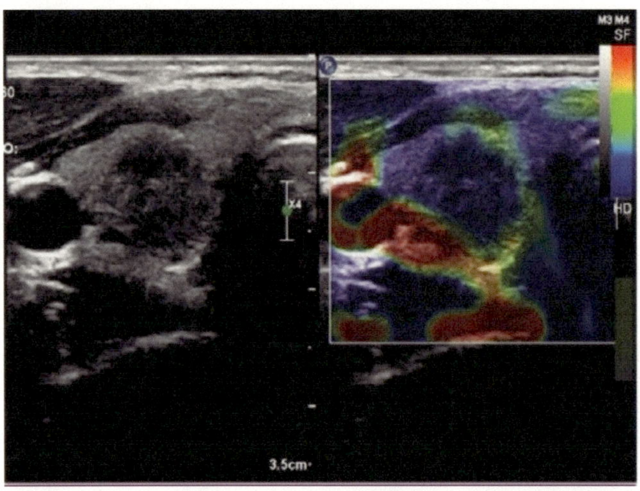

Figure 3. Phillips machine. Image in the left: grey scale US: solid thyroid nodule, transversal section. Image on the right: strain elastography, red – green – blue color map convention, hard nodule: blue nodule.

Also it allows a semiquantitative measurement, with the comparison of tissue strain in the Region of interest (ROI), the nodule, compared with healthy surrounding tissue, with automatic computing of the strain ratio (SR). **Figures 4** and **5** show the way of computer-assisted strain ratio evaluation. Internal pulsation of the carotid artery used in thyroid elastography allows both qualitative images (RTE) and also a semiquantitative evaluation, computing the strain ratio (SR) and the elasticity contrast index, in Samsung devices [28]. The higher the SR, the higher the likelihood of malignancy [29].

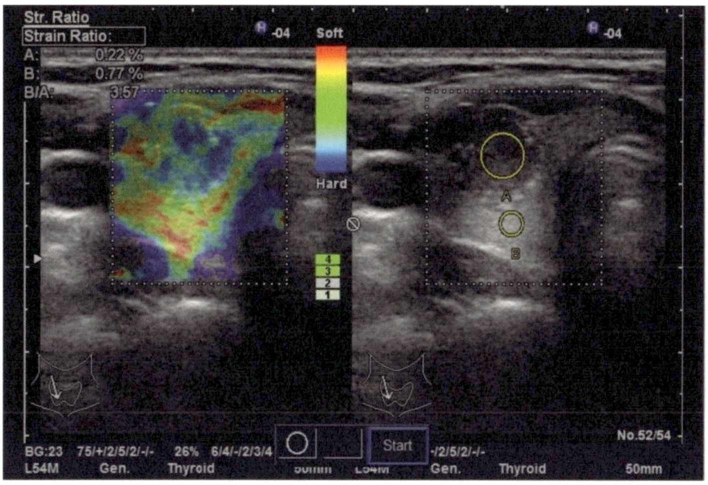

Figure 4. Hitachi device.Image on the left: strain elastography, soft nodule, low strain ratio: average = 3.57. Image on the right: grey scale US: solid thyroid nodule, transversal section.

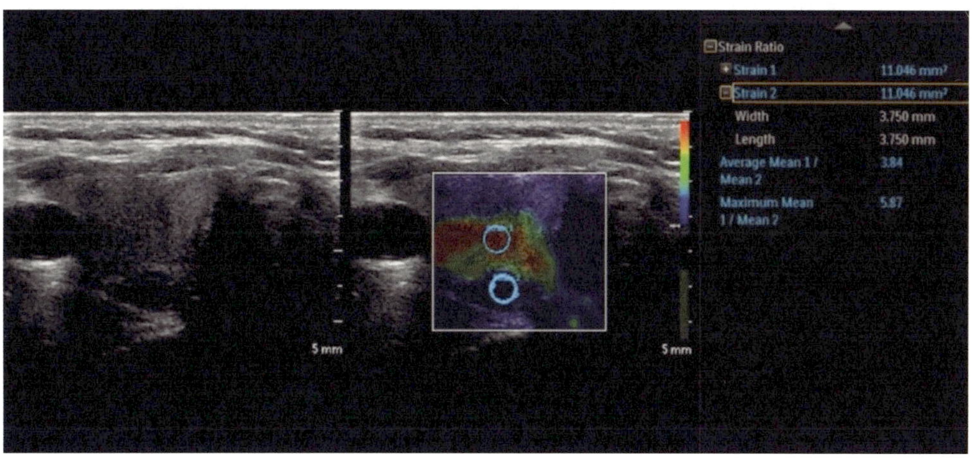

Figure 5. Philips device.Image on the left: grey scale US: solid thyroid nodule, transversal section. Image on the right: strain elastography, hard nodule: red colour (blue-green-red convention map), increased strain ratio: average = 3.84, maximum = 5.87.

The parameters used in strain elastography are strain (colour map), strain ratio geometric measures and elastography to B-mode size ratio (EI/B) ratio [30].

Strain elastography can be performed also by internal force, using transversal displacement of the tissue, without any external compression, secondary to the acoustic radiation force impulse imaging, used by Siemens devices, using the analysis of single images or a predefined time loop but not a real-time evaluation [27].

The following devices using strain elastography: ElaXto (Esaote), RTE (Hitachi Aloka), elastography (General Electric, Philips, Toshiba, Ultrasonix), eSieTocuh: (Samsung, Siemens), respectively, ARFI: VirtualTouch Imaging: (Siemens) are currently present on the commercial ultrasound machine market [30].

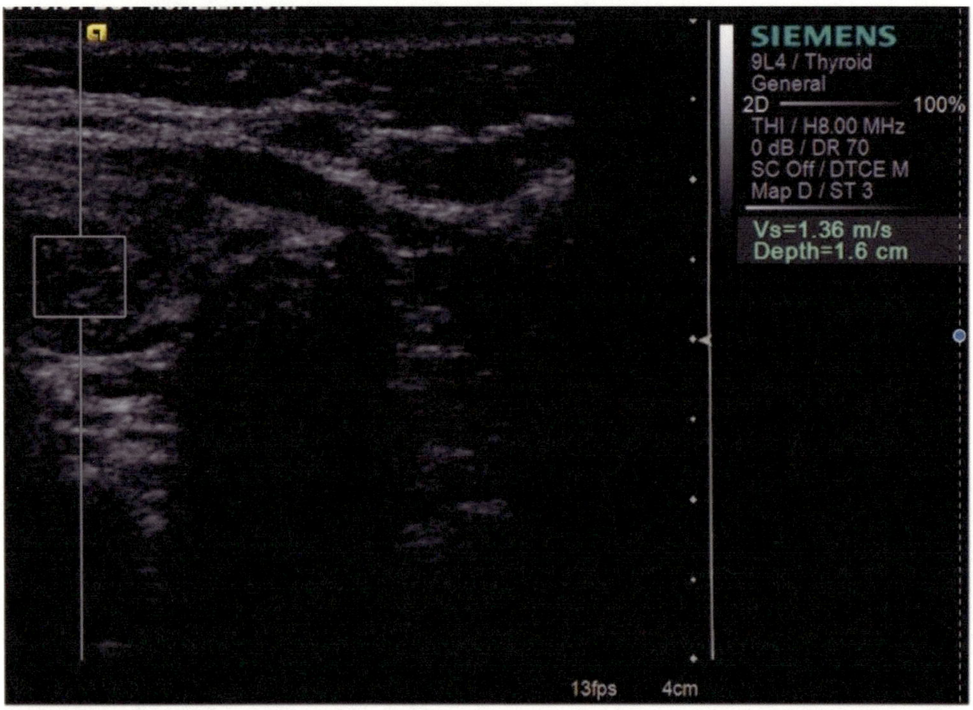

Figure 6. ARFI technique in a solid thyroid nodule: grey scale only evaluation, automatic ROI (1 mm), evaluation of SWE speed (m/s) in the nodule = median value of 10 serial measurements.

It is worth mentioning that the amount of external applied pressure has to be medium and is quantified for each device: for Hitachi machines, the compression scale is displayed always, and the pressure should be between 3 and 4 [31, 32]; in Siemens machines, it should be respectively a quality factor about 50 [33] and for Philips devices, it should maintain a steady pressure level displayed on the screen [34].

http://dx.doi.org/10.5772/64374

2.2. Elastography methods – shear wave elastography

Shear wave elastography assesses the elasticity of the tissues by evaluating the attenuation of the shear waves, which are transverse components of particle displacements, and they move in the tissue, with a speed that is dependent on the stiffness of the tissue [27]. There are two applicable methods: the supersonic shear wave and the acoustic radiation force impulse (ARFI) [35].

Focused ultrasound-induced waves are used in thyroid imaging, the supersonic shear waves, with a measurement of wave velocity (m/s) as the wave attenuates along a perpendicular direction to the transducer, or measuring directly the elasticity of ROI (kilopascals). The colour map displays the soft tissues as blue and hard tissues as red [36].

ARFI uses short-duration acoustic pulses that excite the tissue within the ROI and measures only the speed (m/sec) in these lesions, without any colour-coded images [37]. **Figures 6** and **7** represent ARFI evaluation for solid and cystic thyroid lesion.

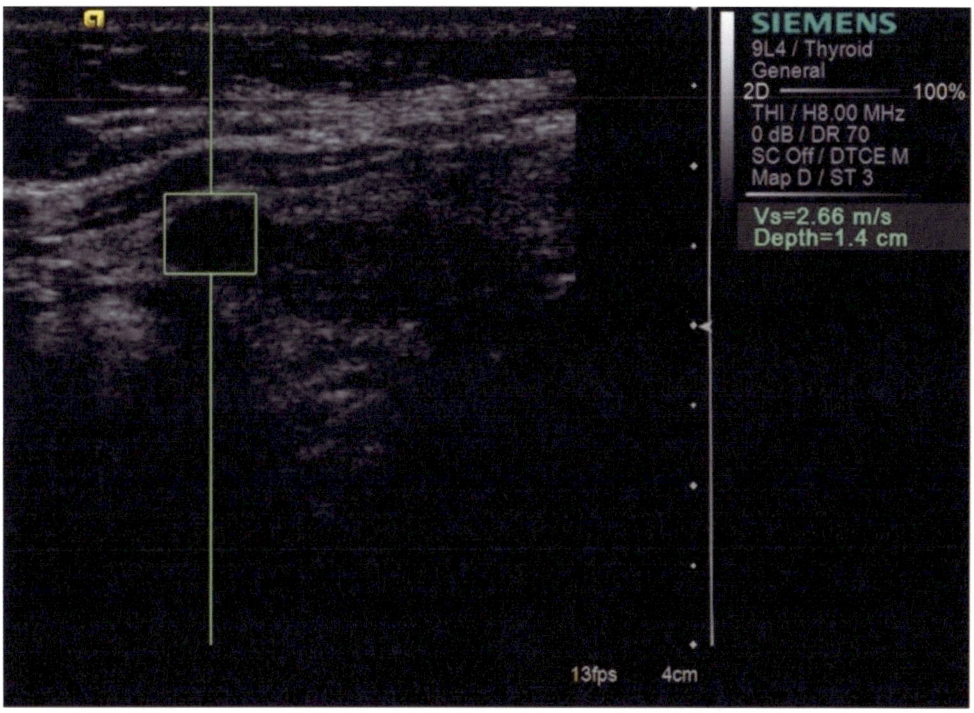

Figure 7. ARFI technique in a solid thyroid nodule: grey scale only evaluation, automatic ROI (1 mm), evaluation of SWE speed (m/s) in the cystic lesion = median value of 10 serial measurements.

The following devices using shear wave elastography are currently present on the market: Virtual Touch (Siemens and Philips) and speed imaging (SuperSonic Image) [30]. Supersonic devices offer, as in strain elastography, both qualitative images: colour map images related to strain of the nodules, respectively, qualitative evaluation, with measurement of the elasticity of the lesion. **Table 1** summaries the qualitative and quantitative SWE information (**Figure 8**).

	Colour	kPa	Type
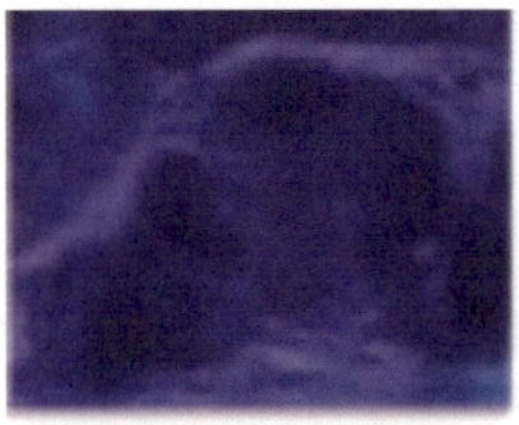	Dark blue	>0–36	Benign
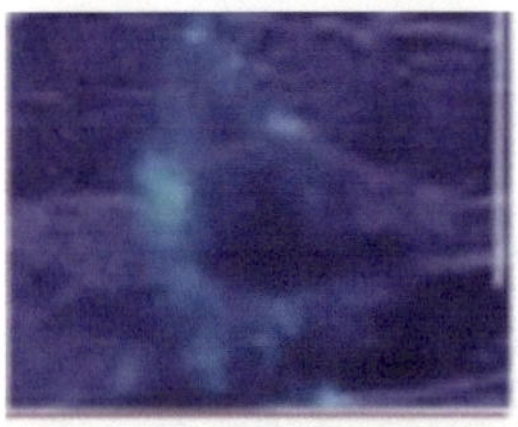	Light blue	>36–72	
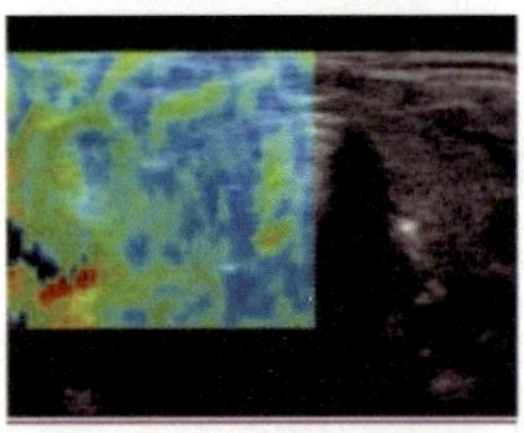	Green	>72–108	
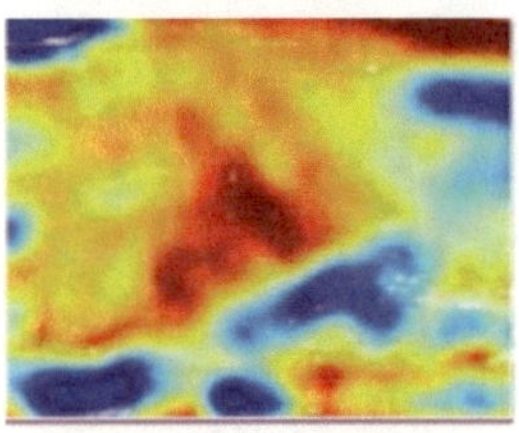	Orange	>108–144	
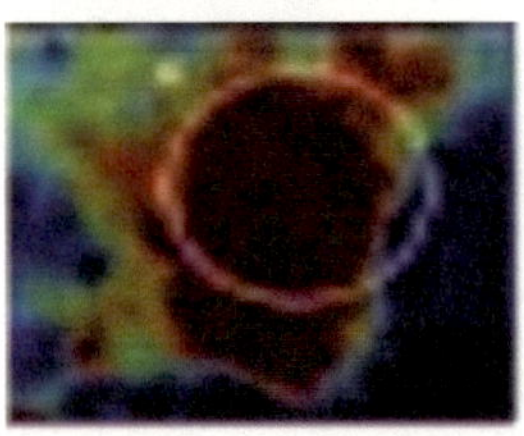	Red	>144–180	Malignant

Table 1. Qualitative (colour map) and quantitative (kPa) results in SWE—SuperSonic Aixplorer Machine.

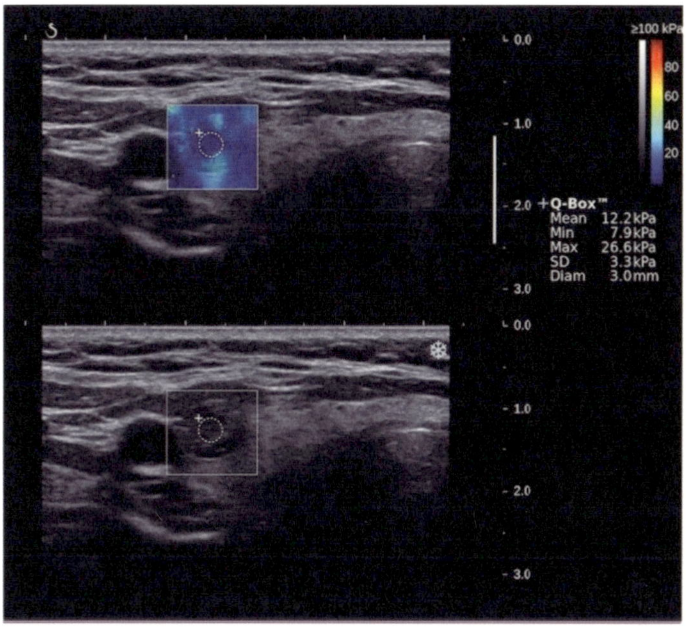

Figure 8. SuperSonic machine.Image below: conventional grey scale evaluation, solid thyroid nodule. Image above: SWE elastography: soft thyroid nodule, 12.2 kPA elasticity = benign lesion. Score 1: even soft elasticity in the whole nodule; Score 2: elasticity in a large part of the nodule; Score 3: elasticity in the peripheral part of the nodule; Score 4: no elasticity in the whole nodule; Score 5: no elasticity in the nodule and the area surrounding the nodule.

2.3. Elastography techniques

2.3.1. Strain elastography

The first information regarding elastography in thyroid nodular pathology came from the Rago group [22] which used the Ueno scale for breast lesions, adapted for thyroid, describing qualitative strain elastography evaluation: score 1 elasticity in the whole lesion, score 2 mostly soft, score 3 soft periphery, score 4 entire hard nodule and score 5 an elasticity beyond the 2B margins of the nodule = infiltration of the surrounding tissue initial described and used by Hitachi Machines (**Figure 9**). Other common colour schemes for thyroid RTE is the Asteria's 4-point scale based on Itoh scale for breast [38]: score 1 = entirely elastic, score 2 = mostly soft nodule, score 3= mostly hard nodule, score 4= entirely hard nodule initial described and used by Hitachi Machines (**Figure 10**). Generally, in RTE elastography, nodules with Rago scores 4 and 5, or Asteria scores 3 or 4 are considered highly suspicious for malignancy [24]. The initial result of the second evaluation showed a sensitivity of 97% and specificity of 100% for Rago's criteria [22], respectively, 94.1 and 81% for Asteria's criteria. Since these first reports, there has been much data describing the quality of RTE, with excellent meta-analysis: Moon [39], Sun [40], Dudea [21] and Wuguo [41] and also suggesting that the elastography evaluation is always made after the grey scale ultrasound and the observer integrates the 2B ultrasound information with the RTE information, for a better diagnostic performance of thyroid cancer [24].

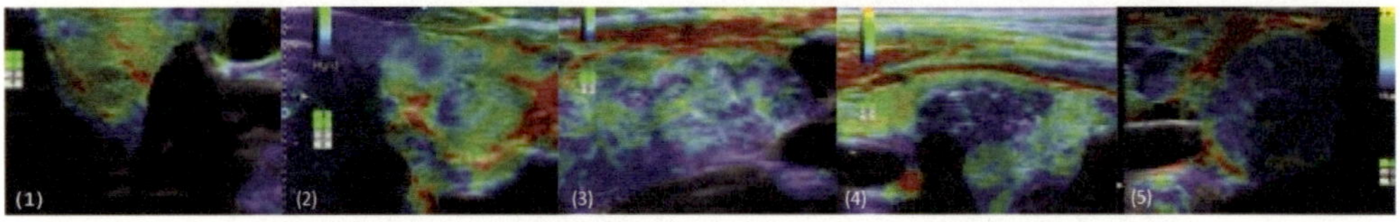

Figure 9. Rago criteria for qualitative strain elastography images. Score 1: even soft elasticity in the whole nodule; Score 2: elasticity in a large part of the nodule; Score 3: elasticity in the peripheral part of the nodule; Score 4: no elasticity in whole nodule; Score 5: no elasticity in the nodule and the area surrounding the nodule.

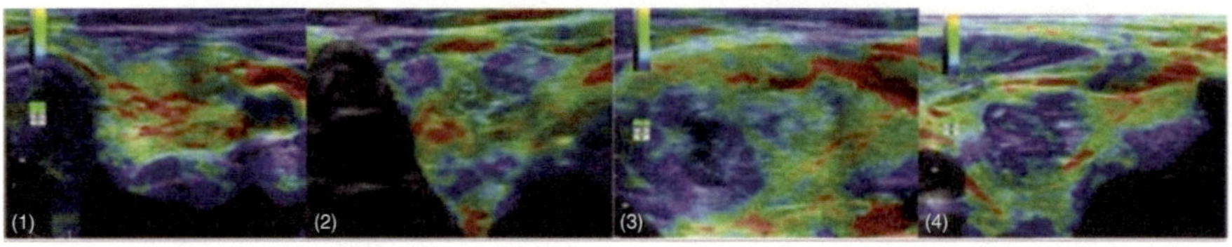

Figure 10. Asteria criteria for qualitative strain elastography images. Score 1: Elasticity in the whole nodule; Score 2: Elasticity in the large part of the nodule; Score 3: Stiffness in the large part of the nodule; Score 4: Nodule without elasticity.

When using the ES system, the diagnostic capacity of differentiating malignant lesions was high, calculated for a group of 4668 patients with 5481 nodules [40] with a pooled sensitivity of 0.79 (95% CI 0.77–0.81) of colour map elastography, confirmed by other more recent meta-analysis: sensitivity of 0.787% (95% CI: 0.793–0.861) and specificity of 0.812 (95% CI: 0.736–0.852) on 10.001 thyroid nodules [41]. The diagnostic results are good also for the ARFI strain elastography devices [20]

The semiquantitative approach of strain elastography was reported from the beginning of the use of this type of elastography in thyroid diseases [42]. The technique uses a comparison of the nodules with the surrounding non-nodular thyroid tissue, similar in depth (difference of depth less than 1 cm) [32]. The strain ratio evaluation, the semiquantitative approach, associates higher diagnostic values compared with qualitative elastography, with a pooled sensitivity of 0.85 (95% CI 0.81–0.89), respectively, a pooled specificity of 0.80 (95% CI 0.77–0.83) [40]. The only problem of the strain approach is the absence of a consensus: the threshold value should be used for the diagnostic.

In the EFSUMB guidelines, different articles are cited with different strain ratio values: 2.0 [43] sensitivity, specificity, positive predictive value (PPV) and NPV of 97.3, 91.7, 87.8 and 98.2%, respectively, value of 0.31 [44] that assures a NPV of 100% and a PPV of 42% using a cutoff of <0.15, respectively, a 2.05 value [31], with the mention that these studies used Q elastography/ARFI strain technique. The most published articles use strain ratio values between 2.5 and 4.5: 3.79 [45]; 2.73 [46]; 3.85 [47]; 4.225 [48]; 4.0 [49]; 4.0 [41], 3.75 [50]. The same values are seen in a recent meta-analysis [40, 41], where the quantitative elastographic approach was better in the cancer risk evaluation than the qualitative color map evaluation. There are some differences when comparing the strain ratio values in different studies: retrospective analysis of confirmed cancer cases of FNAB or pathology reports [40] or previous calculated strain ratio value, specific for each center [51]. There are no specific values for different types of thyroid carcinoma: 5.02 ± 2.07 for papillary carcinoma, 4.95 ± 2.12 for follicular carcinoma, respectively, 6.54 ± 0.55 for undifferentiated carcinoma [52]. But there are correlations between the SR and Bethesda score on FNAB evaluation: mean SR = 1.94 ± 2.12 for Bethesda I + II, versus 7.07 ± 5.46 for Bethesda V + VI [53].

The WFUMB recommendations are yet to be published, but the breast guidelines have not recommended any clear value for strain ratio [30], so it would be difficult to give a universal recommendation.

There are also some other parameters used in strain elastography:

- Area ratio (AR) used in VTI devices, where the area of the nodule is measured and compared with the area of a surrounding thyroid tissue, three different measurements, and the mean value is considered [54]. The described threshold value for AR suggestive for malignancy is a ratio of 1.08 with a sensibility, specificity, PPV and NPV of 91.3, 86.6, 82.3 and 93.4%, respectively [54].
- Hard area ratio measures the ratio of the hard area within the nodule versus the whole nodule area, with a cutoff value of 0.6 suggestive for malignancy: 92.9% sensibility, 91.3% specificity and 92% accuracy [55], with difficulties when the hard area is not compact [46].
- Strain ratio nodule to sternocleidomastoid muscle: the muscle is considered the reference area for strain calculation and not the healthy thyroid tissue, with reasonable results: 90% sensitivity and 50% specificity for a cutoff value of 1.5 [56].
- Strain index is a ratio between the strain from the whole nodule divided with the strain of the soft part of the nodule, with a cutoff value of 2.05 [57].
- Stiffness ratio is a special ratio calculated by the Philips devices by comparing the stiffness of the nodule versus the surrounding apparent healthy tissue, with a described cutoff value of 3.16 [32].
- Systolic thyroid strain index = compares the highest strain near the carotid artery versus the lowest strain in the thyroid nodule, on a special fixed ROI of 2 mm × 2 mm [58]. No clear cut values are described.
- Elasticity contrast index = the technique is specific for Samsung machines—obtains a strain oscillation map, with malignant lesions showing a higher contrast versus a benign lesion [28]. The measurement should be done at least twice, in transverse section, with consideration of the greatest value [20, 28]. The cutoff value described in the literature is between 3, 5 and 4 [20, 59, 60]. It should be considered that the results are influenced by age, atherosclerosis, hypertension and conditions associated with tachycardia [61].

There are some limitations when observing RTE results: calcification, cyst and position of nodules [62], but the data are not clear, since there are other studies describing the excellent value of RTE in nodules with calcifications [20].

The main described limitations/special situations are the following:

- Nodule size: there are some studies suggesting that large nodules, over 3 cm maximum diameter can underestimate the stiffness of the nodule [63]. This aspect is not recognised universally, since there are studies saying that the diagnostic quality of RTE is unaffected by the nodule size [29].

- Position of nodule: profound nodules, especially in overweight patients, are sometimes difficult to be evaluated by strain elastography if the signal is not deep enough because stress transmission is reduced as the distance increases, with false positive hardening of the nodule [63]. Isthmic nodules should be explored with caution, since they are between hard surfaces and longitudinal scans should be used in order to have also healthy thyroid tissue for semiquantitative evaluation [21]. When evaluating thyroid nodules, especially anterior ones, they should be compared with thyroidal tissue and not with surrounding muscles because they can be false negative evaluated as soft [64].

- Compression intensity per se can change the appearance of the nodules. Strain elastography is dependent on the experience of the examiner. The operator has to perform compression that should not only be reliable but also reproducible. Non-uniform compression produces variability [55]. Several compression cycles are required for a stable and reliable result [55, 65, 66].

- Pre-stress compression can change the displayed stiffness of the nodule by a false increase in stiffness [67] so that the operator should not perform any precompression or palpation before RTE examination [67].

- Bull's eye effect is a typical appearance of the cystic lesion (simple or complex), which has been described in breast elastography, but can be seen in large cystic lesions and also in thyroid.

- The healthy thyroid parenchyma, which is used for a comparison of the stiffness of the lesion, should be at least in more than a half with "green colour" in order not to influence the strain ratio. Thyroid atrophy, diffuse fibrotic changes can affect the relative stiffness of the nodule when compared with the surrounding tissue [21].

- Calcifications inside the nodule are associated with increased stiffness. This is considered the rule, regardless whether there are micro calcifications or rim calcifications [22, 66, 68, 69]. Even if this is generally accepted [61] there are some studies that have demonstrated the contrary: elastography is a helpful differential diagnostic tool in calcified thyroid nodules [20].

- Condition associated with tachycardia—in techniques that use internal compression induced by carotid pulsation, the lesion stiffness is changed.

- Observer experience: after all the previous cited data, experience is required in order to reach the correct degree of external compression, to choose the right position and dimension of ROI, although some authors say [33] that the learning curve is not influenced by the diagnostic performance of RTE.

2.3.2. Shear wave elastography

There are two major types of this elastography, with totally different diagnostic characteristics [24]. They use different ways of generation transversally propagating waves that propagate with different speed in the thyroid tissue, proportionally to the stiffness of the tissues: acoustic radiation force impulse quantification techniques and real-time shear wave elastography.

ARFI quantification estimates the stiffness of the tissue by measuring the speed of ultrasound-generated waves [70]. During a pause in breathing, the ARFI option of the device is turned on, the standard ROI (5 mm diameter or 2 cm diameter) is positioned on the nodule in the solid part and the device registers the speed [35]. Five to ten successive measurements are recommended for each nodule in order to obtain a valid evaluation [29, 71]. The normal interval of speed is between 0 and 9 m/sec [35], the higher the speed, the higher the tissue stiffness.

There are some studies evaluating the ARFI diagnostic quality in the differential diagnosis of thyroid nodules. The differences suggested by ARFI between benign and malignant thyroid is the value of speed, with different cutoff described values with a different sensitivity and specificity: 2.75 m/s [72] 2.9 m/s, sensibility of 91.3% and specificity of 85.10% [54], 2.85 m/s sensibility of 94.4% and specificity of 85.3% [72], 2.55 m/s, sensibility of 86.36% and specificity of 94.42 [73] 2.87 with 75% sensibility and 82.2% specificity [35], or 3.1 m/s with a specific of 91% [70]. All the values were retrospectively calculated with no clear recommendation of a used value [61] not even with a recommendation regarding values on the normal population [61]. The European guideline concluded that there was not sufficient data for reaching any conclusion at this time.

The method has some significant technical limitations:

- The dimensions of ROI are fixed, with two options: 5 mm/2cm large window. The majority of the studies are performed in nodules that are larger than 2 cm in diameter [70, 73]. In smaller nodules, not only is the measurement inaccurate [21] but also the velocity of the US wave is not stable [74].

- Nodule composition: inhomogeneity due to calcifications or cystic degenerescense makes the placement of ROI inside the nodule impossible [75].

- The penetration depth of ARFI is a maximum of 5.5 cm or so? Deeper lesion; big goitres or overweight patients are not suitable for ARFI evaluation [76].

- The devices measure speeds with values between 0 and 9 m/s [35]. Higher speed cannot be measured so very stiff nodules cannot be evaluated [29, 35, 77].

- Experienced operators are needed for the evaluation to avoid pressure on the evaluated skin in order not to influence the measurement [24].

ARFI evaluation is a simple evaluation, but further studies are required before considering it a valuable stiffness evaluation tool in nodular thyroid disease.

2.3.3. Real-time shear wave elastography (supersonic elastography SSE)

The SSE is performed like a conventional ultrasound, with a linear probe at the end of the conventional US evaluation, with the patient in apnoea [24]. The procedure was first used in 2010 [78], since then numerous papers have evaluated the diagnostic performance of SSE. The evaluation is operator independent, requires no external compression or no?, generating qualitative information: colour maps with following colour code: blue = soft tissue, red = hard tissue, respectively, quantitative information evaluated by elasticity index (EI) expressed in kilopascal [24, 78]. As strain elastography, SSE is displayed in parallel with grey scale US, with placement of ROI on the nodular lesion. For quantitative evaluation at least three loops should be recorded [79] with no movements of the transducer.

The diagnostic qualities of the qualitative, colour map SSE are fair, with a sensibility of 95.5% and specificity of 45.7% for elasticity II score (predominantly soft), 72.7 and 84.5% for elasticity III score (elastic on edges and rigid middle, respectively, 54.5 and 97.4% for elasticity IV score (markedly increased stiffness) [80].

Most of the studies report different threshold values for EI as a cutoff for differentiating benign versus malignant lesions.

The described cutoff values are comprised between 34.6 and 90.34 kPa without being able to identify a unique cutoff value [81]: 65.0 kPa (sensitivity = 85.20%, specificity of 93.90% [78], 6.00 kPa (sensitivity = 80.0%, specificity = 90.50% [82], 34.50, sensitivity of 76.90% and specificity of 71.10% [78], 90.34 kPa (sensitivity of 90.34% and specificity of 86.89% [80], 45 kPa (sensitivity of 83.30% and specificity of 91.40% [83].

Interestingly enough, one study [80] evaluated the different diagnostic values of SSE using different cutoff values for the same group of cases (cancer prevalence of 21.35%): sensitivity of 95.2%/specificity of 67.1% for hardness ≥50 kPa, sensitivity of 90.5% and specificity of 72.2% for hardness ≥59 kPa, sensitivity of 81.0% and specificity of 77.3% for hardness ≥65 kPa, sensitivity of 85.7 % and specificity of 81.3 % for hardness ≥49 kPa, sensitivity of 90.5% and specificity of 73.5% for hardness ≥42 kPa, respectively, 95.2% sensitivity and 70.3% specificity for a threshold for hardness of ≥38 kPa. This is the best example that there is still a lot to do in respect of unifying the SSE information. Still, increased hardness values are considered independent predictors of thyroid malignancy with high sensitivity (95.0–95.5%) [84]. The European guideline does not offer any clear information regarding SSE [61], only the comment that the higher the EI, the higher the probability of malignancy. There is still no standardised method for measurement of thyroid lesions; no clear EI cutoff value is described, not even for the same machine [78–80].

However, the method can guide the FNAB, avoiding the puncture of benign nodules [85] independent of the coexistence of autoimmune thyroid disease.

There are some limitations described for the SSE technique:

- If external pressure is used, it produces a false positive increase in elasticity with false positive results [79, 86];
- The presence of fluid does not permit the propagation of the shear wave with no information beyond the liquid zone;
- The presence of calcifications alters the accuracy of SSE especially in small nodules [82, 87].
- Vertical artefacts;
- Structure of the neck *per se* can affect the quality of the shear weave; the presence of trachea, carotid artery and surrounding tissue can affect the SSE diagnostic performance [80] especially in deeply located nodules.

More data are still required in order to find the correct location of SSE in nodular thyroid disease evaluation.

2.4. Comparison of strain and shear wave elastography

Regardless of the type of elastography, the used principle and the evaluated parameters, the evaluation of the hardness of lesions is an important aspect that adds diagnostic information and value compared with classical sonography. There are some studies that have attempted to answer the direct question: which elastography technique should be used for a better differential diagnosis of thyroid cancer [41, 72, 88, 89]?

A recent meta-analysis [89] evaluation of 10.001 thyroid nodules showed better diagnostic sensitivity (0.830, 95% CI: 0.793–0.861 versus 0.787, 95% CI: 0.727–0.847) and specificity (0.812, 95% CI: 0.763–0.852 versus 0.805, CI 95%: 0.712–0.873) with better area under receiver operator curve (AUROC) of 0.885 for RTE compared with AUROC of 0.842 for SWE [41].

Another comparative analysis [88] evaluated the diagnostic performance of RTE versus SSE, comparing a Hitachi Ascendus device, with a 5–13 MHz linear probe versus an Aixplorer Device, with a 4–15 MHz linear probe, on the same 49 consecutive patients with thyroid nodular disease. After analysis of the pathology report, the two diagnostic approaches were compared, with similar results for sensitivity, specificity positive and negative predictive value, regardless of the nodule size: below 1 cm, between 1 and 3 cm or bigger. Sensitivity was higher for RTE than for SWE (79.0% versus 68.4%) with better accuracy (82.8% versus 81.3%) and Negative predictive value (90.5% versus 86.7%), but the differences were not statistically significant. Moreover, coarse calcified nodules were false-positive results in RTE and true-negative results in SWE. The limitation of the study was the low number of the cases, the authors recognising that the studied population may not be representative of a screening population [88]. Another head-to-head comparative study, comprised 30 consecutive patients, with the pathology report as the golden standard diagnostic [72], comparing the RTE technique with the ARFI evaluation, using the same machine, Acusson Siemens 2000 device, concluding that the AUROC of ARFI (0.94) was higher than that of RTE (0.78). However, the number of cases was very small, the heterogeneity of the nodules high, uninodular and polynodular goitre were included, with exclusion of nodules smaller than 1 cm, and the results of this study were not confirmed by other studies. The performance of two of the above-mentioned devices,

Hitachi machine and Siemens S 2000, were also compared on a head-to-head evaluation, performed in 80 consecutive patients, also with a pathology report as the golden standard [90]. Elastographic patterns demonstrated a moderate and high degree of consistency for compression elastography (RTE) and VTI (ARFI); there was no conclusive result by measuring absolute velocities (ARFI) with an overlapping of shear wave velocity for malignant nodules with the velocities for benign nodules; shear wave techniques were inferior to strain elastography.

Without being conclusive, till now, evidence suggests that strain elastography seems to be better in the diagnostic of thyroid nodular disease.

3. Conclusion

The estimation for 2019 is that PTC will be the third most common cancer in women [90]; the correct identification of suspect cases and targeted diagnostic for high-risk lesions is still the challenge in thyroid nodular disease. There is substantial evidence showing that elastography indicators are more predictive for malignancy than conventional grey-scale patterns, such as hypoechogeneity, inhomogeneity, microcalcifications, irregular margins, no halo sign, taller than wide or intranodular vascularisation [91]. A positive elastogram, suggestive of malignancy is more useful in the diagnostic than a positive grey-scale ultrasound evaluation [91].

The association of grey scale US and elastography facilitates the evaluation of nodules with intermediate cytology [92]. The appearance of the nodules of elastography can change the attitude towards FNAB. In the cases of soft nodules, without any grey-scale suspicious characteristics, the FNAB can be delayed or postponed [93]. Authors [94] consider that nodules classified as Asteria 1 and Asteria 2 should not undergo FNAB because of the high NPV of elastography. Presence of a hard nodule on an elastogram should indicate the need for FNAB, regardless of the aspect in grey scale US [93].

Thyroid elastography should be considered in conjunction with other ultrasound characteristics, such as in breast cancer. Low risk nodules with increased stiffness should be referred to FNAB, regardless of dimensions or conventional ultrasound characteristics; medium risk nodules with low stiffness should be followed up instead of FNAB, and medium and high risk nodules with increased stiffness should be recommended for FNAB. Elastography increases the specificity of grey scale US; it should be always integrated with its information and should be considered as complementary to conventional US.

Author details

Dana Stoian, Timar Bogdan*, Marius Craina, Mihaela Craciunescu, Romulus Timar and Adalbert Schiller

*Address all correspondence to: timar.bogdan@umft.ro

University of Medicine and Pharmacy: Victor Babes, Timisoara, Romania

References

[1] Moon WJ, Baek JH, Jung SL, Kim DW, Kim EK, Kim JY, Lee JH, Lee JH, Lee YH, Na DG, Park JS, Park SW, Ultrasound and ultrasound based management of thyroid nodules: consensus statement and recommendations. Korean J Radiol 2011;12(1)1–14.

[2] Tunbridge WM, Evered DC, Hall R, Appleton D, Brewis M, Clark F , Evans JG, Young E, Bird T, Smith PA. The spectrum of thyroid disease in a community: the Wickham Survey. Clin Endocrinol (Oxford), 1977;1: 481–493.

[3] Vanderpump MPJ. The epidemiology of thyroid disease. Br Med Bull 2011; 99:39–51. DOI: 10.1093/bmb/ldr030] of thyroid nodules, especially in elderly and female population.

[4] Guth S, Theune U, Aberle J, Galacj A, Bamberger CM. Very high prevalence of thyroid nodules detected by high frequency (13MHz) ultrasound examination. Eur J Clin Invest 2009;39: 699–706.

[5] Pellegriti Frasca F, Regalbuto C, Squatrito S, Vigneri R. Worldwide increasing incidence of thyroid cancer: update on epidemiology and risk factors. J Cancer Epidemiol. 2013; 2013:965212. DOI: 10.1155/2013/965212.

[6] Panini E, Guglielmi R, Bianchini A et al. Risk of malignancy in nonpalpable thyroid nodules: predictive value of ultrasound and color-Doppler features. JCEM 2002;87 (5): 1941–1946.

[7] Mathews W, Forsythe AV, Brady Z, et al. Cancer risk in 680,000 people exposed to computed tomography scans in childhood or adolescence: data linkage study of 11 million Australians. BMJ. 2013; 346:f2360. DOI: 10.1136/bmj.f2360.

[8] Wulaningsih WMichaelsson K, et al. Inorganic phosphate and the risk of cancer in the Swedish AMORIS study. BMC Cancer. 2013; 24 (13):257. DOI: 10.1186/1471-2407-13-257.

[9] Davies L, Welch HG. Current thyroid cancer trends in the United States. JAMA Otolaryngol Head Neck Surg. 2014; 140:317–322.

[10] Cooper DS, Doherty GM, Haugen MD et al. Revised ATA management Guidelines for Patients with thyroid nodules and differentiated thyroid cancer. Thyroid 2009; 19 (11) DOI 10.1089/thy.2009.0110.

[11] Haugen BR, Alexander EK, Bible KC, Doherty GM, Mandel SJ, Nikiforov YE, Pacini F, Randolph GW, Sawka AM, Sclumberger M, Tuttle RM, Wartofsky L. 2015 American Thyroid Association Management Guidelines for adult patients with thyroid nodules and differentiated thyroid cancer. Thyroid. 2015;26(1):1–133. DOI: 10.1089/thy. 2015.0020.

[12] Gharib H, Papini E, Paschke R et al. American Association of Clinical Endocrinologist, Associazione Medici Endocrinologi, and European Thyroid Association medical

guidelines for clinical practice for the diagnosis and management of thyroid nodules. Endocr Pract 2010;16 (suppl 1)1–114.

[13] Moon Wj, Baek JH, Jung SL et al. Korean Society of Radiology. Ultrasound and the ultrasound based management of thyroid nodules: consensus statement and recommendations. Korean J Radiol. 2011; 12:1011.

[14] Perros P, Colley S, Boelaert K, Evans C, Evans RM, Gerrard GE, Gilbert JA, Harrison B, Johnson SJ, Giles TE, Moss L, Lewington V, Newbold KL, Taylor J, Thakker RV, Watkinson J, Williams GR. British Thyroid Association Guidelines for the Management of Thyroid Cancer. 3rd edition. Clin Endocrinol. 2014; 81(Suppl 1):1–136.

[15] Jou VY, Stelow EB, Dustin SM et al. Malignancy risk for fine needle aspiration of thyroid lesions according to the Bethesda System for Reporting Thyroid Cytopathology. Am J Clin Pathol. 2010; 134(3):450–456.

[16] Wang CCH, Friedman L, Kennedy G, et al. A Large Multicenter Correlation Study of thyroid nodule cytopathology and histopathology. Thyroid 2011; 21 (3): 243–251.

[17] Giard RW, Hermans J. Use and accuracy of fine-needle aspiration cytology in histologically proven thyroid carcinoma: an audit using a national anthology database. Cancer 2000;90(6):330–334.

[18] Sandeep GM, Navin M, Prad M. Investigating the value of fine needle aspiration cytology in thyroid cancer. J Cytol 2011;28(4):185–190.

[19] Nell S, Kist J, Debray TP, de Keiser B, van Oostenbrugge TJ, et al. Qualitative elastography can replace thyroid fine needle aspiration in patients with soft thyroid nodules. A systematic review and meta-analysis. Eur J Radiol. 2015; 84(4):652–661.

[20] Kim MH, Luo S, KO SH, Lim DJ, Lim Y. Elastography can effective decrease the number of fine-needle aspiration biopsies in patients with calcified thyroid nodules. Ultrasound Med Biol. 2014; 40(10):2329–2335.

[21] Dudea SM, Botar-Jid C. Ultrasound elastography in thyroid disease. Med Ultrason. 2015; 17(1):74–96.

[22] Rago T, Santini F, Scutari M, Pinchera A, Vitti P. Elastography: new developments in ultrasound for predicting malignancy in thyroid nodules. J Clin Endocrinol Metab. 2007; 92:2917–2922.

[23] Nigthingale KR, McAlveavt SA, Trahey GE. Shear wave generation using acoustic radiation force: in vivo and ex vivo results. Ultrasound Med Biol 2003;29:1715–1723.

[24] Kwak JY, Lim Eun-Kyung. Ultrasound elastography for thyroid nodules: recent advances. Ultrasonography. 2014;33(2):75–82.

[25] Shiima T, Nightingale KR, Palmeri ML, Hall T, BAmber JC, Barr RG, Castera L, Choi BI, Chou YH, Cosgrove D, Dietrich CF, Ding H, Amy D, Farrock A, Ferraioli G, Filice C, Rust MR, Nakashima K, Schafer F, Sporea I, Suzuli S, Wilson S, Kudo M. WFUMB

guidelines and recommendations for clinical use of ultrasound elastography: Part 1: Basic principles and terminology. Ultrasound Med Biol. 2015; 41(8):1126–1147.

[26] Itoh A, Ueno E, Tohno Kamma H, Takahashi H, Shiina T. Breast disease: clinical application of US elastography for diagnosis. Radiology 2006;239:341–350.

[27] Bamber J, Crosgrove D, Dietrich CF et al. EFSUMB guidelines and recommendations on the clinical use of ultrasound elastography. Part 1: Basic principles and technology. Ultraschal Med. 2013;34: 169–184.

[28] Lim DJ, Luo S, Kim MH, KO SH, Kim Y. Interobserver agreement and interobserver reproductibility in thyroid ultrasound elastography. Am J Roentgenol 2012; 198:896–901.

[29] Cantisani V, Grazhdan H, Ricii P, Mortele K, Di Segni M, D'Andrea V, et al. Q elastography of solid thyroid nodules: assessment of diagnostic efficacy and interobserver variability in large patient cohort. Eur Radiol 2014; 24:143–150.

[30] Barr R, Katzutaka N, Amy D, Cosgrove A, Farrock A, et al. WFUMB GUidleines and recommendations for clinical use of ultrasound elastography. Part 2: breast. Ultrasound Med Biol, 2015; 41(5):1148–1160.

[31] Xing P, Wu L, Zhang C, Li S, Liu C, Wu C. Differentiation of benign from malignant thyroid lesions: calculation of strain ratio on thyroid sonoelastography. J Ultrasound Med 2011;30:663–669.

[32] Guazzaroni M, Spinelli A, Coco I, del Giudice C, Girardi V, Simonetti G.. Value of strain ratio on thyroid real time sonoelastography. Radiol Med 2014;119:490155.

[33] Calvete AC, Rodriquez JM, de Dios Berna-Mestre J, Rios A, Abellan-Rivero D, Reus M. Interobserver agreement for thyroid elastography: value of quality factor, J Ultrasound Med 2013;32:495–504.

[34] Eltyib HE, Awad IA, Elsayed NM, Jastaniah SD. Real time ultrasound elastography for the differentiation of benign and malignant thyroid nodules. Open J Med Imaging. 2014;4:38–47.DOI:10.4236/ojmi.2014.41006.

[35] Zhang YF, Xu HY, Liu C, Guo LH, Liu LN, et al. Virtual touch tissue quantification of acoustic radiaton force impunse: a new ultrasound elastic imaging in the diagnostic of thyroid noduels. PLoS One. 2012;7:e49094.

[36] Sebag F, Vaillant'Lombard J, Berbis J, Griser V, Henry JF, Petit P, et al. Shear wave elastography: a new ultrasound imaging mode for the differential diagnosis of benign and malignant thyroid nodules. J Clin Endocrinol Metab. 2010;95:5281–5258.

[37] Bojunga J, Dauth N, Berner C, Meyer G, Holzer K, Voelkl L, et al. Acoustic radiation force impulse imaging for differentiaton of thyroid nodules. PLoS One. 2012;242735.

[38] Asteria C, Giovanardi A, Pizzocaro A, Cozzaglio L, Norabito A, Somalvico F, et al. US-elastography in the differential diagnosis of benign and malignant thyroid nodules. Thyroid 2008;18: 523–531.

[39] Moon HJ, Sung JM, Kim EK, Yoon JH, Ypuk JH, Kwak JY. Diagnostic performance of gray scale US and elastography in solid thyroid nodules. Radiology 2012;262:1002–1013.

[40] Sun J, CAi J, Wang X. Real time ultrasound elastography for differentiation of benign and malignant thyroid nodules. J Ultrasound Med. 2014;33:495–502.

[41] Wuguo T, Shuai M, Jiang W, Shu Z, Lingji SM, Donglin L. Comparison of diagnostic accuracy of real0time elastography and shear wave elastography in differentiation malignant from benign thyroid nodules. Medicine 2015; 94 (52):p3 2312.

[42] Cantisani V, D'Andrea V, Biancari F et al. Prospective evaluation of multiparametric ultrasound and quantitative elastosonography in the differential diagnosis of benign and malignant thyroid nodules: preliminary experience. Eur J Radiol 2012; 81: 2678–2683.

[43] Vorlander C, Wolff J, Saalabian S et al. Real-time ultrasound elastography: a noninvasive diagnostic procedure for evaluating dominant thyroid nodules. Langenbecks Arch Surg 2010; 395: 865–871.

[44] Cantisani V, Ulisse S, Guaitoli E. et al. Q elastography in the presurgical diagnostic of thyroid nodules with intermediate cytology. PLoS One 2012:7:e50725.

[45] Ding J, Cheng H, Ning C, Huang J, Zhang Y. Quantitative measurement for thyroid cancer characterization based on elastography. J Ultrasound Ed 2011; 30:1259–1266.

[46] Wang H, Brylka D, Sun LN, Lin YQ, Sui GQ, Gao J. Comparison of strain ratio with elastography score system in differentiating malignant from benign thyroid nodules. Clin Imaging 2013; 37:50–55.

[47] Ning CP, Jiang SQ, Zhang T, Sun LT, Tian JW. The value of strain ratio ratio in differential diagnosis of thrypod solid nodules. Eur J Radiol 2012; 81:286–291.

[48] Lyshchik A, Higashi T, Asato R et al. Thyroid gland tumor diagnosis at US elastography. Radiology. 2005;237:202–211.

[49] Stoian D, Bogdan T, Derban M, Pantea S, Varcus F, Craina M, Craciunescu M. TIRADSL the impact of quantitative strain elastography for better stratification of cancer risk. Med Ultrason 2015; 17(3):327–332.

[50] Cakal E, Sahin M, Unsal II et al. Elastography in the differential diagnosis of thyroid nodules. Ultrason Imaging 2014; DOI:10.1177/016173461547542.

[51] Stoian D, Cornianu M, Dobrescu A, Lazar F. Nodular thyroid cancer. Diagnostic value of real time elastography. Chirurgia (Bucur.) 2012;107(1):39–46.

[52] Wang HL, Zhang S, Xin XJ et al. Application of real time ultrasound elastography in diagnosing benign and malignant thyroid solid nodules. Cancer Biol Med 2012; 9:124–127.

[53] Kura M, Balarinoa C, Tamagone F, Campagno B, Bertini K, Escalante JG, Vega A, Peresotti B, Vilallonga J, Saubidet A. Relationship between the value of elastography ratio and the Bethesda cutolgical classification in thyroid pathology. Rev Argent Radiol 2014;78(3):128–137.

[54] Zhang FJ, Han RL, Zhao XM. The value of virtual touch tissue imagin (VTI) and virtual touch tissue quantification (VTQ) in the differential diagnosis of thyroid nodules. Eur J Radiol 2014; 83:2033–2040.

[55] Park SH, Kim SJ, Kim EK, Kim MJ, Son EJ, Kwak JY. Interobserver agreement in assessing the sonographic and elastographic features of malignant thyroid nodules. Am J Roentgenol. 2009; 193:W416-W2-423.

[56] Kagoya R, Monobe H, Tojima H. Utility of elastography for differential diagnosis of benign and malignant thyroid nodules. Otolaryngol Head Neck Surg 2010; 143:230–234.

[57] Ciledag N, Arda K, Aribas BK, Aktas E, Kose SK. The utility of ultrasound elastography and micropure imaging in the differentiation of benign and malignant thyroid nodules. Am J Roentgenol. 2012; 198:W244–W249.

[58] Dighe M, Kim J, Luo S, Kim Y. Utility of the ultrasound elastographic systolic thyroid stiffness index in reducing fine-needle aspitrations. J Ultrasound Med 2010; 29:5650574.

[59] Cantisani V, Consorti F, Guerrisi A et al. Prospective comparative evaluation of quantitative elastosonography and contrast enhanced ultrasound for the evaluation of thyroid nodules: preliminary experience. Eur J Radiol. 2013;82:1892–1898.

[60] Cantisani V, Lodise P, di Rocco G et al. Diagnostic accuracy and interobserver agreement of quasistatic ultrasound elastography in the diagnostic of thyroid nodules. Ultraschall Med 2014. DOI:10.1055/s-0034-1366467.

[61] Cosgrove D, Piscaglia F, Bamber J, Bojunga J, Correas J-M, Gilja OH, et al. EFSUMB Guidelines and Recommendations on the clinical use of ultrasound elastography. Part 2: Clinical Applications. Ultraschall Med 2013; 34:238–253.

[62] Shao J, Shen Y, Lu Y, Wang J. Ultrasound scoring in combination with ultrasouns elastography for differentiating benign and malignant thyroid nodules. Clin Endocrinol (Oxf) 2014;19. DOI:10.1111/cen.12589.

[63] Bathia KS, Rasalkar DP, Lee YP, et al. Cystic changes in thyroid nodules. A cofounding factor for real-time qualitative thyroid ultrasound elastography. Clin Radiol 2011; 66:799–807.

[64] Hong Y, Liu X, Yhang X, Chen M, Luo Z. Real time elastography in the differential diagnosis of benign and malignant thyroid nodules. J Ultrasound Med 2009; 28:8610867.

[65] Bojunga J, Herrmann G, Meyer S, Weber S, Zeuzem S, Friedrich-Rust M. Real tine elastography for differentiation of benign and malignant thyroid nodules: a meta-analysis. Thyroid. 2010; 20(10):1145–1150.

[66] Rago T, Scutari M, Santini F, et al. Real time elastography: use fool tool for redefining the presurgical diagnosis in thyroid nodules with intermediate or nondiagnostic cytology. JCEM 2010;95(12):5274–5280.

[67] Havre RF, Waage OH, Gilja S, Odegaard Nesje LB. Real time elastography: strain measurements are influenced by the position of the reference area. Ultraschall Med. 2011; DOI: 10.1055/s-0031-1273247.

[68] Andrioli M, Persani L. Elastographic techniques of the thyroid gland: current status. Endocrine. 2014;46:4550461.

[69] Kim JK, Baek JH, Lee JH et al. Ultrasound elastography for thyroid nodules: a reliable study. Ultrasound Med Bio, 2012;38:15081513.

[70] Friedrich-Rust M, Romenski O, Meyer G, et al. Acoustic radiation force impulse imaging for evaluation of the thyroid gland: a limited patient feasibility of the thyroid gland. A limited patient feasibility study. Ultrasonics 2012;52:69–74.

[71] Bojunga J, Dauth N, Berner C et al. Acoustic radiation force impulse imaging for differentiation of thyroid nodules. PLoS One 2012;7:e42735.

[72] Zhang J, Diao XH, Chai QL, Chen Y. Comparative study of acoustic radiation force impulse imaging with real-time elastography in differentia diagnosis of thyroid nodules. Ultrasound Med Biol. 2013;39:2217–2225.

[73] Gu J, Du L, Bai M, et al. Preliminary study if the diagnostic value of acoustic radiation force impulse technology for differentiating between benign and malignant thyroid nodules. J Ultrasound Med. 2012; 31:763–771.

[74] Fukuhara T, Matsuda E, Fujiwara K et al. Phantom experiment and clinical utility of quantitative shear wave elastography for differentiating thyroid nodules. Endocr J 2014;61:615–621.

[75] Grazhdani H, Catinasi V, Lodise P et al. Prospective evaluation of acoustic radiation force impulse technology in the differentiation of thyroid nodules: accuracy and interobserver variability assessment. J Ultrasound. 2014; 17(1):13-20. doi: 10.1007/s40477-013-0062-5.

[76] Goerts RS, Amann K, Heide R, BErnatik T, Neurath MF, Strobel D. An abdominal and thyroid status with ARFI elastometry: a feasibility study: ARFI elastometry of human organs. Eur J Radiol 2011; 80: e226–e230.

[77] Zhanh YF, Liu C, Xu HX, et al. RFI imaging: a new tool for diagnostic papillary microcarcinoma. Biomed Res Int 2014;14: 416969.

[78] Sebag F, Valillant Lombard J, Berbis J, Griset V, Henry JF, et al. Shear wave elastography: a new ultrasound imaging mode for the differential diagnosis of benign and malignant thyroid nodules. JCEM 2010;95:5281–5258.

[79] Bathia KS, Tong CS, Cho CC, Yuen EH, Lee YY et al. Shear wave elastography of thyroid nodules in routine clinical practice: preliminary observations and utility for detecting malignancy. Eur Radiol 2012; 22: 2397–2406.

[80] Parulska ES, Wolinski K, Stangierski A, et al. Comparison of diagnostic value of conventional ultrasonography and shear wave elastography in the prediction of thyroid lesions malignancy. PLoS One 2013;8(11):e81532.

[81] Zhang B, Xuelei M, Wu N, et al. Shear wave elastography for differentiation of benign and malignant thyroid nodules. a meta-analysis. J Ultrasound Med 2013;32:2163–2169.

[82] Veyrieres JB, Albarel F, Lombard JV, et al. A threshold value in shear wave elastography to rule out malignant thyroid nodules. A reality? Eu Radiol 2012;22:2397–2406.

[83] Huang Y, Wang ZL, Wan WB, Su L, Tang J. Quantitative research on supersonic shear imaging in diagnosis if thyroid nodules by elastography. Chin J Med Ultrasound 2011;8:1282–1288.

[84] Park AY, Son EJ, Han K, Youk JH et al. Shear wave elastography of thyroid nodules for prediction of malignancy in large scale study. Eur J Radiol 2015;84(3):407–412.

[85] Magri F, Cutiris S, Capelli V et al. Shear wave elastography in the diagnosis of thyroid nodules: feasibility in the case of coexistent chronic autoimmune Hashimoto's thyroiditis. Clin Endocrinol. 2012;76:137–141.

[86] Lippolis PV, Tognini S, Materazzi G et al. Is elastography actually useful in presurgical selection of thyroid nodules with intermediate cytology? JCEM 2011;96: E1826–E1830.

[87] Lim I, Kim EK, Yoon JH et al. Quantitative assessment of shear wave ultrasound elastography in thyroid nodules: diagnostic performance for predicting malignancy. Eur Radiol 2013; 23:2532–2537.

[88] Liu BX, Xie XY, Liang HY, et al. Shear wave elastography versus real-time elastography on evaluation thyroid nodules: a preliminary study. Eur J Radiol 2014;83:1135–1143.

[89] Sommer O, LAnz H, Hutter J et al. Elastography predicts thyroid cancer: comparison of two methods. Eur Soc Radiol. 2014 DOI:10.1594/ecr2014/C-1267.

[90] Brito JP, Nofal A, Montori V, Hay ID, Morris JC. The impact of subclinical disease and mechanism of detection on the rise in thyroid cancer incidence: a population-based study in Olmsted County, Minnesota during 1935 through 2012. Thyroid 2015;25: 999–1007.

[91] Razavi SA, Hadduck TA, Sadigh G, Dwamena BA. Comparative effectiveness of elastographic and B-mode ultrasound criteria for diagnostic discrimination of thyroid nodules: a meta-analysis. Am J Roentgenol. 2013;200:1317–1326.

[92] Garino F, Deandrea M, Motta M et al. Diagnostic performance of elastography in cytological intermediate thyroid nodules. Endocrine 2014; DOI:10.1007/s1202-014-438-0.

[93] Mehrota P, McQueen A, Kolla S, Johnson SJ, Richardson DL. Does elastography reduce the need for thyroid FNAs? Clin Endocrinol 2013;78:942–949.

[94] Nell S, Kist JW, Debray TP, et al. Qualitative elastography can replace thyroid nodule fine needle aspiration in patients with soft thyroid nodules. A systematic review and meta-analysis. Eur J Radiol 2015(85):652–661.

Chapter 5

The Advantages and Limitations of Ultrasound Elastography in Diagnosis of Thyroid Carcinoma

Nazan Ciledag, Hidir Kaygusuz, Burcu Sahin,
Elif Aktas, Fatma Gul Buyukbayraktar Imamoglu and
Bilgin Kadri Aribas

Additional information is available at the end of the chapter

http://dx.doi.org/10.5772/64407

Abstract

Thyroid nodules have high prevalence in the general population. Only minorities of thyroid nodules are malignant; nevertheless, still biopsies are performed in differential diagnosis of malignant and benign thyroid nodules. Conventional ultrasound is widely used in diagnosis and characterization of thyroid nodules. There are several suspicious ultrasound features that predict thyroid cancer, such as solid consistence, marked hypoechogenicity, taller-than-wide shape, irregular or microlobulated or spiculated margins, no peripheral hypoechoic halo, and micro- or macrocalcifications. However, none of these signs have high sensitivity or specificity nor high degree of confidence for diagnosis or exclusion of thyroid carcinoma. Ultrasound elastography, recently developed, promising, noninvasive technique that evaluates tissue stiffness, has become one of the main focuses in thyroid imaging. There are two ultrasound elastography methods: strain ultrasound elastography (also known as real-time elastography or qualitative elastography) and shear wave elastography (quantitative elastography and acoustic radiation force impulse imaging). The purpose of this chapter is to present the principles of thyroid application, advantages, and limitations of both ultrasound elastography techniques.

Keywords: malignant thyroid nodules, ultrasound elastography, shear wave elastography, strain ultrasound elastography, acoustic radiation force impulse imaging

1. Introduction

Thyroid nodules are a common medical problem. Although the majority of the thyroid nodules are benign, malignancy has a prevalence of 5–15% [1, 2]. Conventional ultrasound is accurate in the detection of thyroid nodules. There are several suspicious ultrasound features that predict a malignant thyroid nodule, such as hypoechogenicity, marked hypoechogenicity, a microlobulated or spiculated margin, punctate micro- or macrocalcifications, a taller-than-wide shape, and intranodular vascularization [3, 4]. Although conventional ultrasound is an excellent tool for detecting thyroid nodules, it has a relatively low diagnostic performance for the differentiation between benign and malignant nodules [5–7]. For this reason, ultrasound-guided fine-needle aspiration (FNA) is required for the nodules greater than 10 mm or those with suspicious ultrasound signs that have a high specificity for malignancy (60–98%), but FNA cannot be performed for all thyroid nodules because they are extremely common and approximately 5% of them are malignant [8, 9]. Furthermore, even for nodules undergoing ultrasound-guided FNA, the sensitivity for malignancy may be suboptimal (54–90%) because the specimens may be inadequate, nonrepresentative, or indeterminate for histopathologic examination especially in the case of follicular lesions [10–13]. As a result, a significant number of patients eventually receive unnecessary thyroid surgery. Therefore, improvement of a noninvasive diagnostic method for malignant nodules diagnosis is needed.

As the malignancies change, the mechanical properties of the soft tissue, such as tissue hardness and tissue stiffness evaluation, have become a part of nodular characterization. Ultrasound elastography, which was introduced in the 1990s, provides real-time information regarding the tissue elasticity and allows in vivo assessment of the tissue's mechanical properties, mapping of tissue stiffness, and characterization of soft tissue lesions [14]. Ultrasound elastography has become a promising, noninvasive technique to depict malignant nodules. Ultrasound elastography is based on the principle that, under compression, the softer parts of tissues deform easier than the harder parts [15]. The American Thyroid Association guidelines in 2009 stated that ultrasound elastography is an emerging and promising technique that requires additional validation with prospective studies [16]. Real-time strain ultrasound elastography was the first technique used, based on the measurement of the degree of tissue deformation as a response to an external force with a compression induced by the ultrasound probe that was then replaced by carotid internal excitation allowing improvement in sensitivity. Calculated tissue elasticity is displayed as a color map (elastogram) overlay of the conventional B-mode image. Elastograms allow qualitative analysis of the nodule. As a semiquantitative parameter, the strain index or the strain value ratio is calculated from the comparison between the tissue elasticities in the regions of interest (ROI) within a lesion and the surrounding reference tissue therefore providing useful analytic information. However, real-time strain ultrasound elastography has some limitations such as high operator skill dependence, inevitable intra- or inter-observer variability, and the impossibility of quantitative analysis. To overcome these limitations, a new ultrasound elastography technique based on shear wave has been developed. In comparison to the above technique shear wave elastography is a quantitative, operator-independent and reproducible technique. Shear wave ultrasound elastography is based on the propagation of acoustic force impulse induced by ultrasound beams through soft tissue to displace tissue and create shear waves that represent the local viscoelastic properties of the tissue and is displayed as Young's modulus (kPa) [18, 19]. Stiffer tissue exhibits a higher Young's modulus. Shear wave elastography allows quantitative nodules stiffness analysis in kilopascals to reinforce the predictive value of malignancy.

2. Physical principles and technique of ultrasound elastography

2.1. Real-time strain ultrasound elastography

Real-time strain ultrasound elastography is the most widely available type of ultrasound elastography. This is a dynamic imaging technique that reveals the physical properties of soft tissue by characterizing the differences in stiffness between the region of interest and the surrounding tissue through measuring the degree of tissue deformation under the application of external force applied by ultrasound probe or by physiological movements (e.g., carotid pulsation) (**Figure 1**). Tissue deformation occurring after compression and decompression period is calculated semiquantitatively via the Young's modulus and displayed graphically in color code or gray scale in the elastograms. The degree of deformation of the underlying soft tissue is calculated to estimate tissue stiffness with both the strain ratio/strain index values and elastographic maps (elastograms). In this technique, a vertical force should be performed uniformly and repeatedly in a vertical direction with a light pressure, and compression periods are followed by decompression resulting in changes in dimensions and shape, which are then used to calculate the stiffness of the tissue. The quality of the operator's free-hand pressure is

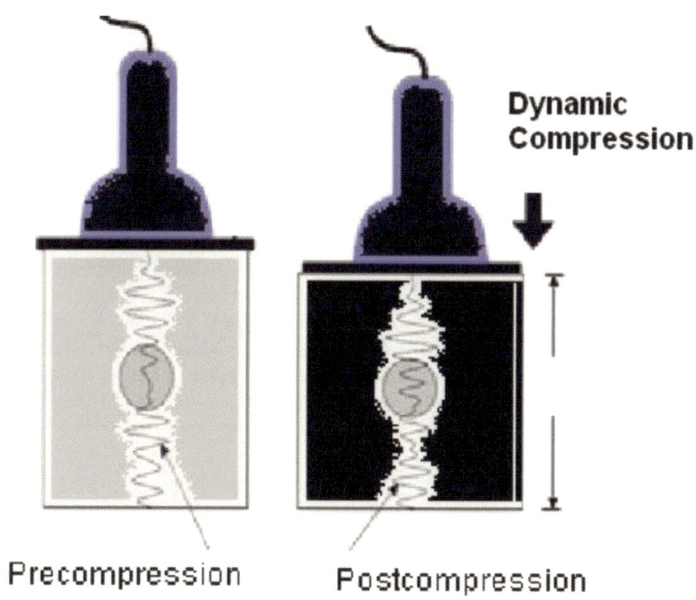

Figure 1. A diagram of the static ultrasound elastography.

visualized on the screen as a sine-wave or displayed with a numerical scale, allowing the operator to assess the validity of the compression cycles in real-time. For computing strain images without noise, a light and cyclic probe pressure must be performed [2, 17]. Stiff, rigid nodules exhibit less displacement compared with elastic, soft ones. An elliptic, or rounded region of interest (ROI), is used, large enough to include the entire nodule as well as a large portion of the surrounding thyroid and perithyroid tissue. This technique allows a qualitative and a semiquantitative assessment of nodule elasticity. Qualitative analysis of a nodule based on the prevalent color in the nodule can be obtained from visual scoring of colors within the color-coded elastographic map (elastogram) [17, 18]. Elastograms may be presented in gray scale or in color by different manufacturers. The hard tissue may be coded in light or red or blue code depending on the manufacturer.

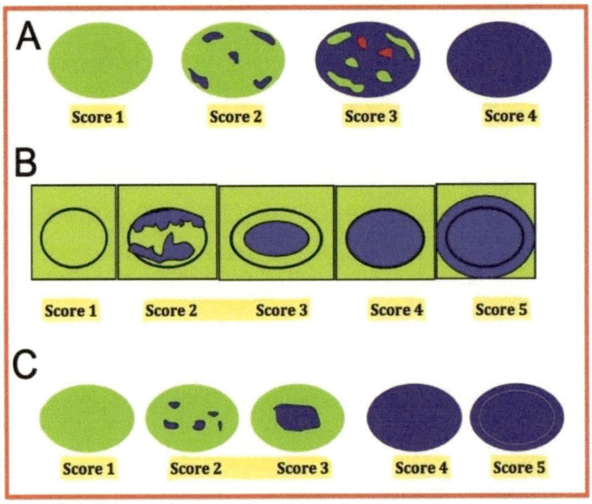

Figure 2. (A) Strain elastographic scores by Asteria et al. [19]. A score of 1 indicated elasticity in the entire examined area. A score of 2 indicated elasticity in a large part of the examined area. A score of 3 indicated stiffness in a large part of the examined area. A score of 4 indicated a nodule without elasticity. (B) Strain elastographic scores by Rago et al. [20]. A score of 1 indicated even elasticity in the whole nodule. A score of 2 indicated elasticity in a large part of the nodule. A score of 3 indicated elasticity only at the peripheral part of the nodule. A score of 4 indicated no elasticity in the nodule. A score of 5 indicated no elasticity in the nodule or in the area showing posterior shadowing. (C) Strain elastographic scores by Ueno et al. [21]. A score of 1 indicated even strain for the entire hypoechoic lesion (i.e., the entire lesion was evenly shaded in green). A score of 2 indicated strain in most of the hypoechoic lesion, with some areas of no strain (i.e., the hypoechoic lesion had a mosaic pattern of green and blue). A score of 3 indicated strain at the periphery of the hypoechoic lesion, with sparing of the center of the lesion (i.e., the peripheral part of lesion was green, and the central part was blue). A score of 4 indicated no strain in the entire hypoechoic lesion (i.e., the entire lesion was blue, but its surrounding area was not included). A score of 5 indicated no strain in the entire hypoechoic lesion or in the surrounding area (i.e., both the entire hypoechoic lesion and its surrounding area were blue).

The three principal scoring systems are those classified by Asteria et al. [19], Rago et al. [19], and Itoh et al. [21] (**Figure 2**). The first scoring system, based on the breast strain real-time ultrasound elastography scale of Itoh et al. [21], includes four different patterns [19]. Asteria's criteria defined a score of 1 as elasticity that is entirely soft in the nodule, 2 as mostly soft in the nodule, 3 as mostly hard in the nodule, and 4 as entirely hard in the nodule [19]. The thyroid nodules with scores 1 and 2 are considered benign and those with scores 3 and 4 are classified as suspicious for malignancy [19]. However, some authors have found that assigning benignity to score 3 further increases the specificity of the method for cancer detection [22].

In Ueno's classification, color coding of elastograms was in five groups [21]. The score 1 indicated strain for the entire lesion (the entire lesion was evenly shaded in soft color code). The score 2 indicated strain in most of the lesion with some areas of no strain (a mosaic color pattern). The score 3 indicated strain at the periphery of the lesion, with sparing of the center of the lesion (the peripheral part of the lesion was soft, and the central part was harder). The score 4 indicated no strain in the entire lesion (the entire lesion was in hard color code, but its surrounding area was not included). The score 5 indicated no strain in the entire lesion or in the surrounding area (both the entire lesion and its surrounding area were in hard color code). Scores of 4 and 5 are classified as suspicious for malignancy.

Rago et al. used five-point scales based on Itoh et al.'s [21] study using strain elastography. A score of 1 defined elasticity that is entirely soft in the nodule, 2 as mostly soft in the nodule, 3 as peripherally soft, 4 as entirely hard in the nodule, and 5 as hard in the area under consideration as well as the entire nodule [20]. The first three scores are considered as suggestive of being benign and scores of 4 and 5 are classified as suspicious for malignancy.

Rubaltelli et al. used a modified Asteria scale for thyroid nodules [23]. It consists of a five-step system that divides Asteria score 3 into patterns 3A and 3B, with a scale description as follows. Pattern 1: the entire nodule section is diffusely elastic. Pattern 2: the formation appears to be largely elastic with the inconstant appearance of inelastic areas during the real-time imaging. Pattern 3: constant presence of large inelastic areas is seen at the periphery (Pattern 3A) or center (Pattern 3B) of the formation. Pattern 4: uniformly displayed inelasticity throughout the whole nodule. Lesions that present Pattern 1 or 2 are classified as probably benign, while Patterns 3 and 4 are indicative of probable malignancy.

For semiquantitative analysis of the elasticity (the strain ratio or strain index), two similar sized regions of interest (ROI) at similar depth from the transducer (depth difference should be less than 10 mm) are drawn over the target region (nodule strain) and the adjacent reference normal parenchyma (the strain of the softest part of the surrounding normal tissue), respectively, then the strain ratio is automatically calculated through the machine. Three different measurements should be undertaken, and their average should be considered as the final value [24].

Main causes of false positive results of strain ratio measurement are transverse scans of the thyroid lobe (due to the interference with carotid artery pulsations); the ROI including the carotid artery or other neighboring tissues (therefore, it is difficult to apply in multinodular goiter); nodules located in the lower pole or in the isthmus are difficult to compress and to compare with normal parenchyma; irregular shaped, large nodules (due to the lack of comparable size reference tissue, nonuniform nodule compression, areas with altering stiffness may lead to false results); performing real-time strain ultrasound elastography with a high pressure may alter results (during whole examination period, slight, constant pressure over tissue should be applied [24]; microcalcifications in benign nodules; subacute thyroiditis; fibrosis and atypical adenoma may induce false positive [25, 26]; microcarcinomas show lower strain ratio values, between 1.74 and 2.96, and may be easily misdiagnosed [24].

Among the cited causes for false negative results of strain ratio are the following: follicular carcinoma, very well-differentiated carcinoma, carcinoma with central necrosis and degeneration, small papillary carcinoma in lymphoma, and microcarcinoma [27].

Lyshchik et al. reported the cutoff value >4 for malignancy yielded sensitivity of 82%, specificity of 96%, and accuracy 92% [27]. Xing et al. reported the cutoff value >3.79 for malignancy yielded sensitivity of 97.8%, specificity of 85.7%, positive predictive value of 88%, and negative predictive value of 97.8% [25]. Ning et al. reported the cutoff value >4.25 for malignancy yielded sensitivity of 81.8%, specificity of 82.9%, and accuracy 88% [25]. Cantisani et al. reported the cutoff value >2.02 for malignancy yielded sensitivity of 93% and specificity of 92% [28].

An alternative approach for strain ratio evaluation of large nodules or thyroiditis cases (the ones with the lack of adjacent reference normal thyroid parenchyma) is the use of nodule to sternocleidomastoid muscle strain value assessment. In this approach, the adjacent muscle at similar depth was used as a reference tissue, instead of the normal thyroid parenchyma. Kagoya et al. [29] reported that, a value >1.5 showed 90% sensitivity and 50% specificity for cancer. Ciledag et al. [30] reported a cutoff value >2.31 provided 85.7% sensitivity, 82.1% specificity, and 82.4% accuracy .

2.2. Shear wave elastography

Shear wave ultrasound elastography is a recently developed imaging technique that is based on the propagation of acoustic force impulse induced by ultrasound beams through soft tissue to displace tissue and create shear waves (**Figure 3**) [31]. Shear waves are the transverse components of particle displacement that are rapidly attenuated by the tissue. These acoustic pulses can be focused at different depths in soft tissue at supersonic speed and enhanced by forming a Mach cone, which increases the shear wave propagation to obtain the Young's modulus. The Young's modulus gives a local assessment of tissue elasticity at the point of interest. It gives a local real-time measurement of tissue elasticity quantitatively in kilopascal units (kPa) as measured in shear wave velocity units (m/sec) and qualitatively in real-time

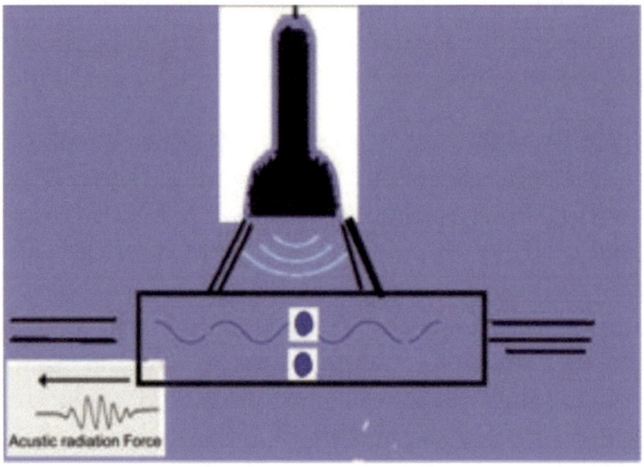

Figure 3. A diagram of the physical interaction of shear wave ultrasound.

http://dx.doi.org/10.5772/64407

color coded elastograms. On an elastogram within a given ROI, a variety of stiffness parameters can be measured, including the mean stiffness (E_{mean}), maximum stiffness (E_{max}), and standard deviation (SD). In both the shear wave imaging techniques, semiquantitative analysis of the elasticity (the strain ratio or the strain index) may be measured.

2.3. Methodology of shear wave elastography

There are two methods for shear wave elastography of the clinical practice of thyroid nodules: the supersonic shear wave and the acoustic radiation force impulse methods. Supersonic shear wave ultrasound elastography uses focused ultrasonic beams that propagate through the entire imaging area. The elasticity is expressed as in meters per second (m/s) and does not display color-coded images for elastography.

The examination is performed with the patient placed in the same manner as for the conventional ultrasound. The acoustic radiation force impulse imaging technique is integrated in a conventional ultrasound system using a 9–12 MHz linear transducer. The shear wave elastography (supersonic shear wave elastography) technique using a linear probe (4–15 MHz). The probe is gently placed on the cervical skin surface with slight pressure on the thyroid. The patient is asked to hold the breath and the quantitative evaluation is turned on. In acoustic radiation force impulse imaging technique, the ROI, should be placed in thyroid tissue or within the solid component of a nodule, avoiding cystic areas or those with calcifications. For the assessment of a nodule, it is recommended not to include the adjacent thyroid parenchyma. The displayed color-coded image shows soft tissue in blue and rigid tissue in red. After acoustic radiation force impulse activation, the velocity is displayed on the screen, with the depth measurement. Five to ten valid measurements should be performed to obtain reliable values. After activation of shear wave elastography, the quantitative information is assessed as the elasticity index in kiloPascal. In shear wave elastography it is important to set the machine for optimal image acquisition and set the elasticity index range on the thyroid preset protocol to 0–180 kPa. For shear wave elastography measurements, the whole nodule should be placed within the Q box with a small amount of surrounding thyroid tissue. Due to the technical limitations on cystic lesions, the shear wave velocity cannot be measured (shear waves do not propagate in fluids). At least three cineloops, lasting 10 s each, for each lesion should be obtained for a reliable evaluation.

The major advantages of this technique are operator independence, reproducibility, and the ability of semiquantitative, quantitative, and qualitative evaluation of tissue elasticity without manual compression artifacts.

Shear wave elastography has been used to evaluate the elasticity values of different tissues such as breast, thyroid, lymph nodes, muscles, and the abdominal organs such as the liver and pancreas.

Limitations and causes of false results of shear wave elastography are the contact and the pressure applied on the neck of the patient via the operator's hand that could alter the measurements (a generous amount of ultrasound gel should be used to avoid this artifact); in shear wave elastography technique, the elasticity of the structures is influenced by the external pressure applied, the stiffness rising with increasing pressure due to the nonlinear elastic effect artifact (due to this artifact, in the isthmic nodule, the stiffness is increased because of the neighboring trachea) [32]; in acoustic radiation force impulse imaging technique, the size of the nodule is a limitation because the ROI size is standard (5 mm × 6 mm or 2 cm × 2 cm) and cannot be changed (in acoustic radiation force impulse imaging technique, ROI contains both nodule and surrounding thyroid parenchyma so that the value of the velocity of the nodule will not be real); nodules with fluid areas or calcifications should be excluded due to the impossibility to place the ROI inside the parenchyma of the nodule [33, 34]. In the acoustic radiation force impulse imaging technique, penetration depth is limited to 5.5 cm, so large thyroids or very large and deep located nodules cannot be properly assessed [35]; the impossibility to measure velocities higher than 9 m/s is another limitation of acoustic radiation force impulse imaging technique, thus very hard nodules will not be measured properly [28].

Zhang et al. showed that for differentiation between benign and malignant nodules, the diagnostic performance of measured ultrasound (US) wave velocity is better for a nodule diameter greater than 20 mm [36]. Zhang et al. [36] reported the cutoff value >2.87 for malignancy yielded sensitivity of 75% and specificity of 82.2%. Han et al. [37] reported that the best cutoff value of velocity for differentiation between benign and malignant is 2.75 m/s.

Veyrieres et al. [34] reported the cutoff value of >66 kPa for malignancy yielded sensitivity of 80%, specificity of 90.5%, positive predictive value of 52.8%, and negative predictive value of 99.3%.

3. Clinical application of elastography in thyroid nodules

In clinical practice, elastography is usually performed as an extension of conventional ultrasound and not as an independent test. Therefore, a comparison of conventional ultrasound with elastography can be meaningless in view of its current clinical utility. The value of elastography should be evaluated by comparing the conventional US with a combination of conventional US and elastography.

4. Basic technique requirements for ultrasound elastography of thyroid nodules

During real-time ultrasound elastography, breath holding and no swallowing are of paramount importance for correct evaluation. A generous amount of gel and slight skin contact are needed. The image focus should be placed at or below the level of the nodule. The examiner applies slight and regular manual axial (anterior-posterior) vibration to the transducer. It is impossible to measure and quantify exactly the initial compression as well as the compression that induces repeated tissue strain.

For standardization of the compression and for the reproducibility, most manufacturers provide a strain quality indicator, either numeric or graphic. On Hitachi machines, the

http://dx.doi.org/10.5772/64407

compression quality scale should indicate levels 3–4. Only images obtained at these quality levels are fit for assessment. On Siemens machines, a quality factor above 50 for 3–4 successive frames has been recommended. Choosing the shortest, the exploratory ultrasound beam path to the nodule is important for optimal ROI placement to avoid strain decay with distance. The elastographic ROI should cover whole nodule. It is also important to exclude from the ROI, as much as possible, the vessels (mainly carotid), the esophagus, trachea, bones, and muscles. It is always important to keep in mind that real-time strain ultrasound elastography displays the relative strain of the structures in the ROI. The absolute value of the strain depends on the initial compression applied by the transducer (variable and nonquantifiable) and on the exploring repeated compression used to produce the images—again, variable. Strain values do not represent the elasticity modulus. As strain changes with the applied compression, its absolute (numeric) value (although measured and displayed by some machines) is completely inappropriate to compare two lesions or two individuals. Quite often there is interference between the pulsations induced by the hand or by the US beam and the ones coming from the carotid artery, which leads to image degradation. On the other hand, lateral systolic expansion of the carotid artery pulsation compresses the thyroid nodule against the trachea and induces anterior-posterior expansion of the gland that may be detected as strain. At least one commercially available application developed by Samsung Medison uses carotid artery pulsations as the sole strain inductor for elastography.

Technical causes of limitations of real-time strain ultrasound elastography of thyroid applications are

Scanning plane and interference with carotid pulsation is one of the limitations of ultrasound elastographic application of thyroid nodules. Transverse scans through the thyroid are more susceptible to interferences from carotid pulsation, and therefore, less suitable for real time strain ultrasound elastography. Longitudinal scans are less susceptible to carotid artery pulsations and also offer larger thyroid reference tissue.

Scan slice thickness should be around 5 mm since a thicker sample volume induces averaging the data of both small nodule and neighboring thyroid tissue, which lead to false elasticity results. This limitation is not an issue for highly focused transducers. Having a ROI as large as possible is important to include in much normal tissue, less than 50% green thyroid reference parenchyma in the ROI may result in false results. On the other hand, if possible, avoiding the inclusion of vessels, bones, and other nonthyroid tissues in ROI is important. Out-of-plane of the nodule during compression and color loss artifact in the nodule are other limitations.

Nodule location is very important in elastographic evaluations. Anterior nodules, protruding to the capsule, may be mislabeled as soft because strap muscles represent the reference tissue, not the thyroid parenchyma. Isthmic nodules are also difficult to assess because of the nodule compression difficulties between the hard planes (transducer and trachea) and lacking reference tissue. Also deeply located nodules present difficulties due to the stress decay phenomenon. Stress transmission is reduced as the distance from the transducer increases. Less tissue dislocation in deep portions of the thyroid will induce a hardening artifact. The nodules located in front of the common carotid artery are the most susceptible to pulsation interferences. Nodules within residual parenchyma lack reference tissue for comparison.

Elastography is not suited for nodules with a diameter less than 5 mm [38, 39], although the exact lower limit of the diameter for real-time strain ultrasound elastography usability is not known [40]. Elastography is also unsuitable for nodules larger than 3 cm or lobar size nodules cannot be encompassed by the reference thyroid tissue and are not suitable for real-time strain ultrasound elastography [40].

Intranodular calcification is associated with increased stiffness irrespective of underlying pathology and results in false elasticity values.

Fibrosis associated with subacute thyroiditis or Hashimoto thyroiditis may increase nodule stiffness [28, 41].

Necrosis, even without liquefaction, may induce soft areas. Intranodular colloid cystic changes: the presence of fluid inside the nodule changes the real-time strain ultrasound elastography appearance of the nodule [28, 38]. Only the solid component of the partially cystic nodules can be assessed accurately with real-time strain ultrasound elastography.

Nodule pathology is highly correlated with real-time strain ultrasound elastographic appearance of nodules. Of all thyroid cancers, mostly the papillary type is expected to appear hard, providing only 7% false negative results [40]. Follicular cancer may appear elastic and as do other types of malignancy. Contrarily, some benign nodules may be hard. Papillary carcinoma is harder than follicular or medullary carcinoma; therefore, there is no optimal cutoff value for predicting microcarcinoma. This leads to lower sensitivity but higher specificity [42]. Carneiro-Pla [43] reported that the majority of microcarcinomas were missed by the shear wave elastography examination.

Additional technical causes of limitations of real-time strain ultrasound elastography are [44] the physicians' skill and experiences, arbitrary selection of a color scale, neighbor arterial pulsation artifacts, using different qualitative scoring systems with lack of standardization, and manual, arbitrary selection of elastograms' representative image leading to subjectivity [28, 45].

In summary, the main causes for false-positive real-time strain ultrasound elastographic diagnoses of thyroid cancer are calcification, fibrosis, thyroiditis (subacute/chronic/Hashimoto thyroiditis), nodules larger than 3 cm or lobar size nodules, and deep location of nodules. Main causes for false negative real-time strain ultrasound elastographic diagnoses of thyroid cancer are follicular/medullary/nondifferentiated/metastatic cancer, anterior subcapsular/isthmic location of nodule, nodules larger than 3 cm, lobar size nodules with the lack of reference normal thyroid parenchyma around the nodule, or necrotic nodules [26].

5. Conclusion

Ultrasound elastography of thyroid nodules is an easy, completely painless, and rapid technique that assesses hardness as an indicator of malignancy. Ultrasound elastography is not an alternative imaging technique to conventional ultrasound, but it is an additional methodology that can be integrated into the conventional ultrasound examination to increase the accuracy, the positive predictive value, and the negative predictive value of conventional ultrasound. The addition of this methodology can reduce the number of patients pursuing unnecessary biopsy. US elastography can also be considered as a reliable screening tool for characterizing thyroid nodules. An elasticity score of 1 is indicative of benign pathology in almost all cases and can be used to exclude many patients from further invasive assessments. Ultrasound elastography has a considerable potential in diagnosis of thyroid malignancies, especially in cytological indeterminate and nondiagnostic nodules.

Author details

Nazan Ciledag[1*], Hidir Kaygusuz[1], Burcu Sahin[1], Elif Aktas[1], Fatma Gul Buyukbayraktar Imamoglu[2] and Bilgin Kadri Aribas[1]

*Address all correspondence to: drnazangokbayrak@yahoo.com.tr

1 Radiology Department, Dr. Abdurrahman Yurtaslan Ankara Oncology Research and Education Hospital, Ankara, Turkey

2 Radiology Department, Ataturk Research and Education Hospital, Ankara, Turkey

References

[1] W.M. Tumbridge, D.C. Evered, R. Hall, D. Appleton, M. Brewis, F. Clark, J.G. Evans, E. Young, T. Bird, and P.A. Smith. The spectrum of thyroid disease in a community: the Whickham survey. Clinical Endocrinology 1997; 7: 481–493.

[2] V. Cantisani, H. Grazhdani, E. Drakonaki, V. D'Andrea, M. Di Segni, E. Kaleshi, F. Calliada, C. Catalano, A. Redler, L. Brunese, F. M. Drudi, A. Fumarola, G. Carbotta, F. Frattaroli, N. Di Leo, M. Ciccariello, M. Caratozzolo, and F. D'Ambrosio. Strain US elastography for the characterization of thyroid nodules: advantages and limitation. International Journal of Endocrinology. 2015, Article ID 908575, pp. 8 http://dx.doi.org/10.1155/2015/908575

[3] KimE.K., Park C.S., Chung W.Y., Oh K.K., Kim D.I., Lee J.T., et al. New sonographic criteria for recommending fine-needle aspiration biopsy of nonpalpable solid nodules of the thyroid. American Journal of Roentgenology 2002;178:687–691.

[4] MoonW.J., Baek J.H., Jung S.L., Kim D.W., Kim E.K., Kim J.Y., Kwak J.Y., Lee J.H., Lee Y.H., Na D.G., Park J.S., and Park S.W. Ultrasonography and the ultrasound-based management of thyroid nodules: consensus statement and recommendations. Korean Journal of Radiology 2011;12:1–14.

[5] J.D. Iannuccilli, J.J. Cronan, and J.M. Monchik. Risk for malignancy of thyroid nodules as assessed by sonographic criteria: the need for biopsy. Journal of Ultrasound in Medicine 2004;23(11): 1455–1464.

[6] J.K. Hoang, K.L. Wai, M. Lee, D. Johnson, and S. Farrell. US features of thyroid malignancy: pearls and pitfalls. Radiographics 2007; 27 (3): 847–860.

[7] H.G. Moon, E.J. Jung, and S.T. Park. Role of ultrasonography in predicting malignancy in patients with thyroid nodules. World Journal of Surgery 2007; 31(7): 1410–1416.

[8] L. Yassa, E.S. Cibas, C.B. Benson, M.C. Frates, P.M. Doubilet, A.A. Gawande, F.D. Moore, B.W. Kim, V. Nose, E. Marquisee, P.R. Larsen, and E.K. Alexander. Long-term assessment of a multidisciplinary approach to thyroid nodule diagnostic evaluation. Cancer. 2007; 111:508–516. Doi: 10.1002/cncr.23116. PMid: 17999413.

[9] L. Falvo, C. D'Ercole, S. Sorrenti, V. D'Andrea, A. Catania, A. Berni, P. Grilli, and E. De Antoni. Papillary microcarcinoma of the thyroid gland: analysis of prognostic factors including histological subtype. European Journal of Surgery Supplement. 2003; 588:28–32.

[10] Y.Y. Tee, A.J. Lowe, C.A. Brand and R.T. Judson, Fine-needle aspiration may miss a third of all malignancy in palpable thyroid nodules: a comprehensive literature review. Annals of Surgery 2007; 246(5): 714–720.

[11] Y. Peng and H.H. Wang. A meta-analysis of comparing fine-needle aspiration and frozen section for evaluating thyroid nodules. Diagnostic Cytopathology 2008; 36(12): 916–920.

[12] Y.C. Oertel, L. Miyahara-Felipe, M.G. Mendoza, and K.Yu. Value of repeated fine needle aspirations of the thyroid: an analysis of over ten thousand FNAs. Thyroid 2007; 17(11): 1061–1066.

[13] G.L. La Rosa, A. Belfiore, D. Giuffrida, C. Sicurella, O. Ippolito, G. Russo, and R. Vingeri. Evaluation of the fine needle aspiration biopsy in the preoperative selection of cold thyroid nodules. Cancer 1991; 67(8): 2137–2141.

[14] S. Franchi-Abella, C. Elie, and J.M. Correas. Ultrasound elastography: advantages, limitations and artifacts of the different techniques from a study on phantom. Diagnostic and Interventional Imaging 2013; 94: 497–501.

[15] B.S. Garra. Elastography: current status, future prospects, and making it work for you. Ultrasound Quarterly 2011; 27(3): 177–186.

[16] J. Ophir, I. Céspedes, H. Ponnekanti, Y. Yazdi, and X. Li. Elastography: a quantitative method for imaging the elasticity of biological tissues.Ultrasonic Imaging 1991; 13(2): 111–134.

[17] E. Ueno and A. Itoh. Diagnosis of breast cancer by elasticity imaging. Eizo Joho Medical 2004; 36(12): 2–6.

[18] D.S. Cooper, G.M. Doherty, and B.R. Haugenetal. Revised American thyroid association management guidelines for patients with thyroid nodules and differentiated thyroid cancer. Thyroid 2009; 19(11): 1167–1214.

[19] C. Asteria, A. Giovanardi, A. Pizzocaro, L. Cozzaglio, A. Morabito, F. Somalvico, A. Zoppo. US-elastography in the differential diagnosis of benign and malignant thyroid nodules. Thyroid 2008; 18(5): 523–531.

[20] T. Rago, F. Santini, M. Scutari, A. Pinchera and P. Vitti. Elastography: new developments in ultrasound for predicting malignancy in thyroid nodules. Journal of Clinical Endocrinology and Metabolism 2007; 92(8): 2917–2922.

[21] A. Itoh, E. Ueno, E. Tohno, H. Kamma, H. Takahashi, T. Shiina, M. Yamakawa, and T. Matsumura. Breast disease: clinical application of US elastography for diagnosis. Radiology 2006; 39(2): 341–350.

[22] G. Azizi, J. Keller, M. Lewis, D. Puett, K. Rivenbark, and C. Malchoff, Performance of elastography for the evaluation of thyroid nodules: a prospective study. Thyroid 2013; 23(6): 734–740.

[23] L. Rubaltelli, S. Corradin, A. Dorigo, M. Stabilito, A. Tregnaghi, S. Borsato, and R. Stramare. Differential diagnosis of benign and malignant thyroid nodules at elastosonography.Ultraschall in der Medizin 2009; 30(2): 175–179.

[24] C.P. Ning, S.Q. Jiang, T. Zhang, L.T. Sun, Y.J. Liu, and J.W. Tian. The value of strain ratio in differential diagnosis of thyroid solid nodules. European Journal of Radiology 2012; 81: 286–291.

[25] P. Xing, L. Wu, C. Zhang, S. Li, C. Liu, and C. Wu. Differentiation of benign from malignant thyroid lesions. Calculation of the strain ratio on thyroid sonoelastography. Journal of ultrasound in medicine 2011; 30: 663–669.

[26] S.M. Dudea and C. Botar-Jid. Ultrasound elastography in thyroid disease. Medical Ultrasonography 2015; 17: 74–96. DOI: 10.11152/mu.2013.2066.171.smd

[27] A. Lyshchik, T. Higashi, R. Asato, S. Tanaka, J. Ito, J.J. Mai, C. Pellot-Barakat, M.F. Insana, A.B. Brill, T. Saga, M. Hiraoka, and K. Togashi. Thyroid gland tumor diagnosis at US elastography. Radiology 2005; 237: 202–211.

[28] V. Cantisani, P. Lodise, H. Grazhdani, E. Mancuso, E. Maggini, G. Di Rocco, F. D'Ambrosio, F. Calliada, A. Redler, P. Ricci, and C. Catalano. Ultrasound elastography in the evaluation of thyroid pathology. Current status. European Journal of Radiology 2014; 83: 420–428.

[29] R. Kagoya, H. Monobe, and H. Tojima. Utility of elastography for differential diagnosis of benign and malignant thyroid nodules. Otolaryngology—Head and Neck Surgery 2010; 143: 230–234.

[30] N. Çiledag, K. Arda, B.K. Aribas, E. Aktas, and S.K. Köse. The utility of ultrasound elastography and micropure imaging in the differentiation of benign and malignant thyroid nodules. American Journal of Roentgenology 2012; 198: W244–W249.

[31] J Bamber, D. Cosgrove, C. F. Dietrich, J. Bojunga, F. Calliada, V. Cantisani, J.M. Correas, M. D'Onofrio, E.E. Drakonaki, M. Fink, M. Friedrich-Rust, O.H. Giljia, R.F. Havre, C. Jenssen, A.S. Klauser, R. Ohlinger, A. Saftioiu, F. Schaefer, I. Sporea, F. Piscaglia. EFSUMB guide-lines and recommendations on the clinical use of ultrasound elastography. Part 1. Basic principles and technology. Ultraschall in der Medizin 2013; 34(2): 169–184.

[32] F. Magri, S. Chytiris, V. Capelli, S. Alessi, E. Nalon, M. Rotondi, S. Cassibba, F. Calliada, L. Chiovato. Shear wave elastography in the diagnosis of thyroid nodules: feasibility in the case of coexistent chronic autoimmune Hashimoto's thyroiditis. ClinEndocrinol 2012; 76: 137–141.

[33] H. Grazhdani, V. Cantisani, P. Lodise, G. Di Rocco, M.C. Proietto, E. Fioravanti, A. Rubini, A. Redler. Prospective evaluation of acoustic radiation force impulse technology in the differentiation of thyroid nodules: accuracy and interobserver variability assessment. J Ultrasound 2014; 17: 13–20.

[34] J.B. Veyrieres, F. Albarel, J.V.Lombard, J. Berbis, F. Sebag, C. Oliver, P. Petit. A threshold value in Shear Wave elastography to rule out malignant thyroid nodules: a reality? Eur J Radiol 2012; 81: 3965–3972.

[35] R.S. Goertz, K. Amann, R. Heide, T. Bernatik, M.F. Neurath, D. StrobelD. An abdominal and thyroid status with Acoustic Radiation Force Impulse Elastometry feasibility study: Acoustic Radiation Force Impulse Elastometry of human organs. Eur J Radiol 2011; 80: e226–e230.

[36] Y.F. Zhang, H.X. Xu, Y. He, C. Liu, L.H. Guo, L.N. Liu, J.M. Xu. Virtual touch tissue quantification of acoustic radiation force impulse: a new ultrasound elastic imaging in the diagnosis of thyroid nodules. PLoS One 2012; 7: e49094.

[37] R. Han, F. Li, Y. Wanga, Z. Ying, Y. Zhang. Virtual touch tissue quantification (VTQ) in the diagnosis of thyroidnodules with coexistent chronic autoimmune Hashimoto's thyroiditis: A preliminary study. Eur J Radiol 2015; 84: 327–331.

[38] Y. Hong, X. Liu, Z. Li, X. Zhang, M. Chen, Z. Luo. Real-time ultrasound elastography in the differential diagnosis of benign and malignant thyroid nodules. J Ultrasound Med 2009; 28: 861–867.

[39] Y.R. Hong, Y.L. Wu, Z.Y. Luo, N.B. Wu, X.M. Liu. Impact of nodular size on the predictive values of gray-scale, color-Doppler ultrasound and sonoelastography for assessment of thyroid nodules. J Zhejiang Univ-Sci B (Biomed & Bio- technol) 2012; 13: 707–716.

[40] Oliver C, Vaillant-Lombard J, Albarel F, J. Berbis, JB. Veyrieres , F. Sebag, P. Petit. What is the contribution of elastography to thyroid nodules evaluation? Ann Endocrinol (Paris) 2011; 72: 120–124.

[41] C. Shuzhen. Comparison analysis between conventional ultrasonography and ultrasound elastography of thyroid nodules. Eur J Radiol 2012; 81: 1806–1811.

[42] A.Y. Park, E.J. Son, K. Han, J.H. Youk, J. Kim, C.S. Park. Shear wave elastography of thyroid nodules for the prediction of malignancy in a large-scale study. Eur J Radiol 2015; 84: 407–412.

[43] D. Carneiro-Pla. Ultrasound elastography in the evaluation of thyroid nodules for thyroid cancer. CurrOpin On- col 2013; 25: 1–5.

[44] Kim JK, Baek JH, Lee JH, J.L. Kim, E.J. Ha, T.Y. Kim, W. Bae Kim, Y.K. Shong. Ultrasound elastography for thyroid nodules: a reliable study? Ultrasound Med Biol 2012; 38: 1508–1513.

[45] D.J. Lim, S. Luo, M.H. Kim, S.H. Ko, Y. Kim. Interobserver agreement and intraobserver reproducibility in thyroid ultrasound elastography. American Journal of Roentgenology 2012; 198: 896–901.

Chapter 6

FDG PET in Thyroid Cancer

Irina Wimmer and Robert Pichler

Additional information is available at the end of the chapter

http://dx.doi.org/10.5772/64110

Abstract

Thyroid malignancies are relatively rare cancer types but have a substantially high incidence in the group of all endocrine malignancies. Most thyroid cancer patients have differentiated thyroid cancer and prognosis is generally favourable. Tumour growth tends to be slow and radioiodine therapy is successful in differentiated cell tumour type with the ability to accumulate iodine. So, where can ^{18}F-fluorodeoxyglucose positron emission tomography (FDG PET) imaging be applied? The role of FDG PET in differentiated thyroid cancer starts with the development of metastatic diseases, which are not responsive to radioiodine therapy anymore. FDG accumulates in tumour lesions that are missed by iodine scintigraphy. FDG PET is more sensitive in patients with an aggressive histological subtype, including Hürthle cell. Thyroid cancer is definitely not the role model indication for FDG PET imaging, but for the management of differentiated thyroid cancer with metastases and more aggressive types of malignancies of the thyroid, FDG PET proves to be clinically useful. Incidental detection of malignancy in FDG-avid thyroid nodules has to be taken into consideration when FDG PET examinations have been conducted for reasons unrelated to the thyroid.

Keywords: thyroid cancer, FDG PET, incidentaloma, iodine, DOPA PET

1. Introduction

1.1. Thyroid cancer

Thyroid malignancies are relatively rare cancer types but have a substantially high incidence in the group of all endocrine malignancies [1]. Most thyroid cancer patients have differentiated thyroid cancer (i.e. the papillary and the follicular type), and prognosis is generally favourable [1]. Tumour growth tends to be slow and radioiodine therapy is successful in differentiated cell tumour type with the ability to accumulate iodine. Therefore, where can ^{18}F-fluorodeoxyglucose positron emission tomography (FDG PET) imaging be applied?

2. FDG PET in thyroid cancer

In the last two decades, PET and PET/CT have proven to show a substantial diagnostic role in most human cancer entities. The development was related to FDG, a glucose derivate labelled with F18, showing avidity in cancer types with high tumour-related metabolism and upregulation of the glucose transporter system [2]. Imaging with positron emitting isotopes has the advantage of higher spatial resolution compared to gamma cameras. That enables quantification and hybrid imaging with CT, which provides precise morphological data. However, what appears to be useful for patients with melanoma or high-grade lymphoma must not be useful in the case of thyroid cancer. Here, nuclear medicine provides the possibility of specific gamma camera imaging with iodine 131 (^{131}I) or 123 (^{123}I) and recently also by PET with iodine 124 (^{124}I).

2.1. FDG PET in differentiated thyroid cancer

There exists a consensus that FDG PET has no objective in the primary evaluation of differentiated thyroid cancer—routine preoperative FDG PET scanning is not recommended by the American Thyroid Association (ATA) Management Guidelines [3]. A primary cancer lesion of the thyroid can easily be missed by FDG PET [1, 4]. In general, the suspicion of thyroid malignancy leads to thyroidectomy and by this to histologically based diagnosis, including eventually some form of cervical lymph node surgery. If there is some indication, the next step is to perform radioiodine ablation, which results additionally in providing post-therapeutic iodine scan images. For the follow-up examinations, thyroglobulin (Tg) is considered a strong marker of persistent or recurrent disease [5]. The role of FDG PET starts with the development of metastatic diseases, which are not responsive to radioiodine therapy any more. FDG accumulates in tumour lesions that are missed by iodine scintigraphy [1, 4]. A German group of Tübingen explained these findings as early as 1995 [6]. Highly differentiated thyroid cancer (DTC) cells still express the sodium-iodide symporter (NIS), which enables iodine uptake in the thyroid. This ability gets lost when cells become less differentiated. On the contrary, FDG is internalised to the cell by a transporter protein (glut-1), which is overexpressed in malignant cell types. Inverse alterations of either iodine or FDG uptake in metastases are called the flip-flop phenomenon. Feine et al. presented a group of 34 patients showing FDG and/or ^{131}I uptake, 30 of whom exhibited the flip-flop phenomenon. Five per cent of the metastases had both FDG and ^{131}I uptake [4]. Since then, there has been knowledge of the coexistence of functionally more differentiated tumour cells with retained iodine trapping mechanism and low glucose metabolism, and more undifferentiated carcinoma cells that have lost their iodine trapping mechanism and have a high glucose uptake [7].

A meta-analysis by Dong et al. in 2009 covered 571 patients who had recurrent or metastatic DTC and a radioiodine-negative whole-body scan (WBS) [8]. FDG-PET was proven to be especially effective in detecting metastases in patients with elevated Tg levels and normal

http://dx.doi.org/10.5772/64110

radioiodine WBS. A pooled patient-based sensitivity and specificity of about 84% each was found for FDG PET.

Optimal initial therapy is mandatory for favourable patient outcome, but can only be performed if all non-avid tumour lesions are known before treatment planning. Rosenbaum-Krumme et al. found that the TNM stage was changed due to the FDG PET results in 21% of the patients. The authors concluded that FDG PET in high-risk patients with DTC nowadays has been established as an initial-staging modality [7] (**Figure 1**).

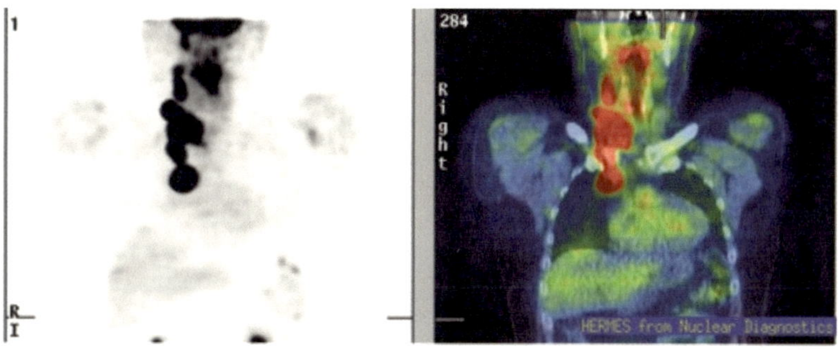

Figure 1. A 47-year-old man presented with sensomotoric deficit of the left arm at the Neurological Clinic in Linz (Austria). Further diagnosis revealed a thyroid malignoma infiltrating the cervical vertebral column and adjacent soft tissue (as can be seen FDG-avid on FDG PET/CT images). The next step was a combined operation of the malignant goiter and the tumour masses infiltrating to the bone. As histology still presented papillary differentiation (Ki-67 was 4%), the patient was sent to radioiodine therapy further on.

FDG PET has a high negative-predictive value (NPV) about 90% in DTC patients regarding recurrence-free follow-up after 3 years. FDG PET should be performed in all high-risk DTC patients—after the first radioiodine therapy—to improve patient management and risk stratification [9]. A prognostic relevance of FDG imaging is therefore presumed. Also, the volume of FDG-positive malignant tissue is of relevance, Wang et al. showed that volumes of ≤125 ml were associated with a 3-year survival of 96% compared to 18% of patients with higher volumes [10].

Elevated Tg levels are an indicator for FDG-positive lesions [11], but it has been demonstrated that high Tg levels are not related to FDG positivity alone, but also to iodine positivity [7]. It was recognised that about 10–15% of patients have elevated serum Tg levels despite negative iodine WBS [12]. In respect to the clinical value of Tg measurement, it has to be considered that Tg autoantibodies interfere with the measurement and may mask the presence of recurrent or metastatic disease [13]. In this condition, patient surveillance is complicated and some of the restrictions might be overcome with routinely practised FDG PET in this patient group, additionally to neck ultrasound and other diagnostic modalities provided by nuclear medicine.

In total, ATA guidelines strongly recommend considering FDG PET scanning in high-risk DTC patients with elevated serum Tg (generally >10 ng/ml) when negative radioiodine imaging is expressed [3]. As the availability of PET/CT scanners and cyclotrons has become satisfactory at least in central Europe, we advocate combined imaging with iodine and FDG whenever thyroid hormone withdrawal or stimulation with recombinant human thyroid stimulating hormone (TSH) has been conducted. Although there have been conflicting reports regarding the additional advantage for FDG PET imaging, a possible modest benefit due to TSH stimulation can be assumed [11]. Such a procedure has been successfully introduced in our institutions located in Austria.

2.2. FDG PET in subtypes of DTC and anaplastic thyroid cancer

Aggressive histologic subtypes of thyroid cancer carry a worse prognosis [14]. The clinical usefulness for FDG-PET may be more robust for Hürthle cell thyroid cancer (3–4% of DTC) as opposed to papillary and follicular DTC [15]. Generally, FDG PET is more sensitive in patients with an aggressive histological subtype, including Hürthle cell, but also poorly differentiated

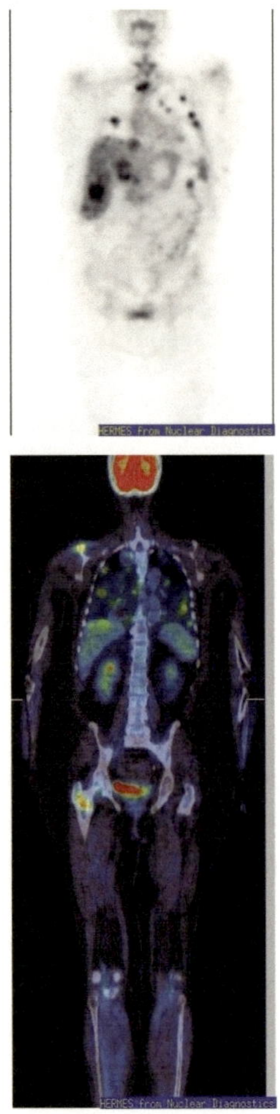

Figure 2. This 72-year-old woman originally presented with multiple lung metastases incidentally detected at the Hospital of Wels (Austria). The primary tumour was localised in the thyroid gland and histology revealed poorly differentiated thyroid carcinoma (Ki67 25%, TTF-1 and Tg positive). For post-operative restaging, FDG PET was arranged and presented multiple metastases of lung, liver and bone.

carcinoma, tall cell [3] and insular cell variants. Accurate localisation of disease is essential in Hürthle cell thyroid cancer because surgery and external beam radiation therapy may be beneficial. Hürthle cell thyroid cancer tends to be FDG-avid and all patients should undergo FDG PET in the post-operative setting onwards [15].

Poorly differentiated thyroid carcinoma represents a distinct stage in the progression from well-differentiated to anaplastic carcinoma [14]. When primary dedifferentiation with high Ki67 values can be observed and especially in the case of anaplastic thyroid cancer (which represents about 1.5% of all thyroid malignancies), the usefulness of iodine scanning tends to be low. This emphasises the importance of FDG PET in this setting (**Figure 2**). Approximately 20–50% of patients with early tumour dissemination are positive for distant metastases [16]. Unfortunately, the relevance for monitoring the disease is limited because of the bad prognosis of anaplastic thyroid cancer. Anaplastic carcinoma usually shows intense FDG uptake, and in selected cases FDG PET may be helpful in directing or evaluating treatment [14]. Here, nuclear medicine can provide somatostatin receptor imaging as well (to evaluate therapeutic options as radiopeptide therapy [17]), but monitoring the disease would still be the task of FDG PET.

It is worth noting that the role for FDG PET in staging and restaging of primary lymphoma of the thyroid gland is evidentially present [18].

2.3. FDG PET in medullary thyroid cancer

Medullary thyroid cancer (MTC) is a rare form of thyroid cancer (about 4–5%), descending from calcitonin-producing C-cells not related to iodine-capture processes and thyroid hormone production. Ultrasound, serum calcitonin screening, genetics of multiple endocrine neoplasia (MEN) syndromes, cytology and histology with immunohistochemistry for calcitonin, and various diagnostic tools of radiology play an important role for diagnosis and disease monitoring.

In regard to nuclear medicine, the impact of FDG and DOPA PET as well as somatostatin receptor imaging—and the order in which those methods should be applied—is still a matter of debate.

A PET study may be requested in patients with high serum calcitonin and/or carcinoembryonic antigen (CEA) levels after surgery. FDG PET is not a meaningful test in patients with low to moderate calcitonin levels and can occasionally be negative even at very high calcitonin levels of >1000 pg/ml [14]. Archier et al. recently reported experiences with a relatively large group of 86 MTC patients. DOPA PET/CT was positive in 65 patients (sensitivity of 76%), and distant metastatic disease was observed in 29 patients [19]. Beheshti et al. compared FDG and DOPA PET in the same patients with MTC and showed superiority of DOPA to detect metastases. However, lymph node metastases, which were only seen on FDG PET, were also described [20]. We suggest to use DOPA PET on the first run and to save FDG PET imaging for inconclusive or DOPA PET-negative cases. An illustrative case can be seen in **Figure 3**.

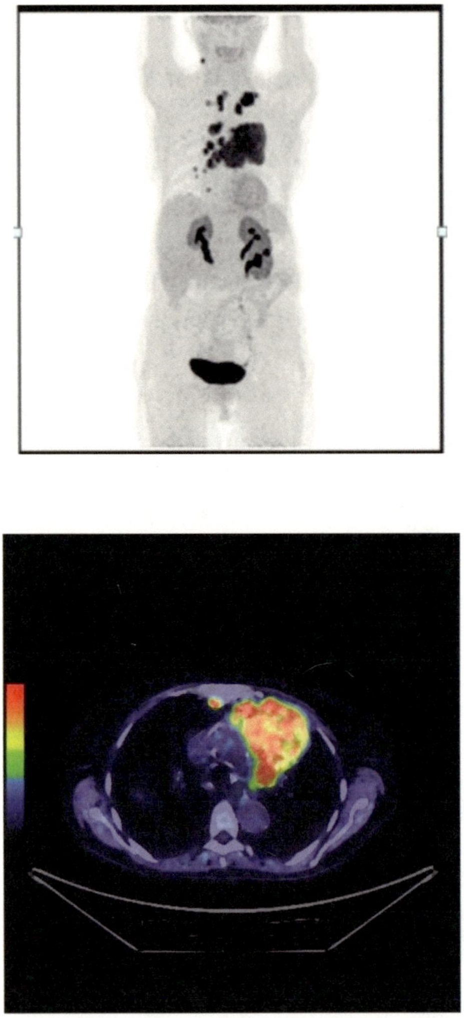

Figure 3. Medullary thyroid carcinoma was identified in 2008 at a metastatic stage yet. In 2015, the 74-year-old patient was sent to the University Hospital St. Pölten (Austria) for restaging by L-3,4-Dihydroxyphenylalanin (is an amino acid) (DOPA) PET (serum calcitonin of >3000 ng/dl). She also presented with diarrhoea as an associated endocrine symptom. The DOPA PET images revealed inoperability with cervical tumour masses and extensive thoracic lymph node metastases. The endocrine clinic ameliorated by the use of somatostatin analogues.

3. FDG PET in thyroid incidentalomas

Meanwhile, there are abundant data consisting of patients who underwent FDG PET/CT for (mostly oncological) reasons unrelated to pathologies. Then, the finding of a focal FDG uptake in a thyroid nodule generally merits further examination, and thyroid surgery with histological verification is necessary in many cases. The intensity of FDG uptake measured by SUV

http://dx.doi.org/10.5772/64110

(standard uptake value) cannot discriminate with certainty benign and malignant thyroid nodules. The risk to find a malignant entity can be estimated at 25–50%. Of course, these data depend upon the characteristics of the patient group as age and iodine supply of the home country are contributing factors. Diffuse-elevated FDG uptake in the thyroid can be found when Hashimoto´s thyroiditis is present. Focal uptake is limited to nodules of the thyroid. A prevalence of 1.5–3% for FDG-avid incidentaloma can be expected [21–23].

4. Conclusion

Thyroid cancer is definitely not the role model indication for FDG PET imaging, but for the management of differentiated thyroid cancer with metastases and more aggressive types of malignancies of the thyroid, FDG PET proves to be clinically useful. Incidental detection of malignancy in FDG-avid thyroid nodules has to be taken into consideration when FDG PET examinations have been conducted for reasons unrelated to the thyroid.

Author details

Irina Wimmer[1] and Robert Pichler[2,3,4*]

*Address all correspondence to: Robert.Pichler@gespag.at

1 Department of Internal Medicine and Institute of Nuclear Medicine, Karl Landsteiner Medical University, University Hospital St. Pölten, St. Pölten, Austria

2 Institute of Nuclear Medicine, Kepler University Hospital, Neuromed Campus, Linz, Austria

3 Institute of Nuclear Medicine, LKH Steyr, Steyr, Austria

4 Department of Radiology, Institute of Nuclear Medicine, Medical University Graz, Graz, Austria

References

[1] Haslerud T, Brauckhoff K, Reisæter L, Küfner-Lein R, Heinecke A, Varhaug JE, Biermann M. F18-FDG-PET for recurrent differentiated thyroid cancer: a systematic meta-analysis. Acta Radiol. 2015 Jul 9. pii: 0284185115594645.

[2] Ell PJ, Gambhir SS (eds.). Nuclear medicine in clinical diagnosis and treatment. 3rd ed., Churchill Livingston; Edinburgh, 2004.

[3] Haugen BR, Alexander EK, Bible KC, Doherty GM, Mandel SJ, Nikiforov YE, Pacini F, Randolph GW, Sawka AM, Schlumberger M, Schuff KG, Sherman SI, Sosa JA, Steward DL, Tuttle RM, Wartofsky L. 2015 American Thyroid Association management guidelines for adult patients with thyroid nodules and differentiated thyroid cancer: the American Thyroid Association Guidelines task force on thyroid nodules and differentiated thyroid cancer. Thyroid. 2016; 1:1–133. doi: 10.1089/thy.2015.0020.

[4] Feine U, Lietzenmayer R, Hanke JP, Held J, Wöhrle H, Müller-Schauenburg W. Fluorine-18-FDG and iodine-131-iodide uptake in thyroid cancer. J Nucl Med. 1996;37:1468–72.

[5] Bournaud C, Raverot V. Follow-up of differentiated thyroid carcinoma. Ann Endocrinol (Paris). 2015;76(1 Suppl 1):1S27–33. doi: 10.1016/S0003-4266(16)30011-7.

[6] Feine U, Lietzenmayer R, Hanke JP, Wöhrle H, Müller-Schauenburg W. 18FDG whole-body PET in differentiated thyroid carcinoma. Flipflop in uptake patterns of 18FDG and 131I. Nuklearmedizin. 1995;34:127–34.

[7] Rosenbaum-Krumme SJ, Görges R, Bockisch A, Binse I. ^{18}F-FDG PET/CT changes therapy management in high-risk DTC after first radioiodine therapy. Eur J Nucl Med Mol Imaging. 2012;39:1373–80. doi: 10.1007/s00259-012-2065-4.

[8] Dong MJ, Liu ZF, Zhao K, Ruan LX, Wang GL, Yang SY, Sun F, Luo XG. Value of 18F-FDG-PET/PET-CT in differentiated thyroid carcinoma with radioiodine-negative whole-body scan: a meta-analysis. Nucl Med Commun. 2009;30:639–50. doi: 10.1097/MNM.0b013e32832dcfa7.

[9] Ruhlmann M, Binse I, Bockisch A, Rosenbaum-Krumme SJ. Initial [18F]FDG PET/CT in high-risk DTC patients. A three-year follow-up. Nuklearmedizin. 2016 Feb 2;55(3).

[10] Wang W, Larson SM, Fazzari M, Tickoo SK, Kolbert K, Sgouros G, Yeung H, Macapinlac H, Rosai J, Robbins RJ. Prognostic value of [18F]fluorodeoxyglucose positron emission tomographic scanning in patients with thyroid cancer. J Clin Endocrinol Metab. 2000;85:1107–13.

[11] Kloos RT. Approach to the patient with a positive serum thyroglobulin and a negative radioiodine scan after initial therapy for differentiated thyroid cancer. J Clin Endocrinol Metab. 2008;93:1519–25. doi: 10.1210/jc.2007-2357.

[12] Alzahrani AS, Mohamed G, Al Shammary A, Aldasouqi S, Abdal Salam S, Shoukri M. Long-term course and predictive factors of elevated serum thyroglobulin and negative diagnostic radioiodine whole body scan in differentiated thyroid cancer. J Endocrinol Invest. 2005;28:540–6.

[13] Liu Y. The role of 18F-FDG PET/CT in the follow-up of well-differentiated thyroid cancer with negative thyroglobulin but positive and/or elevated antithyroglobulin antibody. Nucl Med Commun. 2016 Jan 25. Nucl Med Commun. 2016;37:577-82. doi: 10.1097/MNM.0000000000000480. [Epub ahead of print]

[14] Abraham T, Schöder H. Thyroid cancer – indications and opportunities for positron emission tomography/computed tomography imaging. Semin Nucl Med. 2011;41:121–38. doi: 10.1053/j.semnuclmed.2010.10.006.

[15] Pryma DA, Schöder H, Gönen M, Robbins RJ, Larson SM, Yeung HW. Diagnostic accuracy and prognostic value of 18F-FDG PET in Hürthle cell thyroid cancer patients. J Nucl Med. 2006;47:1260–6.

[16] Kobayashi M, Itabashi H, Ikeda T, Yamazaki N, Kaji T, Takagane A. Simultaneous occurrence of distant metastases to the small intestine and the thoracic esophagus from anaplastic thyroid carcinoma: a case report. Surg Case Rep. 2015;1:63. doi: 10.1186/s40792-015-0066-9.

[17] Lapa C, Werner RA, Schmid JS, Papp L, Zsótér N, Biko J, Reiners C, Herrmann K, Buck AK, Bundschuh RA. Prognostic value of positron emission tomography-assessed tumor heterogeneity in patients with thyroid cancer undergoing treatment with radiopeptide therapy. Nucl Med Biol. 2015;42:349–54. doi: 10.1016/j.nucmedbio.2014.12.006.

[18] Naswa N, Sharma P, Nazar AH, Mohapatra TK, Bal C, Kumar R. 18F-FDG PET/CT for initial assessment and response monitoring in a case of high grade primary lymphoma of the thyroid gland: a case report and review of literature. Indian J Nucl Med. 2014;29:94–6. doi: 10.4103/0972-3919.130291.

[19] Archier A, Heimburger C, Guerin C, Morange I, Palazzo FF, Henry JF, Schneegans O, Mundler O, Abdullah AE, Sebag F, Imperiale A, Taïeb D. 18F-DOPA PET/CT in the diagnosis and localization of persistent medullary thyroid carcinoma. Eur J Nucl Med Mol Imaging. 2015 Oct 24. 2016;43:1027-33. doi: 10.1007/s00259-015-3227-y. [Epub ahead of print]

[20] Beheshti M, Pöcher S, Vali R, Waldenberger P, Broinger G, Nader M, Kohlfürst S, Pirich C, Dralle H, Langsteger W. The value of 18F-DOPA PET-CT in patients with medullary thyroid carcinoma: comparison with 18F-FDG PET-CT. Eur Radiol. 2009;19:1425–34. doi: 10.1007/s00330-008-1280-7.

[21] Cohen MS, Arslan N, Dehdashti F, Doherty GM, Lairmore TC, Brunt LM, Moley JF. Risk of malignancy in thyroid incidentalomas identified by fluorodeoxyglucose-positron emission tomography. Ann Surg. 2001;235:648–54.

[22] Are C, Hsu JF, Schoder H, Shah JP, Larson SM, Shaha AR. FDG-PET detected thyroid incidentalomas: need for further investigation? Ann Surg Oncol. 2007;14:3210–5.

[23] Adas M, Adas G, Koc B, Ozulker F. Incidental thyroid lesions on FDG-PET/CT: a prevalence study and proposition of management. Minerva Endocrinol. 2015;40:169–75.

Chapter 7

^{124}I PET: Pretherapeutic Staging, Detection of Recurrent Thyroid Cancer and Dosimetry

Marcus Ruhlmann, Verena Ruhlmann,
Walter Jentzen and Andreas Bockisch

Additional information is available at the end of the chapter

http://dx.doi.org/10.5772/63671

Abstract

Radioiodine therapy (RIT) is an integral component in the treatment of differentiated thyroid cancer (DTC). Patients usually undergo RIT as initial therapy or later in the case of recurrent or persistent disease. The most important requirement for a successful RIT is the ability of metastases and thyroid (remnant) tissue to accumulate radioiodine. In order to calculate the achievable absorbed radiation dose for a lesion, volume and iodine kinetics in the lesion need to be determined. Pretherapeutic imaging and dosimetry with ^{124}I PET provide the methodology to answer these questions.

Keywords: 124I PET/CT, thyroid cancer, staging, recurrence, dosimetry

1. Introduction

Thyroid cancer is divided into differentiated thyroid cancer (DTC) and undifferentiated thyroid cancer. In contrast to the undifferentiated thyroid cancer, the vast majority of the DTC accumulates iodine in the tumour cells. Utilizing this characteristic, DTC patients can undergo radioiodine therapy (RIT). RIT of DTC patients provides a very effective therapy with only minimal side effects using standard activities, which is established for more than half a century. Patients are treated according to their tumour stage. Low-risk patients usually undergo a single RIT with activities up to 4 GBq ^{131}I. High-risk patients undergo at least one or several RIT with higher activities [1, 2]. While performing RIT with high activities of ^{131}I, the organs at risk need specific attention. These are the bone marrow and the lung, especially in case of multiple metastases. The amount of ^{131}I activity and the number of RIT depend on the results of the first RIT: if metastases were detected in the posttherapeutic scan, further RIT may be necessary for an effective treatment of metastases. Therefore, a pretherapeutic diagnostic, which detects iodine avid metastases, is desirable. The same holds for the first RIT for patients with a high likelihood for metastases. The pretherapeutic risk stratification is one of the greatest challenges in treating DTC patients. Although the overall prognosis for the most DTC patients is excellent [3], unfortunately, some DTC patients suffer from recurrences or persistent disease. These patients have already undergone RIT. In cases of recurrent or persistent disease, the cancer cells often show less up to none radioiodine uptake. Patients with low or missing radioiodine uptake would not or would only slightly benefit from an additional RIT [4]. Therefore, the knowledge of the localization and the radioiodine uptake level of lesions have great influence on therapy decision and the amount of therapeutic activity.

Pretherapeutic imaging of DTC patients can be performed with different radioiodine isotopes and the corresponding imaging modalities. ^{131}I as diagnostic isotope is used since decades. Usually, activities up to 185 MBq ^{131}I are administered [5]. Another radioiodine isotope for pretherapeutic imaging is ^{123}I, which is hardly used due to its lower imaging sensitivity and higher costs [5]. Both isotopes can be visualized by planar scintigraphies with a gamma camera or as 3D imaging with a single photon emission tomography (SPECT) camera. Compared to positron emission tomography (PET), the spatial resolution of gamma cameras is lower. However, radioiodine diagnostics using ^{131}I prior to intended RIT is not advisable mainly for two reasons. First, until today it is not possible to derive reliable lesion dosimetry data from ^{131}I scans. Second, ^{131}I imaging needs relative high activities resulting in high radiation doses. It is well known, that this leads to a so called stunning and, thus, reduces the response of subsequent RIT [6].

^{124}I PET in combination with computed tomography (CT) overcomes both problems. It offers optimal imaging to detect radioiodine uptake in tumour cells before patients undergo RIT, while only low ^{124}I activities are required compared to ^{131}I imaging [7–11]. Stunning is unlikely and was not reported yet [5]. In addition, pretherapeutic ^{124}I diagnostic provides, in comparison with ^{131}I and ^{123}I, a higher quantitative capacity to perform a reliable lesion dosimetry. This enables a tailor-made RIT with optimized absorbed tumour doses and an ^{131}I activity, which is considered to be safe for the patient, based on the blood dosimetry.

2. Patient preparation, ^{124}I application and PET(/CT) imaging

There are two important requirements for a successful performance of ^{124}I PET(/CT) diagnostics or RIT: First, all patients are put on a low iodine diet. This is important to increase the radioiodine uptake of the tumour cells. After performing a CT scan with contrast agents containing iodine, for example, the tumour cells are saturated with iodine and would show only a low radioiodine uptake. Therefore, any iodine contamination has to be avoided to ensure a good radioiodine uptake during diagnostic imaging or therapy. Second, the tumour cells have to be stimulated to achieve a high radioiodine uptake. The increase of the thyroid stimulating hormone (TSH) can be reached on two ways: endogenous or exogenous stimulation. The endogenous stimulation is usually chosen after initial thyroidectomy. Patients have to stay on hormone withdrawal for about 4 weeks, until the TSH serum concentration exceeds 30 mU/l [2, 5]. During this time, patients may experience hypothyroid symptoms such as fatigue, listlessness, depression and concentration disorders. The other way is an exogenous stimulation with recombinant human TSH (rhTSH). The rhTSH is administered via an intramuscular injection two and one day before diagnostic imaging or treatment. The exogenous stimulation spares patients having the hypothyroid symptoms. Moreover, a lower blood dose was reported in rhTSH stimulated patients [12, 13] compared to endogenous stimulation. However, the equivalence of therapeutic efficiency concerning tumour elimination under rhTSH stimulation is not proven.

^{124}I is a positron emitting nuclide with a half-life of 4.2 days. Like many other positron emitting nuclides, ^{124}I is produced in a cyclotron. Under endogenous or exogenous TSH stimulation, ^{124}I can be administered in two different ways: orally or intravenously. The amount of administered ^{124}I activities reported in the literature is between 25 MBq and 74 MBq [7, 14, 15].

In the time of combined PET/CT scanners, it is much easier to locate focal radioiodine uptake for example in the neck [16]. The new scanner generation provides fast scans with an acquisition time of e.g. 15 min for a scan from thigh to head. Besides the scan parameters and the scanner properties, the time point of scan is very important. In the beginning of ^{124}I PET(/CT) imaging, multiple scans were performed at 4, 24, 48, 72, and ≥96 h after ^{124}I application. This time and resource consuming approach has been optimized and the necessary scans could be reduced to 2 time points: 24 and 96 h after ^{124}I application [14]. The first scan 24 h after ^{124}I application enables the detection of focal pathological iodine uptake as correlate for metastases or local relapse. This scan is sufficient for diagnostic purpose. The first and second scans are mainly needed for lesion dosimetry to estimate the lesion absorbed (radiation) dose during RIT (details see below). However, occasionally, weakly radioiodine accumulating metastases only show uptake in the late scan.

3. ^{124}I PET(/CT) in initial DTC staging

The RIT is crucial for an effective treatment of DTC [17, 18]. Patients with higher initial tumour stage or advanced disease with lymph node or distant metastases routinely undergo RIT with higher ^{131}I activities or several RIT. The knowledge of metastases prior to first RIT would be beneficial for therapy planning. If no metastases are present, lower activities of ^{131}I would be reasonable. Patients with many metastases, especially bone or pulmonary metastases, should be treated carefully because of bone marrow toxicity and the risk of radiation-related pneumonitis or lung fibrosis [19, 20].

Another advantage of pretherapeutic ^{124}I PET is the re-staging and especially up-staging in patients with suspect findings in sonography. Shortly before RIT (about three weeks after thyroidectomy) patients should undergo sonography of the neck. If conspicuous lymph nodes are present, additional clarification is necessary to adapt therapy management. In this process, ^{124}I PET offers the possibility to detect focal iodine uptake in case of lymph node metastases and therapy activity of ^{131}I can be adapted. If no radioiodine uptake was found in conspicuous lymph nodes, it might be a reactive lymph node or a radioiodine negative lymph node metastasis; both will not be affected by the RIT.

During the first RIT, there is usually focal radioiodine uptake in the thyroid bed in accordance with thyroid remnant tissues. Other focal radioiodine uptake located beyond the thyroid bed is suspicious for malignancy, for example in the neck is typical for lymph node metastases.

4. ^{124}I PET(/CT) in patients with persisting or recurrent thyroid cancer

In the clinical course of patients with DTC, some patients suffer from tumour persistence after initial RIT or experience a relapse of DTC at a later stage. These patients mostly present an elevated and/or increasing serum level of thyroglobulin. Sometimes new tissue in the thyroid bed or suspect lymph nodes can be detected in sonography of the neck as a correlate. The most preferable therapy option would be an additional RIT in these cases. Unfortunately, thyroid cancer cells can dedifferentiate and partially or completely lose the ability to accumulate iodine. These patients with the so-called radioiodine negative metastases do not or only slightly profit from additional RIT. Other therapies such as surgery or external beam radiotherapy would be the therapy of choice in radioiodine negative metastases. But not all patients are radioiodine negative in case of recurrent disease. Therefore, a selection must be performed prior to futile RIT.

After initial RIT and thyroid remnant ablation, no pathological focal iodine uptake should be visible. Therefore, every focal uptake, for example in the neck or lung, is highly suspect for metastases or local relapse (except physiological uptake, e.g. in the salivary glands).

5. ^{124}I PET/MRI

Within the last years, simultaneous PET/MRI (PET/magnetic resonance imaging) has been successfully implemented into scientific and clinical imaging, demonstrating its excellent diagnostic potential, mainly in oncologic imaging. Based on its excellent soft tissue contrast, MRI is known to provide superior assessment of head and neck tumours and with the increasing implementation of integrated whole-body PET/MR devices, combining the strength of PET as well as morphological and functional MRI. In this assessment, it could be of great advantage in the localization of focal iodine uptake. The first publication about simultaneous ^{124}I PET/MRI showed promising results [21].

http://dx.doi.org/10.5772/63671

6. ^{124}I Dosimetry

The ^{124}I dosimetry deals with the determination of tumour lesion dose per administered ^{131}I activity (LDpA) and the estimation of the so-called maximum tolerable activity (MTA) of ^{131}I. The LDpA can help in the decision process if an additional RIT is a promising approach. If a prescribed lesion dose seems to be reachable, the RIT is combined with a significant chance of cure [22–24]. Due to the heterogeneity of metastases of a patient, there may be a significant spread of LDpA in the different metastases. In consequence, RIT might be helpful in some metastases and the other metastases need to be treated by surgery or external beam radiotherapy.

The MTA derived from blood dosimetry is the ^{131}I activity that results in 2 Gy blood dose, which is used as a surrogate for the bone marrow dose. Blood doses below 2 Gy are expected to be tolerable without relevant side effects [19]. Furthermore, it is possible to evaluate the risk of radiation-related fibrosis in patients with or without disseminated lung metastases [19, 20]. The blood dosimetry is based on blood sample (BS) and whole-body counter (WC) measurements (see **Figures 1-3**).

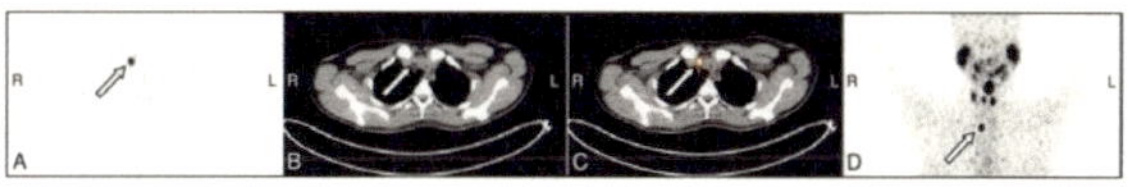

Figure 1. ^{124}I PET/CT in initial staging. A: axial PET. B: axial CT. C: axial PET/CT fusion. D: PET MIP (maximum intensity projection). 19-year-old female patient with a papillary pT2 pN1 DTC, 4 weeks after thyroidectomy. The arrows mark a radioiodine positive lymph node metastasis dorsal of the right clavicle. Moreover, another radioiodine positive lymph node metastasis right cervical, thyroid remnant tissue in the thyroid bed and a lobus pyramidalis are visible.

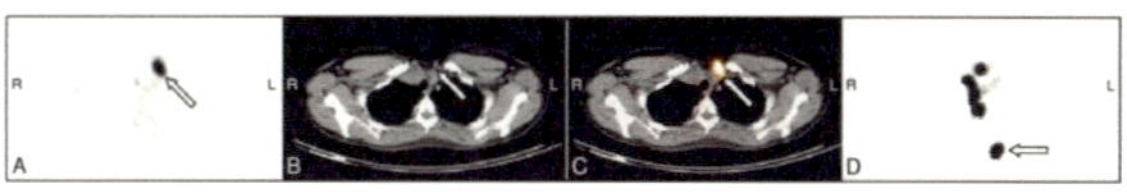

Figure 2. ^{124}I PET/CT in recurrent DTC. A: axial PET. B: axial CT. C: axial PET/CT fusion. D: PET MIP. 22-year-old female patient with a papillary pT4 pN1 DTC, 5 years after thyroidectomy and RIT with 10.0 GBq ^{131}I. The arrows mark a radioiodine positive lymph node metastasis in the jugulum left. Moreover, further radioiodine positive lymph node metastases right cervical are visible on image D.

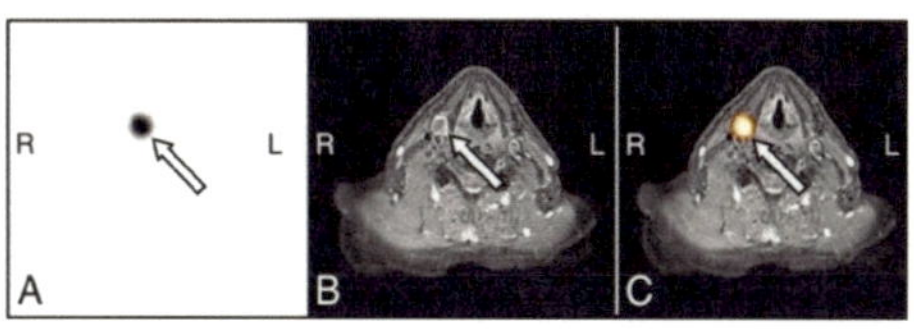

Figure 3. ^{124}I PET/MRI of the neck in recurrent DTC. A: axial PET. B: axial T1-W TSE sequence after contrast agent. C: axial PET/MR fusion. 71-year-old male patient with a follicular pT2 pN0 DTC, 8 years after thyroidectomy and RIT with 6.0 GBq ^{131}I. The arrows mark a lymph node metastasis right cervical.

The lesion and blood dosimetry consists of measurements at different time points after application of ^{124}I to determine the iodine kinetics. The lesion dosimetry requires a minimum of two PET(/CT) scans at 24 and ≥96 h after ^{124}I application. The blood dosimetry by the EANM dosimetry committee uses a comprehensive protocol with measurements over at least 4 days [25], which was optimized and shortened by Jentzen et al. [26]. For the optimized blood dosimetry protocols, patients are divided into the groups prior to first RIT and after first RIT. Prior to initial RIT, more measurements are recommended due to the presence of thyroid tissue. After the first RIT, only three time points are sufficient. In **Figure 4**, the required measurements are visualized. Further details on the calculations of lesion and blood dosimetry can be found in Jentzen et al. [14, 26] (see examples in **Figures 5** and **6**).

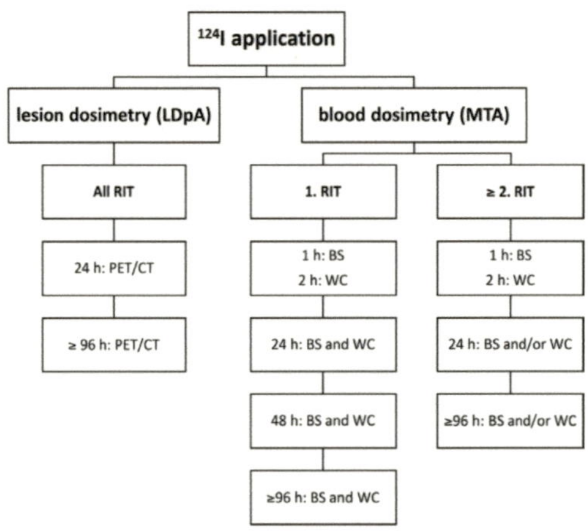

Figure 4. Flowchart of ^{124}I lesion and blood dosimetry. BS: blood sample; WC: whole-body counter.

7. Examples

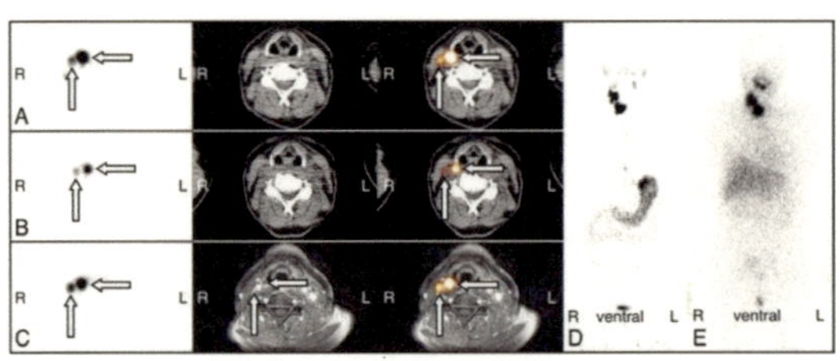

Figure 5. ^{124}I PET/CT and ^{124}I PET/MRI in initial staging. A: axial ^{124}I PET/CT (after 24 h). B: axial ^{124}I PET/CT (after 96 h). C: axial ^{124}I PET/MRI (after 24 h). D: ^{124}I PET MIP (after 24 h). E: Whole-body scan after RIT with 7.0 GBq ^{131}I (after 8 days). 47-year-old female patient with a papillary thyroid carcinoma (pT3 pN1a), 4 weeks after thyroidectomy. The arrows mark two lymph node metastases right cervical. On images D and E, cervical lymph node metastases and thyroid remnant tissue are visible. The blood dosimetry revealed a MTA of 18 GBq ^{131}I, until the blood dose of 2 Gy is reached. The lesion dosimetry estimated a LDpA ranging from 12 to 120 Gy/GBq ^{131}I.

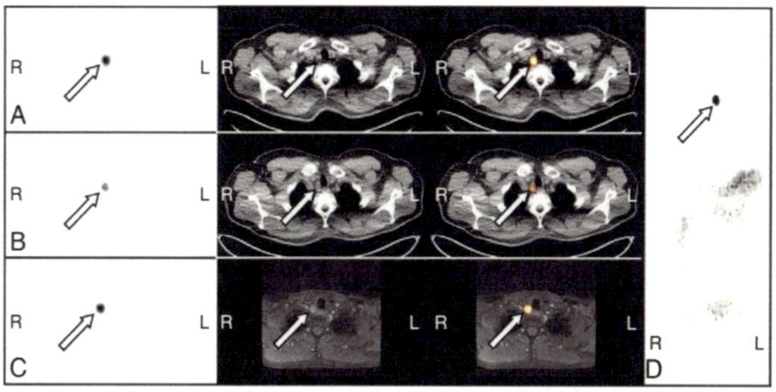

Figure 6. ^{124}I PET/CT and ^{124}I PET/MRI in restaging. A: axial ^{124}I PET/CT (after 24 h). B: axial ^{124}I PET/CT (after 96 h). C: axial ^{124}I PET/MRI (after 24 h). D: ^{124}I PET MIP (after 24 h). 44-year-old male patient with a papillary thyroid carcinoma (pT3 pN1b), 1 year after thyroidectomy and RIT with 6.0 GBq ^{131}I. Thyroglobulin increased without correlate in sonography of the neck. Therefore, a ^{124}I PET dosimetry was performed for restaging. The arrows mark one lymph node metastases right cervical paratracheal. On image D stomach, gastrointestinal tract and urinary bladder are visible. The blood dosimetry revealed a MTA of 37 GBq ^{131}I, until the blood dose of 2 Gy is reached. The lesion dosimetry estimated a LDpA of 14 Gy/GBq ^{131}I.

Author details

Marcus Ruhlmann*, Verena Ruhlmann, Walter Jentzen and Andreas Bockisch

*Address all correspondence to: marcus.ruhlmann@uk-essen.de

University Duisburg-Essen, Department of Nuclear Medicine, Essen, Germany

References

[1] Dietlein M, Dressler J, Eschner W, Grünwald F, Lassmann M, Leisner B, et al. Procedure guidelines for radioiodine therapy of differentiated thyroid cancer (version 3). Nuklearmedizin. ISSN: 0029-5566. 2007;(46):213–219 2007;(5): (155-231) DOI: http://dx.doi.org/10.1160/nukmed-0286.

[2] Haugen BR, Alexander EK, Bible KC, Doherty G, Mandel SJ, Nikiforov YE, et al. 2015 American thyroid association management guidelines for adult patients with thyroid nodules and differentiated thyroid cancer. Thyroid Off J Am Thyroid Assoc. 2016 Jan; 26(1):1-133. doi: 10.1089/thy.2015.0020. 2015.

[3] Mazzaferri EL, Jhiang SM. Long-term impact of initial surgical and medical therapy on papillary and follicular thyroid cancer. Am J Med. 1994;97(5):418–28.

[4] Woodrum DT, Gauger PG. Role of ^{131}I in the treatment of well differentiated thyroid cancer. J Surg Oncol. 2005;89(3):114–21.

[5] Luster M, Clarke SE, Dietlein M, Lassmann M, Lind P, Oyen WJG, et al. Guidelines for radioiodine therapy of differentiated thyroid cancer. Eur J Nucl Med Mol Imaging. 2008;35(10):1941–59.

[6] Morris LF, Waxman AD, Braunstein GD. Thyroid stunning. Thyroid. 2003;13(4):333–40.

[7] Phan HTT, Jager PL, Paans AMJ, Plukker JTM, Sturkenboom MGG, Sluiter WJ, et al. The diagnostic value of ^{124}I-PET in patients with differentiated thyroid cancer. Eur J Nucl Med Mol Imaging. 2008;35(5):958–65.

[8] Pettinato C, Spezi E, Nanni C, Grassetto G, Monari F, Allegri V, et al. Pretherapeutic dosimetry in patients affected by metastatic thyroid cancer using ^{124}I PET/CT sequential scans for ^{131}I treatment planning. Clin Nucl Med. 2014;39(8):e367–74.

[9] Pettinato C, Monari F, Nanni C, Allegri V, Marcatili S, Civollani S, et al. Usefulness of ^{124}I PET/CT imaging to predict absorbed doses in patients affected by metastatic thyroid cancer and treated with ^{131}I. Q J Nucl Med Mol Imaging. 2012;56(6):509–14.

[10] Beijst C, Kist JW, Elschot M, Viergever M, Hoekstra OS, de Keizer B, et al. Quantitative comparison of I-124 PET/CT and I-131 SPECT/CT detectability. J Nucl Med. J Nucl Med. 2016 Jan;57(1):103-8. doi: 10.2967/jnumed.115.162750. Epub 2015 Oct 22. 2015.

[11] Ruhlmann M. High level of agreement between pretherapeutic ^{124}I PET and intratherapeutic ^{131}I Images in detecting iodine-positive thyroid cancer metastases. JNM. 2016. [pub ahead of print] J Nucl Med. 2016 May 5. pii: jnumed.115.169649. [Epub ahead of print] http://www.ncbi.nlm.nih.gov/pubmed/27151981?dopt=Abstract

[12] Luster M, Lippi F, Jarzab B, Perros P, Lassmann M, Reiners C, et al. rhTSH-aided radioiodine ablation and treatment of differentiated thyroid carcinoma: a comprehensive review. Endocr Relat Cancer. 2005;12(1):49–64.

[13] Hänscheid H, Lassmann M, Luster M, Thomas SR, Pacini F, Ceccarelli C, et al. Iodine biokinetics and dosimetry in radioiodine therapy of thyroid cancer: procedures and results of a prospective international controlled study of ablation after rhTSH or hormone withdrawal. J Nucl Med. 2006;47(4):648–54.

[14] Jentzen W, Freudenberg L, Eising EG, Sonnenschein W, Knust J, Bockisch A. Optimized ^{124}I PET dosimetry protocol for radioiodine therapy of differentiated thyroid cancer. J Nucl Med. 2008;49(6):1017–23.

[15] Kist JW, de Keizer B, van der Vlies M, Brouwers AH, van der Zant FM, Hermsen R, et al. ^{124}I PET/CT to predict the outcome of blind ^{131}I treatment in patients with biochemical recurrence of differentiated thyroid cancer; results of a multicenter diagnostic cohort study (THYROPET). J Nucl Med Off Publ Soc Nucl Med. J Nucl Med. 2016 May;57(5): 701-7. doi: 10.2967/jnumed.115.168138. Epub 2015 Nov 25 2015.

[16] Freudenberg LS, Antoch G, Jentzen W, Pink R, Knust J, Görges R, et al. Value of ^{124}I-PET/CT in staging of patients with differentiated thyroid cancer. Eur Radiol. 2004;14(11):2092–8.

[17] Mazzaferri EL, Kloos RT. Clinical review 128: Current approaches to primary therapy for papillary and follicular thyroid cancer. J Clin Endocrinol Metab. 2001;86(4):1447–63.

[18] Eustatia-Rutten CFA, Corssmit EPM, Biermasz NR, Pereira AM, Romijn JA, Smit JW. Survival and death causes in differentiated thyroid carcinoma. J Clin Endocrinol Metab. 2006;91(1):313–9.

[19] Benua RS, Cicale NR, Sonenberg M, Rawson RW. The relation of radioiodine dosimetry to results and complications in the treatment of metastatic thyroid cancer. Am J Roentgenol Radium Ther Nucl Med. 1962;87:171–82.

[20] Benua R, Leeper R. A method and rationale for treating metastatic thyroid carcinoma with the largest safe dose of 131I. In: Medeiros-Neta GE, Gaitan E, editors. Frontiers in Thyroidology. Plenum Medical; New York, NY: 1986. pp. 1317-1321.

[21] Eur J Nucl Med Mol Imaging. 2016 Jun;43(6):1011-7. doi: 10.1007/s00259-015-3288-y. Epub 2015 Dec 19. Imaging with (124)I in differentiated thyroid carcinoma: is PET/MRI superior to PET/CT? Binse I1, Poeppel TD2, Ruhlmann M2, Gomez B2, Umutlu L3, Bockisch A2, Rosenbaum-Krumme SJ2.

[22] Maxon HR, Thomas SR, Hertzberg VS, Kereiakes JG, Chen I-W, Sperling MI, et al. Relation between effective radiation dose and outcome of radioiodine therapy for thyroid cancer. N Engl J Med. 1983;309(16):937–41.

[23] Maxon HR, Englaro EE, Thomas SR, Hertzberg VS, Hinnefeld JD, Chen LS, et al. Radioiodine-131 therapy for well-differentiated thyroid cancer—a quantitative radiation dosimetric approach: outcome and validation in 85 patients. J Nucl Med. 1992;33(6):1132–6.

[24] Jentzen W, Hoppenbrouwers J, van Leeuwen P, van der Velden D, van de Kolk R, Poeppel TD, et al. Assessment of lesion response in the initial radioiodine treatment of differentiated thyroid cancer using ^{124}I PET imaging. J Nucl Med. 2014;55(11):1759–65.

[25] Lassmann M, Hänscheid H, Chiesa C, Hindorf C, Flux G, Luster M, et al. EANM dosimetry committee series on standard operational procedures for pre-therapeutic dosimetry I: blood and bone marrow dosimetry in differentiated thyroid cancer therapy. Eur J Nucl Med Mol Imaging. 2008;35(7):1405–12.

[26] Jentzen W, Bockisch A, Ruhlmann M. Assessment of simplified blood dose protocols for the estimation of the maximum tolerable activity in thyroid cancer patients undergoing radioiodine therapy using ^{124}I. J Nucl Med. 2015;56(6):832–8.

Chapter 8

Differentiated Thyroid Carcinoma with Elevated Thyroglobulin and Negative Radioiodine Whole-Body Scan Metastases

Chao Ma

Additional information is available at the end of the chapter

http://dx.doi.org/10.5772/64356

Abstract

Serum thyroglobulin (Tg) and Tg antibody (TgAb) levels, together with neck ultrasonography and ^{131}I whole-body scintigraphy (WBS), are diagnostic tools for postoperative follow-up of patients with differentiated thyroid carcinoma (DTC). Generally, good correlation is seen between Tg and WBS in follow-up studies for DTC after thyroid remnant ablation. Undetectable serum Tg with negative WBS results suggests complete remission, whereas detectable, or elevated, serum Tg is associated with radioiodine uptake in local or distant metastases. Patients with thyroid cancer cells lacking radioiodine uptake despite an elevated serum Tg level have been referred to as WBS-negative, Tg-positive patients, who represent 10–15% of cases. ^{18}F-FDG PET (FDG-PET) scanning should be considered in high-risk DTC patients with negative WBS and positive Tg. The preferred therapeutic hierarchy for Tg-positive and WBS-negative metastases is surgical excision of loco-regional disease, ^{131}I therapy for radioiodine-responsive disease, external beam radiation, TSH suppression, and systemic therapy with kinase inhibitors. If FDG-PET diagnostic results are negative, one course of ^{131}I treatment may be considered in high-risk patients and individualized. No further ^{131}I therapy is indicated for patients with a negative post-therapy WBS.

Keywords: differentiated thyroid carcinoma, thyroglobulin, whole-body scan, radioiodine

1. Introduction

Serum thyroglobulin (Tg) is a tissue-specific 660 kDa protein that serves as a precursor in thyroid hormone biosynthesis [1]. It is synthesized by both thyroid follicular cells and differentiated cancer cells. Monitoring of serum Tg and Tg antibody (TgAb) levels, together with neck ultrasonography and ^{131}I whole-body scintigraphy (WBS), is used as a diagnostic tool in postoperative follow-up for patients with differentiated thyroid carcinoma (DTC) [2]. Generally, good correlation is seen between Tg and WBS in follow-up studies for DTC after thyroid remnant ablation [3]. Undetectable serum Tg with negative WBS results suggests complete remission, whereas detectable, or elevated, serum Tg is associated with radioiodine uptake in local or distant metastases. Patients with thyroid cancer cells lacking radioiodine uptake despite their elevated serum Tg level have been referred to as WBS-negative, Tg-positive patients [3]. The possible explanations and management for the discordant finding are discussed in this chapter.

2. Description of DTC with elevated Tg level and negative WBS

Tg is a thyroid tissue-specific antigen produced by thyroid follicular cells. Its measurement is the best sign of detecting thyroid tissue, including metastasis of DTC. After a total thyroidectomy and radioiodine ablation, any detectable Tg is interpreted as recurrent disease. Although it is a highly sensitive and specific marker of recurrence, Tg measurement cannot locate the recurrent DTC [4, 5]. Imaging technologies, including WBS, ultrasonography, computed tomography (CT), and magnetic resonance imaging (MRI), play great role in locating the DTC metastases. Tg is a very sensitive marker for thyroid malignancy, and it is not uncommon to encounter patients who show at initial follow-up, detectable Tg levels with negative imaging studies [6]. Patients with thyroid cancer cells lacking radioiodine uptake on WBS despite their elevated serum Tg level have been referred to as WBS-negative, Tg-positive patients; they represent 10–15% of patients with DTC at follow-up. Due to its inferior sensitivity, the routine WBS has been supplanted by serum Tg and neck ultrasonography, CT and/or MRI. The reasons for raised Tg and negative scan results have been summarized previously [7]. The elevated Tg level and negative WBS are classified into "true-negative WBS with false-positive Tg" and "false-negative WBS and true-positive Tg." Because of the low sensitivity of WBS, cervical ultrasonography plays more important role in the follow-up of DTC patients. Therefore, a new challenging scenario has emerged: the ultrasonography-negative, Tg-positive patient [8].

2.1. True-iodine negative and false-positive Tg

(1) Tg assays interference

The possibility of a false-positive serum Tg because of assay interference is rare but should be considered. And serum Tg has a lower false-negative rate than WBS after stimulation of thyroid stimulating hormone (TSH) either by thyroid hormone withdrawal or by recombinant human thyroid stimulating hormone (rhTSH) [9–13]. Optimal follow-up requires remnant ablation, and TSH-stimulated Tg testing [4]. The sensitivities and specificities of various Tg assays vary widely between laboratories, even with the use of an international standard (CRM 457) [14, 15], which have potential to disrupt serial monitoring and prompt inappropriate clinical decisions [9]. Additionally, undetectable serum Tg became detectable in a significant percentage of DTC patients by changing assays [16–18]. Therefore, Tg should be dynamically monitored using the same assay performed in the same laboratory. If possible, patient's serum is frozen and saved for recovery test to assess the reliability of Tg when there is a change in Tg assay [19]. As the sensitivity of commercially available Tg assays improves, TSH-stimulated Tg may not be necessary in patients with low and intermediate risk of recurrence [9].

(2) Circulating TgAb and HAb interferences

A major problem that hampers accurate Tg measurement is the interference by TgAb and HAb resulting in either an under- or overestimation of the serum Tg concentration [19–21]. Depending on the population studied and the assay used, up to 25–30% of patients with DTC have a positive test for TgAb at the time of initial diagnosis [22, 23]. In addition, a small to moderate percentage of patients (in the literature ranging from <1 to >10%) show HAb interference in Tg measurement, an integral tool in the management of DTC patients. These antibodies typically falsely lower the Tg value in immuno-chemiluminometric assays and immuno-radiometric assays, while raising the value in radio-immunoassay.

Therefore, TgAb should be measured in the same serum sample taken for Tg assay [15, 24]. Although for clinical purposes the measurement of Tg and TgAb before thyroidectomy for a suspected or proven DTC is not recommended, a pre-thyroidectomy Tg and TgAb measurement might be used as an "in vivo" recovery test in order to assess the reliability of Tg for use as a postoperative tumor marker [19, 25]. In DTC patients, the limit of quantitation (LoQ) of a given TgAb assay should be regarded as the upper normal limit for the presence of TgAb [25]. Thyroid laboratories should report two reference ranges for TgAb: one based on the presence of TgAb in a population free of thyroid disease, which should be used for the diagnosis of autoimmune thyroid disorders, and the LoQ which should be used as the upper normal limit in DTC patients. A proposed algorithm for follow-up in TgAb-positive patients with DTC was listed in **Figure 1** from Verburg et al. [25].

Persistence of Tg-Ab for more than 1 year after thyroidectomy and ^{131}I ablation probably indicates the presence of residual thyroid tissue and possibly and/or DTC recurrence [22, 24, 26]. A recent study also showed that TSH receptor mRNA accurately predicted disease status in 68% of DTC patients [27].

(3) Benign sources of Tg secretion

Apart from their ability to interfere with Tg assays, benign lesions (possibly with foci of thyroiditis) in persistent residual thyroid tissue or non-thyroidal tissue producing Tg may also result in false-positive Tg in DTC patients. However, residual occult disease is usually the source of post-operative Tg elevations [28–30]. Rarely, TSH-stimulated thymus may produce Tg [6].

Rarely, ectopic thyroid tissue may persist at the base of the tongue or, more often, at any other position along the thyroglossal tract, with the potential to elevate serum Tg levels. The thyroglossal tract is the most common location for ectopic thyroid tissue. This tissue retains

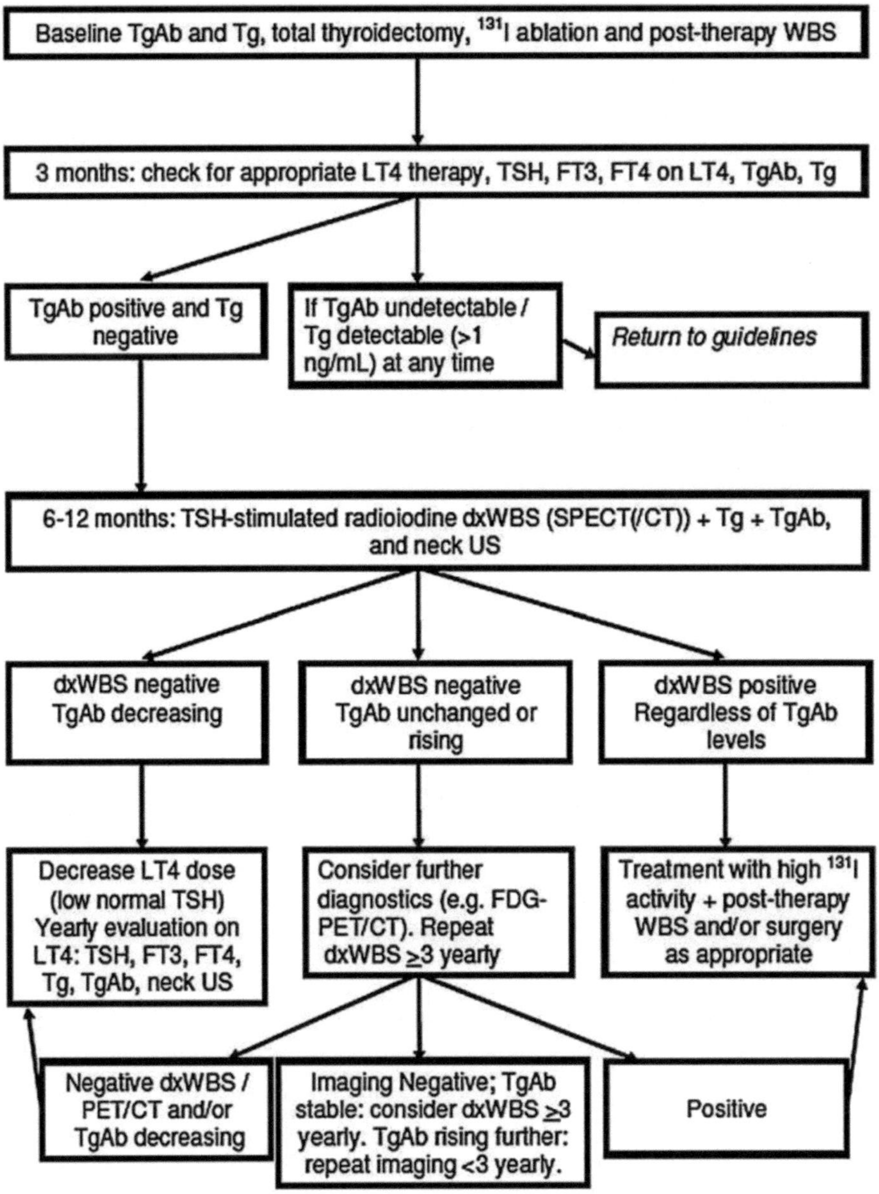

Figure 1. The algorithm for treatment and follow-up in Tb-Ab positive differentiated thyroid cancer patients from Verburg et al. [25].

not only the ability to concentrate iodine, but also to produce Tg and release it into the bloodstream [28, 31, 32]. The iodine metabolism-related proteins such as human sodium/iodide symporter (hNIS) [33], TSH receptor at both mRNA and protein level [6] are present in non-thyroidal tissues, including the thymus. Usually, these functions are dormant, but they may be activated by TSH stimulation [34]. Interestingly, these extra-thyroidal foci may be resistant to multiple ^{131}I treatments [28, 31, 32]. In a series of 548 consecutive diagnostic WBS, ectopic thyroid tissue in the tongue or in the upper part of the thyroglossal duct was visualized in five patients (0.9%) [28]. However, in another study of 60 patients, 19/60 (31.7%) had a linear or focal radioactivity at the superior midline of the neck, suggesting thyroglossal duct remnant [29]. The absence of metastases in the thymus despite high Tg levels was confirmed in five cases [33, 35]. Rare cases of thyroid tissue ectopy has been summarized in some locations such as struma ovarii, the heart (struma cordis), the submandibular, parotid and salivary glands, the duodenum, the adrenal glands, the liver and gallbladder, the pancreas, the axilla, and iris of the eye [6].

In summary, interference with Tg assays by TgAb and HAb, benign lesions (possibly containing thyroiditis) in persistent residual thyroid tissue or nonthyroidal tissue producing Tg may also result in false-positive Tg in DTC patients.

2.2. False-negative WBS and true-positive Tg

The possible causes of false-negative WBS are mentioned below.

(1) Defect of iodine-trapping mechanism such as acquired inactivation mutation of NIS, TPO gene, pendrin, and TSHR

Thyroid hormone synthesis starts with the active uptake of iodine from the circulation via NIS. This process, known as iodine trapping, is stimulated directly by TSH and more circuitously by iodine deficiency. Other proteins, including TPO, TSHR, and pendrin, also play an important role in the thyroid metabolism of iodine. Any defect in NIS, TPO, Tg, and TSHR will contribute to false-negative WBS [7].

(2) De-differentiation of tumor such that it can still produce Tg but has lost its iodine-trapping ability

Various molecular changes within papillary thyroid cancer cells, such as RET/PTC rearrangements, RAS and BRAF mutations [36], β-catenin mutations, PAX8/PPARã, histone acetylation factors involved in angiogenesis including overexpression of vascular endothelial growth factor (VEGF) and EGF receptor (EGFR) underlie the loss of iodide uptake ability [37]. The dedifferentiated DTC cells lost the ability to concentrate iodine but may retain Tg synthesizing capability [3, 7], which underlines the phenomenon of Tg-positive and WBS-negative lesions.

(3) Dispersed microscopic metastases, which are too small to be visualized

(4) Improper patient preparation before WBS

When it is determined that an elevation of Tg is real, if WBS is negative, false-negative scan such as stable iodine contamination and inadequate TSH elevation should be considered [7]. TSH levels should be elevated to at least 30 mIU/L before concluding that a negative WBS is meaningful. This can be achieved either by withdrawal of thyroxine or by rhTSH administration. rhTSH is as effective as thyroid hormone withdrawal on ^{131}I thyroid remnant ablation for

DTC patients with significant benefits in decreased whole-body radiation exposure and health-related quality of life [38, 39]. A summary of appropriate patient preparation for WBS in the hypothyroid state is presented in **Table 1** from Ma et al. [7].

Withdrawal of L-T4 for 4–6 weeks or of triiodothyronine for 2 weeks.
A strict low-iodine diet (50 g iodine per day) followed for 7–14 days before WBS and continuing throughout period of imaging.
Avoidance of iodine-containing medications (e.g., iodinated contrast medium, amiodarone, betadine), iodine-rich foods (e.g., kelp), and possible additives of iodine in vitamin and electrolyte supplements.
TSH > 30 mIU/L.
A mild laxative sometimes administered on the evening before WBS to simplify image interpretation.
Information relating to patient's compliance with low-iodine diet, TSH level, history of thyroid hormone withdrawal, measurement of Tg, history of prior administration of contrast medium or iodine-containing drugs (e.g., amiodarone), menstrual history/pregnancy test, nursing/lactation history, etc.
Measurement of urinary iodine in doubtful cases to rule out iodine contamination; repeated WBS 4–6 weeks after iodine depletion regimen such as diuretic program.
Rule out women with pregnancy and breast feeding.

Table 1. A summary of appropriate patient preparation for WBS from reference by Ma et al.

3. Management of DTC patients with positive Tg and negative WBS

3.1. Other diagnostic modalities for DTC in this setting

In the clinical setting, the precise location of WBS-negative recurrent DTC is mandatory because surgery is the only curative treatment option and metastases that are unable to concentrate ^{131}I are associated with more aggressive clinical behavior [40]. Cervical ultrasonography, CT and MRI, ^{124}I PET/CT have limited roles in the diagnosis of DTC metastases with positive Tg and negative WBS. Non-iodine imaging agents—such as ^{201}Tl, ^{99m}Tc-sestamibi, ^{99m}Tc-tetrofosmin, somatostatin receptor (SRS) scan have reasonable accuracy [41]. However, they have been replaced by ^{18}F-FDG in the follow-up algorithm of DTC patients with positive Tg and negative WBS.

(1) Cervical ultrasonography

Cervical ultrasonography has high sensitivity in detecting recurrence in the thyroid bed and nodal metastases of DTC in the neck [42, 43]. It has been used as first-line diagnostic imaging in DTC follow-up [44, 45]. However, neck ultrasonography has limitations: one is that it does not reveal DTC recurrences in other body sites. It is also difficult for cervical ultrasonography to differentiate scar tissue and locally recurring fibrosis and between nonspecific nodal enlargements and nodal metastases [46]. Therefore, the other limitation of ultrasonography is the low specificity in DTC patients of altered anatomy after thyroid surgery.

(2) CT and MRI

In patients with elevated or rising Tg or TgAb and no evidence of disease on neck ultrasonography or WBS (if performed), CT imaging of the neck and chest should be considered [47]. Diagnostic CT scan may complement neck ultrasonography for the detection of macrometastases in the central compartment, in the mediastinum and behind the trachea [48–50], and is the most sensitive tool for the detection of micro-metastases in the lungs. MRI has also been advocated for imaging the neck and the mediastinum. It is performed without and with injection of gadolinium chelate as contrast medium and does not require any injection of iodine contrast medium. Brain and skeletal MRI and/or CT, or abdominal MRI may be performed in high-risk DTC patients with elevated Tg (generally >10 ng/mL) and negative WBS or ultrasonography, who have systemic symptoms related to those organs, or who will have ^{131}I therapy and may be at risk for complications of tumor swelling [51]. MRI is less sensitive than CT scan for the detection of lung micronodules [47].

(3) ^{18}F-FDG-PET/CT or PET/MRI

The iodine-negative DTC lesions were found to have increased expression of the glucose transporter-1, and often have FDG uptake [52]. Therefore, ^{18}F-FDG-PET is particularly useful in the detection of recurrent or metastatic DTC in patients with positive Tg and negative WBS, allowing detection of metastases not detected by other imaging modalities [53]. In a recent meta-analysis, the combined sensitivity and specificity for FDG-PET/CT were 93 and 81%, respectively [54].

Factors influencing PET/CT sensitivity include tumor de-differentiation, larger tumor burden and to a lesser extent, TSH stimulation [47]. PET is more sensitive in patients with an aggressive histological subtype, including poorly differentiated, tall cell, and Hürthle cell thyroid cancer. The sensitivity of PET (ranging from less than 10–30%) is low in patients with a TSH-stimulated Tg < 10 ng/mL. It is therefore recommended to consider ^{18}F-FDG-PET only in DTC patients with a stimulated Tg level ≥10 ng/mL [47]. A meta-analysis of seven prospective controlled clinical trials indicated that FDG-PET under TSH stimulation either by thyroid hormone withdrawal or by rhTSH had slightly improved diagnostic performance in detecting Tg-positive and WBS-negative DTC lesions. FDG-PET/CT is useful in staging, response assessment after chemotherapy, targeted therapies, or radiotherapy and prognostic assessment for patients with cancer [55]. Therefore, PET/CT imaging should be performed as first-line, with empiric ^{131}I treatment being considered only for those patients with no detectable FDG uptake [51]. PET/CT can also identify lesions with high FDG uptake (SUV) that may be more aggressive and should have multi-targeted kinase inhibitors or close monitoring. A study observed that elevated Tg, but normal PET exists as a definitive entity in DTC. Positive Tg with negative PET was regarded as a favorable prognostic indicator to predict symptom-free status during the follow-up period [56].

However, false positives occur with PET imaging with or without TSH stimulation [50]. The frequency of false-positive lesions varies among series from 0 to 39%, and this high number justifies a fine-needle aspiration (FNA) biopsy with cytology and Tg measurement in the aspirate fluid in cases where surgery is planned, based on PET results.

FDG-PET/CT is useful in staging, response assessment after chemotherapy, targeted therapies, or radiotherapy and prognostic assessment for patients with cancer [55]. PET/CT imaging is more sensitive and should be performed as first-line, with empiric ^{131}I treatment being considered only for those patients with no detectable FDG uptake [51]. PET/CT can also identify lesions with high FDG uptake (SUV) that may be more aggressive and should have multi-targeted kinase inhibitors or close monitoring. A study observed that elevated Tg, but normal PET exists as a definitive entity in DTC. Positive Tg with negative PET was regarded as a favorable prognostic indicator to predict symptom-free status during the follow-up period [56].

(4) ^{124}I PET/CT

^{124}I emits positrons, allowing PET/CT imaging in DTC patients. It is used as for dosimetry and also as a diagnostic tool to localize DTC metastases. ^{124}I PET/CT accurately measures the volume, uptake, and half-life of ^{124}I in each DTC lesion, therefore permitting a reliable individual dosimetric assessment for DTC metastases [47]. ^{124}I-PET has higher sensitivity in detecting the residual thyroid tissue and/or DTC metastases than that of WBS (99% vs. 66%) [57–61]. The combination of ^{124}I and FDG-PET/CT affords a valuable diagnostic method that can be used to make therapeutic decisions in patients with positive Tg and negative WBS [57, 61]. ^{124}I-PET/CT with thyroid hormone withdrawal was found to detect significantly more foci of metastases of DTC [59]. However, it is unclear whether and to what extent patient preparation with rhTSH rather than thyroid hormone withdrawal affects the diagnostic accuracy of ^{124}I PET/CT [57]. ^{124}I is not yet widely available for clinical use and is primarily a research tool at this time.

(5) Somatostatin receptor scan (SRS)

Thyroid tumors are known to express SRS, and therefore, ^{111}In-pentetreotide (somatostatin analog) can visualize non-iodine avid DTC metastases with high concentration of SRS. A case of negative WBS recurrent metastatic papillary thyroid carcinoma with positive ^{111}In-pentetreotide scan was reported [62]. Technetium-99m labeled somatostatin analog, ^{99m}Tc-Hynic-TOC scintigraphy had a sensitivity of 88.46% (23/26), specificity of 100% (2/2), and an accuracy of 89.2% (25/28) [41]. SRS scintigraphy may be useful both in the staging and monitoring of patients with WBS-negative DTC metastases. ^{68}Gallium-somatostatin analogs PET/CT is currently a promising method to study well-differentiated neuroendocrine tumor which has a better sensitivity and therefore is superior to ^{99m}Tc or ^{111}In labeled SRS [63, 64]. SRS scan positive patients are potential candidates for SRS-targeted therapy.

http://dx.doi.org/10.5772/64356

In addition, ^{68}Gallium-somatostatin analogs PET/CT is currently a promising method to study well-differentiated neuroendocrine tumor which has a better sensitivity and therefore is superior to ^{99m}Tc or 111In labeled SRS [63, 64]. ^{18}F-FLT and ^{11}C-MET may also have a diagnostic roles in this clinical setting [65].

(6) Fine-needle aspiration (FNA)

FNA biopsy for cytology and Tg measurement in the aspirate fluid is performed for suspicious lymph nodes >8–10 mm in their smallest diameter. Non-suspicious and small nodes (<8–10 mm in the smallest diameter) can be monitored with neck ultrasonography [47]. Ultrasonography guidance aspiration may improve the results of FNA biopsy, in particular for small lymph nodes and those located deep in the neck. The measurement of Tg in the FNA biopsy washout fluid (FNAB-Tg) is the more accurate tool to detect DTC recurrences and metastases in the neck [66, 67]. However, the application of FNA biopsy Tg is currently hindered by the absence of methodological standardization, a lack of definite cutoff points, and the ongoing debate regarding its accuracy in nonthyroidectomized patients, those with elevated serum Tg, and those with circulating TgAb [66, 67]. A Tg concentration in the aspirate fluid between 1 and 10 ng/mL is moderately suspicious for malignancy [47]; above 10 ng/mL are highly suspicious of DTC metastases [68–70].

In summary, in patients with elevated or rising Tg (>10 ng/mL) or TgAb and no evidence of disease on neck ultrasonography or WBS (if performed), CT imaging of the neck and chest, MRI of the neck and abdomen may be considered. ^{18}F-FDG-PET/CT also plays an important role in the detecting DTC metastases with positive Tg (>10 ng/mL) and negative WBS, and negative conventional imaging. The result of ^{18}F-FDG-PET/CT is helpful in guiding the treatment strategy. FNA biopsy and Tg measurement in washout fluid are helpful in the confirmation of foci detected by ^{18}F-FDG-PET/CT.

3.2. Treatments for Tg-positive and WBS-negative DTC metastases

3.2.1. Empiric ^{131}I treatment

Thyroid hormone withdrawal induces substantial short- and long-term morbidity, decreased quality of life due to associated hypothyroidism.^{131}I therapy may cause early and late sialoadenitis in up to 30% which can lead to xerostomia, dental caries, and stomatitis [71, 72], with a majority of patients suffering from significant changes in physical, psychological, and social well-being [73, 74]. Therefore, the pros and cons of empiric ^{131}I treatment should be well-balanced justified.

The management of elevated serum Tg and radioiodine-negative scans was outlined by Ma et al. [3]. Of 438 patients from 16 studies who were treated empirically with ^{131}I for iodine-negative and Tg-positive DTC disease, 267 (62%) displayed pathological uptakes in the thyroid bed, lungs, bone, mediastinum and lymph nodes. In studies in which data were available for serum Tg levels during TSH suppression therapy or TSH withdrawal, 56% (188/337) patients showed decreased Tg. Of 242 patients from 5 studies who received no specific treatment for iodine-negative and Tg-positive DTC disease, 44% (106/242) showed spontaneous normalization and a significant decrease in serum Tg. Thus, high doses of ^{131}I have therapeutic effects if the Tg level is considered an index of tumor burden, at least in the short term, and could also localize previously undiagnosed recurrences. Therefore, empiric^{131}I treatment may be justified in high-risk patients with serum Tg > 10 ng/mL and a negative WBS and FDG-PET scan results [3, 75, 76]. Pulmonary metastases may be found only on post-therapy WBS [77]. In a study of 283 DTC patients treated with 100mCi (3.7 GBq) of ^{131}I, 6.4% had lung and bone metastases detected after treatment that had been suspected based on high serum Tg alone but had not been detected after 2mCi (74 MBq) ^{131}I WBS [78].

However, most studies in this area have limited reliability as they lacked control groups and an adequate follow-up period [3]. Still missing from our knowledge are long-term survival rates, changes in mass sizes on post-therapy imaging, and radiation-induced side-effects of ^{131}I therapy. Although the tumor burden may be diminished, most patients with negative WBS and positive Tg are not rendered disease free by ^{131}I therapy [79]. Nearly half of patients with Tg-positive and WBS-negative DTC show spontaneous normalization and significant reduction in serum Tg without any specific treatment, ^{131}I therapy should be individualized according to the clinical characteristics and imaging features. A five-year follow-up of 29 patients with elevated Tg (>2 ng/mL) and negative ^{131}I WBS found that 24/29 patients showed Tg decreasing trend without ^{131}I therapy, of whom only one patient recurred; the other 5/29 patients showed a rising trend and all recurred [5].

Therefore, additional diagnostic techniques are strongly recommended for patients with Tg-positive and WBS-negative metastases. If these diagnostic results are positive, treatment options such as surgery, external radiotherapy and tumor embolization can be considered. Empiric ^{131}I therapy is more commonly considered for those with distant metastases or inoperable local disease. If FDG-PET result is negative, one course of ^{131}I treatment may be considered in high-risk patients with. Repeated ^{131}I therapy may be given to patients who had persistent non-resectable DTC metastases and iodine uptake, and there are significant therapeutic benefits until the lesion has been eradicated or the lesion no longer responds to treatment. The risk of repeated therapeutic doses of RAI must be balanced against uncertain long-term benefits. In the case of negative post-therapy WBS, the patient should be considered to have radioiodine-refractory disease and no further ^{131}I therapy should be administered.

3.2.2. Re-differentiation strategies

(1) Retinoic acids (RA) and lithium

RA are active metabolites of vitamin A able to regulate growth and differentiation of many cell types by binding to specific nuclear receptors, the RA receptors, and the retinoid X receptors (RXR) [80]. Lithium increases the residence time of ^{131}I in the thyroid tissue [37, 81, 82]. RA and lithium [82] were used to redifferentiate metastatic DTC and render them responsive to ^{131}I therapy. However, they only yielded a limited clinical benefit.

(2) Iodine-trapping-related gene transfection

hNIS protein is a membrane glycoprotein that transports iodide ions into thyroid cells. This process, known as iodine trapping, is stimulated directly by TSH. Other proteins, including thyroperoxidase (TPO) and pendrin, also play an important role in the thyroid metabolism of iodine [83]. Strategies of gene transfection focused on NIS; TPO has been studied to enhance tumor uptake iodine [84, 85]. Co-transfection of the hNIS and hTPO genes can lead to longer retention of radio iodine [85]. Targeted NIS gene transfer, by viral and non-viral vectors, followed by radionuclide ^{131}I, ^{188}Re, ^{211}At therapy, has been recently suggested for the treatment of advanced or WBS-negative DTC metastases. In thyroid cells, TSH stimulates NIS synthesis [86]. Therefore, hTSHR transfection was investigated in FTC-133 thyroid cells, which improved the expression of thyroid-specific molecules including TSHR, NIS, TPO, and Tg and radioiodide uptake [87, 88]. Iodine-trapping-related gene transfection has not been used clinically yet.

(3) MAPK kinase inhibitor

Mitogen-activated protein kinase (MAPK) signaling inhibits the expression of thyroid hormone biosynthesis genes, including the NIS and TPO, which facilitate iodine uptake and organification, respectively [89, 90]. Inhibition of the MAPK pathway may renew the therapeutic efficacy of ^{131}I by enhancing uptake in patients with thyroid cancer that is refractory to ^{131}I [82]. MAPK1-2 inhibitor selumetinib (AZD6244, ARRY-142886), orally administered at a dose of 75 mg twice daily increased the uptake of ^{124}I in 12 of 20 patients. Selumetinib enhanced ^{131}I uptake in eight patients with advanced DTC. After ^{131}I treatment, partial responses were achieved in 5, stable disease in 3. No severe adverse events were observed [82].

In summary, strategy of re-differentiation of iodine-negative DTC metastases by RA has limited clinical benefit. Iodine-trapping-related protein transfection remains experimental. MAPK kinase inhibitor needs to be confirmed in large population.

3.2.3. Multi-targeted kinase inhibitors

Both sorafenib (BAY 43-9006) and lenvatinib are multi-kinase inhibitors with potent activity against RAF, VEGF receptors, fibroblast growth factor receptors, PDGF receptor, c-KIT and RET kinases [37, 88, 91]. Sorafenib and lenvatinib are both FDA approved for iodine refractory DTC metastases [92]. They achieved clinical benefits in terms of partial response of 12.5–38%, progression-free survival from 9 to 24 months in radioiodine-refractory DTC metastases [37, 91]. The therapeutic effects of other tyrosine kinase inhibitors including sunitinib, imatinib, vandetanib were also summarized [37] and a dozen ongoing trials currently listed in the ClinicalTrials.gov database, evaluating 12 kinase-inhibiting drugs [93].

Adverse effects occurred in 98.6% patients receiving sorafenib: the most frequent were hand-foot skin reactions, diarrhea, alopecia, and rash or desquamation [94].

Selection of a targeted agent should depend on disease trajectory, side effect profile, and goals of therapy. Kinase inhibitor therapy should be considered in radioiodine-refractory DTC metastases, rapidly progressive, symptomatic and/or imminently threatening disease not otherwise amenable to local control using other approaches. Patients who are candidates for kinase inhibitor therapy should be thoroughly counseled on the potential risks and benefits of this therapy as well as alternative therapeutic approaches including best supportive care [47].

3.2.4. Other treatments

(1) TSH suppression

TSH suppression is considered essential in the treatment of patients with positive Tg and negative WBS, because TSH is a trophic hormone that can stimulate the growth of cells derived from thyroid follicular epithelium [45, 95, 96]. Therefore, the recommended TSH level is below 0.1 mU/L, or slightly below or slightly above the lower reference range [9].

(2) Surgery and stereotactic radiotherapy (SBRT)

Most recurrent DTCs respond well to surgery and SBRT [45, 97]. The isolated skeletal metastasis of DTC is recommended for surgery or SBRT [9]. Neurosurgery or SBRT is preferred treatments for solitary brain metastases of DTC [98, 99]. SBRT is considered for loco-regional recurrence that is not surgically resectable, or with extra-nodal extension or involvement of soft tissues, in particular in patients with no evidence of distant disease, but has no role in most patients with resectable lymph node metastases [47].

(3) Chemotherapy

Systematic chemotherapy can be considered for DTC lesions with positive Tg and negative WBS that are not surgically resectable, not responsive to ^{131}I, not amenable to EBRT treatment, or not responsive to multi-targeted kinase inhibitors, and have clinically significant structural disease progression during the last 6–12 months. Two of 49 (3%) patients with DTC metastases had a response to five chemotherapy protocols [100]. In a review by Ahuja et al., 38% of patients with thyroid cancer had reduction in tumor mass to doxorubicin [101]. Combination chemotherapy does not show clear superiority to doxorubicin therapy alone [102]. Therefore, the traditional chemotherapy has limited effects on iodine refractory DTC metastases [9, 103].

(4) Other treatments

Other treatments include percutaneous ethanol injection (PEI), radiofrequency, or laser ablation.

PEI for patients with metastatic DTC in lymph node is promising as a nonsurgical-directed therapy [104, 105]. Most of the studies limited PEI to patients who had undergone previous neck dissections and ^{131}I treatment, those who had FNA-proven DTC in the lymph node and those with no known distant metastases [106]. A general consensus from studies and reviews is that PEI could be considered in patients who are poor surgical candidates [47]. Radiofrequency ablation has been associated with a mean volume reduction that ranges between approximately 55–95% [107, 108], and 40–60% complete disappearance of the DTC metastases in the treatment of recurrent thyroid cancer [108, 109]. More recently, preliminary findings using ultrasonography-guided laser ablation for treatment of cervical lymph node metastases have been reported [110].

In summary, true-negative WBS with positive Tg may be due to benign thyroid remnants (possibly containing thyroiditis) or, rarely, nonthyroidal tissue producing Tg. False-negative WBS with positive Tg can be caused by a defective of acquired iodine-trapping inactivation;

http://dx.doi.org/10.5772/64356

dedifferentiation of tumor which can still produce Tg but has lost its iodine-trapping ability; small dispersed microscopic metastases. Other radioisotopes and additional diagnostic options play an important role in the ascertainment of patients with negative WBS and Tg-positive DTC metastases. FDG-PET/CT should be considered in high-risk DTC patients with negative WBS and positive Tg. If FDG-PET diagnostic results are negative, one course of ^{131}I treatment may be considered in high-risk patients and individualized. No further ^{131}I therapy is indicated for patients with a negative post-therapy WBS. The preferred hierarchy of treatment for Tg-positive and WBS-negative metastases is surgical excision of loco-regional disease in potentially curable patients, ^{131}I therapy for residual radioiodine-responsive disease, external beam radiation or other directed treatment modalities such as thermal ablation, TSH suppression for patients with stable or slowly progressive asymptomatic disease, and systemic therapy with multi-kinase inhibitors, especially for patients with significantly progressive macroscopic refractory disease.

Author details

Chao Ma

Address all correspondence to: mc_7419@hotmail.com

Nuclear Medicine, Affiliated Xinhua Hospital School of Medicine, Shanghai Jiaotong University, Shanghai, China

References

[1] Ringel MD and Ladenson PW. Controversies in the follow-up and management of well-differentiated thyroid cancer. *Endocrine-Related Cancer*. 2004;11:97–116.

[2] Shammas A, Degirmenci B, Mountz JM, McCook BM, Branstetter B, Bencherif B, Joyce JM, Carty SE, Kuffner HA and Avril N. 18F-FDG PET/CT in patients with suspected recurrent or metastatic well-differentiated thyroid cancer. *Journal of Nuclear Medicine: Official Publication, Society of Nuclear Medicine*. 2007;48:221–226.

[3] Chao M. Management of differentiated thyroid cancer with rising thyroglobulin and negative diagnostic radioiodine whole body scan. *Clinical Oncology (Royal College of Radiologists (Great Britain))*. 2010;22:438–447.

[4] Eustatia-Rutten CF, Smit JW, Romijn JA, van der Kleij-Corssmit EP, Pereira AM, Stokkel MP and Kievit J. Diagnostic value of serum thyroglobulin measurements in the follow-up of differentiated thyroid carcinoma, a structured meta-analysis. *Clinical Endocrinology*. 2004;61:61–74.

[5] Gupta M, Choudhury PS, Nag S and Gupta P. Stimulated high serum thyroglobulin with negative whole body imaging do not warrant an aggressive diagnostic and therapeutic approach in differentiated thyroid cancer patients: a follow-up of 5 years or till recurrence. *Hellenic Journal of Nuclear Medicine*. 2015;18:207–214.

[6] Zanotti-Fregonara P, Keller I, Calzada-Nocaudie M, Al-Nahhas A, Devaux JY, Grass-etto G, Marzola MC, Rubello D and Hindie E. Increased serum thyroglobulin levels and negative imaging in thyroid cancer patients: are there sources of benign secretion? A speculative short review. *Nuclear Medicine Communications*. 2010;31:1054–1058.

[7] Ma C, Kuang A, Xie J and Ma T. Possible explanations for patients with discordant findings of serum thyroglobulin and 131I whole-body scanning. *Journal of Nuclear Medicine: Official Publication, Society of Nuclear Medicine*. 2005;46:1473–1480.

[8] Kloos RT. Approach to the patient with a positive serum thyroglobulin and a negative radioiodine scan after initial therapy for differentiated thyroid cancer. *The Journal of Clinical Endocrinology and Metabolism*. 2008;93:1519–1525.

[9] Haddad RI, Lydiatt WM, Ball DW, Busaidy NL, Byrd D, Callender G, Dickson P, Duh QY, Ehya H, Haymart M, Hoh C, Hunt JP, Iagaru A, Kandeel F, Kopp P, Lamonica DM, McCaffrey JC, Moley JF, Parks L, Raeburn CD, Ridge JA, Ringel MD, Scheri RP, Shah JP, Smallridge RC, Sturgeon C, Wang TN, Wirth LJ, Hoffmann KG and Hughes M. Anaplastic thyroid carcinoma, version 2.2015. *Journal of the National Comprehensive Cancer Network: JNCCN*. 2015;13:1140–1150.

[10] Pacini F, Lari R, Mazzeo S, Grasso L, Taddei D and Pinchera A. Diagnostic value of a single serum thyroglobulin determination on and off thyroid suppressive therapy in the follow-up of patients with differentiated thyroid cancer. *Clinical Endocrinology*. 1985;23:405–411.

[11] Haugen BR, Pacini F, Reiners C, Schlumberger M, Ladenson PW, Sherman SI, Cooper DS, Graham KE, Braverman LE, Skarulis MC, Davies TF, DeGroot LJ, Mazzaferri EL, Daniels GH, Ross DS, Luster M, Samuels MH, Becker DV, Maxon HR, 3rd, Cavalieri RR, Spencer CA, McEllin K, Weintraub BD and Ridgway EC. A comparison of re-combinant human thyrotropin and thyroid hormone withdrawal for the detection of thyroid remnant or cancer. *The Journal of Clinical Endocrinology and Metabolism*. 1999;84:3877–3885.

[12] Kloos RT and Mazzaferri EL. A single recombinant human thyrotropin-stimulated serum thyroglobulin measurement predicts differentiated thyroid carcinoma metasta-ses three to five years later. *The Journal of Clinical Endocrinology and Metabolism*. 2005;90:5047–5057.

[13] Castagna MG, Brilli L, Pilli T, Montanaro A, Cipri C, Fioravanti C, Sestini F, Capezzone M and Pacini F. Limited value of repeat recombinant human thyrotropin (rhTSH)-stimulated thyroglobulin testing in differentiated thyroid carcinoma patients with

previous negative rhTSH-stimulated thyroglobulin and undetectable basal serum thyroglobulin levels. *The Journal of Clinical Endocrinology and Metabolism*. 2008;93:76–81.

[14] Spencer CA, Takeuchi M and Kazarosyan M. Current status and performance goals for serum thyroglobulin assays. *Clinical Chemistry*. 1996;42:164–173.

[15] Spencer CA and Lopresti JS. Measuring thyroglobulin and thyroglobulin autoantibody in patients with differentiated thyroid cancer. *Nature Clinical Practice Endocrinology and Metabolism*. 2008;4:223–233.

[16] Phan HT, Jager PL, Paans AM, Plukker JT, Sturkenboom MG, Sluiter WJ, Wolffenbuttel BH, Dierckx RA and Links TP. The diagnostic value of 124I-PET in patients with differentiated thyroid cancer. *European Journal of Nuclear Medicine and Molecular Imaging*. 2008;35:958–965.

[17] Hufner M, Pfahl H, Bethauser H, Heilig B and Georgi P. Comparative plasma thyroglobulin measurements with three non-cross-reactive monoclonal antibodies in metastatic thyroid cancer patients. *Acta Endocrinologica*. 1988;118:528–532.

[18] Schulz R, Bethauser H, Stempka L, Heilig B, Moll A and Hufner M. Evidence for immunological differences between circulating and thyroid tissue-derived thyroglobulin in men. *European Journal of Clinical Investigation*. 1989;19:459–463.

[19] Giovanella L, Suriano S, Ceriani L and Verburg FA. Undetectable thyroglobulin in patients with differentiated thyroid carcinoma and residual radioiodine uptake on a postablation whole-body scan. *Clinical Nuclear Medicine*. 2011;36:109–112.

[20] Giovanella L, Keller F, Ceriani L and Tozzoli R. Heterophile antibodies may falsely increase or decrease thyroglobulin measurement in patients with differentiated thyroid carcinoma. *Clinical Chemistry and Laboratory Medicine*. 2009;47:952–954.

[21] Verburg FA, Waschle K, Reiners C, Giovanella L and Lentjes EG. Heterophile antibodies rarely influence the measurement of thyroglobulin and thyroglobulin antibodies in differentiated thyroid cancer patients. *Hormone and Metabolic Research = Hormon- und Stoffwechselforschung = Hormones et metabolisme*. 2010;42:736–739.

[22] Chiovato L, Latrofa F, Braverman LE, Pacini F, Capezzone M, Masserini L, Grasso L and Pinchera A. Disappearance of humoral thyroid autoimmunity after complete removal of thyroid antigens. *Annals of Internal Medicine*. 2003;139:346–351.

[23] Pacini F, Mariotti S, Formica N, Elisei R, Anelli S, Capotorti E and Pinchera A. Thyroid autoantibodies in thyroid cancer: incidence and relationship with tumour outcome. *Acta Endocrinologica*. 1988;119:373–380.

[24] Spencer CA, Takeuchi M, Kazarosyan M, Wang CC, Guttler RB, Singer PA, Fatemi S, LoPresti JS and Nicoloff JT. Serum thyroglobulin autoantibodies: prevalence, influence on serum thyroglobulin measurement, and prognostic significance in patients with differentiated thyroid carcinoma. *The Journal of Clinical Endocrinology and Metabolism*. 1998;83:1121–1127.

[25] Verburg FA, Luster M, Cupini C, Chiovato L, Duntas L, Elisei R, Feldt-Rasmussen U, Rimmele H, Seregni E, Smit JW, Theimer C and Giovanella L. Implications of thyroglobulin antibody positivity in patients with differentiated thyroid cancer: a clinical position statement. *Thyroid: Official Journal of the American Thyroid Association*. 2013;23:1211–1225.

[26] Chung JK, Park YJ, Kim TY, So Y, Kim SK, Park DJ, Lee DS, Lee MC and Cho BY. Clinical significance of elevated level of serum antithyroglobulin antibody in patients with differentiated thyroid cancer after thyroid ablation. *Clinical Endocrinology*. 2002;57:215–221.

[27] Aliyev A, Soundararajan S, Bucak E, Gupta M, Hatipoglu B, Nasr C, Siperstein A and Berber E. The utility of peripheral thyrotropin receptor mRNA in the management of differentiated thyroid cancer. *Surgery*. 2015;158:1089–1093; discussion 1093–1094.

[28] Zanotti-Fregonara P, Hindie E, Keller I, Calzada-Nocaudie M and Devaux JY. Scintigraphic visualization of glossal thyroid tissue during the follow-up of thyroid cancer patients. *Clinical Nuclear Medicine*. 2007;32:911–914.

[29] Mohamed Sayed MH, Saleh Farghaly HR and Fadl FA. Rate of thyroglossal duct remnant visualization after total thyroidectomy for differentiated thyroid carcinoma and its impact on clinical outcome of radioactive iodine (I-131) ablation. *Indian Journal of Nuclear Medicine: IJNM: The Official Journal of The Society of Nuclear Medicine, India*. 2015;30:116–121.

[30] Lee M, Lee YK, Jeon TJ, Chang HS, Kim BW, Lee YS, Park CS and Ryu YH. Frequent visualization of thyroglossal duct remnant on post-ablation 131I-SPECT/CT and its clinical implications. *Clinical Radiology*. 2015;70:638–643.

[31] Li D, Meng Z, Zhang G, Yu T, Tan J and Dong F. Visualization of thyroglossal duct cyst in differentiated thyroid cancer patient. *Clinical Nuclear Medicine*. 2010;35:499–504.

[32] Basaria S, Westra WH and Cooper DS. Ectopic lingual thyroid masquerading as thyroid cancer metastases. *The Journal of Clinical Endocrinology and Metabolism*. 2001;86:392–395.

[33] Abhyankar A and Basu S. Thymus uptake of 131I in patients with differentiated thyroid carcinoma: three different case scenarios and patterns of uptake and the importance of its recognition in thyroid cancer practice. *Journal of Cancer Research and Therapeutics*. 2015;11:648.

[34] Sauk JJ, Jr. Ectopic lingual thyroid. *The Journal of Pathology*. 1970;102:239–243.

[35] Arce MB, Molina TC, Hernandez TM, de la Cinta Calvo Moron M, Herrero CH, De La Riva Perez PA and Montano JC. Thymic uptake after high-dose I-131 treatment in patients with differentiated thyroid carcinoma: a brief review of possible causes and management. *Endocrinologia y nutricion: organo de la Sociedad Espanola de Endocrinologia y Nutricion*. 2015;62:19–23.

[36] Antonelli A, Ferri C, Ferrari SM, Sebastiani M, Colaci M, Ruffilli I and Fallahi P. New targeted molecular therapies for dedifferentiated thyroid cancer. *Journal of Oncology*. 2010;2010:921682.

[37] Fallahi P, Mazzi V, Vita R, Ferrari SM, Materazzi G, Galleri D, Benvenga S, Miccoli P and Antonelli A. New therapies for dedifferentiated papillary thyroid cancer. *International Journal of Molecular Sciences*. 2015;16:6153–6182.

[38] Ma C, Tang L, Fu H, Li J and Wang H. rhTSH-aided low-activity versus high-activity regimens of radioiodine in residual ablation for differentiated thyroid cancer: a meta-analysis. *Nuclear Medicine Communications*. 2013;34:1150–1156.

[39] Ma C, Xie J, Liu W, Wang G, Zuo S, Wang X and Wu F. Recombinant human thyrotropin (rhTSH) aided radioiodine treatment for residual or metastatic differentiated thyroid cancer. *The Cochrane Database of Systematic Reviews*. 2010:10:Cd008302.

[40] Schlumberger MJ. Papillary and follicular thyroid carcinoma. *The New England Journal of Medicine*. 1998;338:297–306.

[41] Shinto AS, Kamaleshwaran KK, Mallia M, Korde A, Samuel G, Banerjee S, Velayutham P, Damodharan S and Sairam M. Utility of (99m)Tc-Hynic-TOC in 131I whole-body scan negative thyroid cancer patients with elevated serum thyroglobulin levels. *World Journal of Nuclear Medicine*. 2015;14:101–108.

[42] Alzahrani AS, Alsuhaibani H, Salam SA, Al Sifri SN, Mohamed G, Al Sobhi S, Sulaiman O and Akhtar M. Diagnostic accuracy of high-resolution neck ultrasonography in the follow-up of differentiated thyroid cancer: a prospective study. *Endocrine Practice: Official Journal of the American College of Endocrinology and the American Association of Clinical Endocrinologists*. 2005;11:165–171.

[43] Torlontano M, Crocetti U, Augello G, D'Aloiso L, Bonfitto N, Varraso A, Dicembrino F, Modoni S, Frusciante V, Di Giorgio A, Bruno R, Filetti S and Trischitta V. Comparative evaluation of recombinant human thyrotropin-stimulated thyroglobulin levels, 131I whole-body scintigraphy, and neck ultrasonography in the follow-up of patients with papillary thyroid microcarcinoma who have not undergone radioiodine therapy. *The Journal of Clinical Endocrinology and Metabolism*. 2006;91:60–63.

[44] Pacini F, Castagna MG, Brilli L and Pentheroudakis G. Thyroid cancer: ESMO Clinical Practice Guidelines for diagnosis, treatment and follow-up. *Annals of Oncology: Official Journal of the European Society for Medical Oncology/ESMO*. 2012;23(Suppl 7):vii110–vii109.

[45] Cooper DS, Doherty GM, Haugen BR, Kloos RT, Lee SL, Mandel SJ, Mazzaferri EL, McIver B, Pacini F, Schlumberger M, Sherman SI, Steward DL and Tuttle RM. Revised American Thyroid Association management guidelines for patients with thyroid nodules and differentiated thyroid cancer. *Thyroid: Official Journal of the American Thyroid Association*. 2009;19:1167–1214.

[46] Galloway RJ and Smallridge RC. Imaging in thyroid cancer. *Endocrinology and Metabolism Clinics of North America*. 1996;25:93–113.

[47] Haugen BR, Alexander EK, Bible KC, Doherty GM, Mandel SJ, Nikiforov YE, Pacini F, Randolph GW, Sawka AM, Schlumberger M, Schuff KG, Sherman SI, Sosa JA, Steward DL, Tuttle RM and Wartofsky L. 2015 American Thyroid Association Management Guidelines for adult patients with thyroid nodules and differentiated thyroid cancer: The American Thyroid Association Guidelines Task Force on thyroid nodules and differentiated thyroid cancer. *Thyroid: Official Journal of the American Thyroid Association*. 2016;26:1–133.

[48] Ahn JE, Lee JH, Yi JS, Shong YK, Hong SJ, Lee DH, Choi CG and Kim SJ. Diagnostic accuracy of CT and ultrasonography for evaluating metastatic cervical lymph nodes in patients with thyroid cancer. *World Journal of Surgery*. 2008;32:1552–1558.

[49] Choi JS, Kim J, Kwak JY, Kim MJ, Chang HS and Kim EK. Preoperative staging of papillary thyroid carcinoma: comparison of ultrasonography imaging and CT. *AJR American Journal of Roentgenology*. 2009;193:871–878.

[50] Leboulleux S, Schroeder PR, Busaidy NL, Auperin A, Corone C, Jacene HA, Ewertz ME, Bournaud C, Wahl RL, Sherman SI, Ladenson PW and Schlumberger M. Assessment of the incremental value of recombinant thyrotropin stimulation before 2-[18F]-Fluoro-2-deoxy-D-glucose positron emission tomography/computed tomography imaging to localize residual differentiated thyroid cancer. *The Journal of Clinical Endocrinology and Metabolism*. 2009;94:1310–1316.

[51] Rosario PW, Mourao GF, dos Santos JB and Calsolari MR. Is empirical radioactive iodine therapy still a valid approach to patients with thyroid cancer and elevated thyroglobulin? *Thyroid: Official Journal of the American Thyroid Association*. 2014;24:533–536.

[52] Grunwald F, Kalicke T, Feine U, Lietzenmayer R, Scheidhauer K, Dietlein M, Schober O, Lerch H, Brandt-Mainz K, Burchert W, Hiltermann G, Cremerius U and Biersack HJ. Fluorine-18 fluorodeoxyglucose positron emission tomography in thyroid cancer: results of a multicentre study. *European Journal of Nuclear Medicine*. 1999;26:1547–1552.

[53] Altenvoerde G, Lerch H, Kuwert T, Matheja P, Schafers M and Schober O. Positron emission tomography with F-18-deoxyglucose in patients with differentiated thyroid carcinoma, elevated thyroglobulin levels, and negative iodine scans. *Langenbeck's Archives of Surgery/Deutsche Gesellschaft fur Chirurgie*. 1998;383:160–163.

[54] Caetano R, Bastos CR, de Oliveira IA, da Silva RM, Fortes CP, Pepe VL, Reis LG and Braga JU. Accuracy of positron emission tomography and positron emission tomography-CT in the detection of differentiated thyroid cancer recurrence with negative (131) I whole-body scan results: A meta-analysis. *Head and Neck*. 2016;38:316–327.

[55] Grewal RK, Ho A and Schoder H. Novel Approaches to Thyroid Cancer Treatment and Response Assessment. *Seminars in Nuclear Medicine*. 2016;46:109–118.

[56] Ranade R, Kand P and Basu S. Value of 18F-FDG PET negativity and Tg suppressibility as markers of prognosis in patients with elevated Tg and 131I-negative differentiated thyroid carcinoma (TENIS syndrome). *Nuclear Medicine Communications*. 2015;36:1014–1020.

[57] Kist JW, de Keizer B, van der Vlies M, Brouwers AH, van der Zant FM, Hermsen R, Huysmans D, Stokkel MP, Hoekstra OS and Vogel WV. 124I PET/CT to predict the outcome of blind 131I treatment in patients with biochemical recurrence of differentiated thyroid cancer; results of a multicenter diagnostic cohort study (THYROPET). *Journal of Nuclear Medicine: Official Publication, Society of Nuclear Medicine*. 2015.

[58] Phan HT, Jager PL, van der Wal JE, Sluiter WJ, Plukker JT, Dierckx RA, Wolffenbuttel BH and Links TP. The follow-up of patients with differentiated thyroid cancer and undetectable thyroglobulin (Tg) and Tg antibodies during ablation. *European Journal of Endocrinology/European Federation of Endocrine Societies*. 2008;158:77–83.

[59] Van Nostrand D, Khorjekar GR, O'Neil J, Moreau S, Atkins FB, Kharazi P, Mete M, Chennupati SP, Burman KD and Wartofsky L. Recombinant human thyroid-stimulating hormone versus thyroid hormone withdrawal in the identification of metastasis in differentiated thyroid cancer with 131I planar whole-body imaging and 124I PET. *Journal of Nuclear Medicine: Official Publication, Society of Nuclear Medicine*. 2012;53:359–362.

[60] Khorjekar GR, Van Nostrand D, Garcia C, O'Neil J, Moreau S, Atkins FB, Mete M, Orquiza MH, Burman K and Wartofsky L. Do negative 124I pretherapy positron emission tomography scans in patients with elevated serum thyroglobulin levels predict negative 131I posttherapy scans? *Thyroid: Official Journal of the American Thyroid Association*. 2014;24:1394–1399.

[61] Lee J, Nah KY, Kim RM, Oh YJ, An YS, Yoon JK, An GI, Choi TH, Cheon GJ, Soh EY and Chung WY. Effectiveness of [(124)I]-PET/CT and [(18)F]-FDG-PET/CT for localizing recurrence in patients with differentiated thyroid carcinoma. *Journal of Korean Medical Science*. 2012;27:1019–1026.

[62] Usmani S, Esmail A, Marafi F, Al Deen S, Abu Huda F and Al Kandari F. 111In-pentetreotide scintigraphy and 18F FDG PET-CT in differentiated thyroid carcinoma metastases with negative whole body radioiodine scan. *The Gulf Journal of Oncology*. 2015;1:7–13.

[63] Ambrosini V, Nanni C and Fanti S. The use of gallium-68 labeled somatostatin receptors in PET/CT imaging. *PET Clinics*. 2014;9:323–329.

[64] Taieb D, Garrigue P, Bardies M, Abdullah AE and Pacak K. Application and Dosimetric Requirements for Gallium-68-labeled Somatostatin Analogues in Targeted Radionuclide Therapy for Gastroenteropancreatic Neuroendocrine Tumors. *PET Clinics*. 2015;10:477–486.

[65] Lauri C, Di Traglia S, Galli F, Pizzichini P and Signore A. Current status of PET imaging of differentiated thyroid cancer with second generation radiopharmaceuticals. *The*

Quarterly Journal of Nuclear Medicine and Molecular Imaging: Official Publication of the Italian Association of Nuclear Medicine (AIMN) [and] the International Association of Radiopharmacology (IAR), [and] Section of the So. 2015;59:105–115.

[66] Giovanella L, Bongiovanni M and Trimboli P. Diagnostic value of thyroglobulin assay in cervical lymph node fine-needle aspirations for metastatic differentiated thyroid cancer. *Current Opinion in Oncology*. 2013;25:6–13.

[67] Torres MR, Nobrega Neto SH, Rosas RJ, Martins AL, Ramos AL and da Cruz TR. Thyroglobulin in the washout fluid of lymph-node biopsy: what is its role in the follow-up of differentiated thyroid carcinoma? *Thyroid: Official Journal of the American Thyroid Association*. 2014;24:7–18.

[68] Boi F, Baghino G, Atzeni F, Lai ML, Faa G and Mariotti S. The diagnostic value for differentiated thyroid carcinoma metastases of thyroglobulin (Tg) measurement in washout fluid from fine-needle aspiration biopsy of neck lymph nodes is maintained in the presence of circulating anti-Tg antibodies. *The Journal of Clinical Endocrinology and Metabolism*. 2006;91:1364–1369.

[69] Snozek CL, Chambers EP, Reading CC, Sebo TJ, Sistrunk JW, Singh RJ and Grebe SK. Serum thyroglobulin, high-resolution ultrasonography, and lymph node thyroglobulin in diagnosis of differentiated thyroid carcinoma nodal metastases. *The Journal of Clinical Endocrinology and Metabolism*. 2007;92:4278–4281.

[70] Grani G and Fumarola A. Thyroglobulin in lymph node fine-needle aspiration washout: a systematic review and meta-analysis of diagnostic accuracy. *The Journal of Clinical Endocrinology and Metabolism*. 2014;99:1970–1982.

[71] Van Nostrand D. Sialoadenitis secondary to (1)(3)(1)I therapy for well-differentiated thyroid cancer. *Oral Diseases*. 2011;17:154–161.

[72] Fard-Esfahani A, Emami-Ardekani A, Fallahi B, Fard-Esfahani P, Beiki D, Hassanzadeh-Rad A and Eftekhari M. Adverse effects of radioactive iodine-131 treatment for differentiated thyroid carcinoma. *Nuclear Medicine Communications*. 2014;35:808–817.

[73] Schroeder PR, Haugen BR, Pacini F, Reiners C, Schlumberger M, Sherman SI, Cooper DS, Schuff KG, Braverman LE, Skarulis MC, Davies TF, Mazzaferri EL, Daniels GH, Ross DS, Luster M, Samuels MH, Weintraub BD, Ridgway EC and Ladenson PW. A comparison of short-term changes in health-related quality of life in thyroid carcinoma patients undergoing diagnostic evaluation with recombinant human thyrotropin compared with thyroid hormone withdrawal. *The Journal of Clinical Endocrinology and Metabolism*. 2006;91:878–884.

[74] Luster M, Felbinger R, Dietlein M and Reiners C. Thyroid hormone withdrawal in patients with differentiated thyroid carcinoma: a one hundred thirty-patient pilot survey on consequences of hypothyroidism and a pharmacoeconomic comparison to recombinant thyrotropin administration. *Thyroid: Official Journal of the American Thyroid Association*. 2005;15:1147–1155.

[75] Ma C, Kuang A and Xie J. Radioiodine therapy for differentiated thyroid carcinoma with thyroglobulin positive and radioactive iodine negative metastases. *The Cochrane Database of Systematic Reviews*. 2009:Cd006988.

[76] Ma C, Xie J and Kuang A. Is empiric 131I therapy justified for patients with positive thyroglobulin and negative 131I whole-body scanning results? *Journal of Nuclear Medicine: Official Publication, Society of Nuclear Medicine*. 2005;46:1164–1170.

[77] Schlumberger M, Mancusi F, Baudin E and Pacini F. 131I therapy for elevated thyroglobulin levels. *Thyroid: Official Journal of the American Thyroid Association*. 1997;7:273–276.

[78] Schlumberger M, Tubiana M, De Vathaire F, Hill C, Gardet P, Travagli JP, Fragu P, Lumbroso J, Caillou B and Parmentier C. Long-term results of treatment of 283 patients with lung and bone metastases from differentiated thyroid carcinoma. *The Journal of Clinical Endocrinology and Metabolism*. 1986;63:960–967.

[79] Pineda JD, Lee T, Ain K, Reynolds JC and Robbins J. Iodine-131 therapy for thyroid cancer patients with elevated thyroglobulin and negative diagnostic scan. *The Journal of Clinical Endocrinology and Metabolism*. 1995;80:1488–1492.

[80] Coelho SM, Vaisman M and Carvalho DP. Tumour re-differentiation effect of retinoic acid: a novel therapeutic approach for advanced thyroid cancer. *Current Pharmaceutical Design*. 2005;11:2525–2531.

[81] Yamazaki CA, Padovani RP, Biscolla RP, Ikejiri ES, Marchetti RR, Castiglioni ML, Matsumura LK, Maciel RM and Furlanetto RP. Lithium as an adjuvant in the postoperative ablation of remnant tissue in low-risk thyroid carcinoma. *Thyroid: Official Journal of the American Thyroid Association*. 2012;22:1002–1006.

[82] Ho AL, Grewal RK, Leboeuf R, Sherman EJ, Pfister DG, Deandreis D, Pentlow KS, Zanzonico PB, Haque S, Gavane S, Ghossein RA, Ricarte-Filho JC, Dominguez JM, Shen R, Tuttle RM, Larson SM and Fagin JA. Selumetinib-enhanced radioiodine uptake in advanced thyroid cancer. *The New England Journal of Medicine*. 2013;368:623–632.

[83] Carvalho DP and Ferreira AC. The importance of sodium/iodide symporter (NIS) for thyroid cancer management. *Arquivos brasileiros de endocrinologia e metabologia*. 2007;51:672–682.

[84] Chung T, Youn H, Yeom CJ, Kang KW and Chung JK. Glycosylation of Sodium/Iodide Symporter (NIS) Regulates Its Membrane Translocation and Radioiodine Uptake. *PloS One*. 2015;10:e0142984.

[85] Li W, Tan J, Wang P and Wu P. Cotransfected sodium iodide symporter and human tyroperoxidase genes following human telomerase reverse transcriptase promoter for targeted radioiodine therapy of malignant glioma cells. *Cancer Biotherapy and Radiopharmaceuticals*. 2011;26:443–451.

[86] Dohan O, De la Vieja A, Paroder V, Riedel C, Artani M, Reed M, Ginter CS and Carrasco N. The sodium/iodide Symporter (NIS): characterization, regulation, and medical significance. *Endocrine Reviews*. 2003;24:48–77.

[87] Cheng W, Fu H, Feng F, Ma C, Li J, Chen S and Wang H. Efficacy of lentiviral-mediated transfection of hTSHR in poorly differentiated thyroid carcinoma cell line. *Nuclear Medicine and Biology*. 2013;40:576–580.

[88] Feng F, Wang H, Hou S and Fu H. Re-induction of cell differentiation and (131)I uptake in dedifferentiated FTC-133 cell line by TSHR gene transfection. *Nuclear Medicine and Biology*. 2012;39:1261–1265.

[89] Durante C, Puxeddu E, Ferretti E, Morisi R, Moretti S, Bruno R, Barbi F, Avenia N, Scipioni A, Verrienti A, Tosi E, Cavaliere A, Gulino A, Filetti S and Russo D. BRAF mutations in papillary thyroid carcinomas inhibit genes involved in iodine metabolism. *The Journal of Clinical Endocrinology and Metabolism*. 2007;92:2840–2843.

[90] Liu D, Hu S, Hou P, Jiang D, Condouris S and Xing M. Suppression of BRAF/MEK/MAP kinase pathway restores expression of iodide-metabolizing genes in thyroid cells expressing the V600E BRAF mutant. *Clinical Cancer Research: An Official Journal of the American Association for Cancer Research*. 2007;13:1341–1349.

[91] Ye X, Zhu Y and Cai J. Relationship between toxicities and clinical benefits of newly approved tyrosine kinase inhibitors in thyroid cancer: A meta-analysis of literature. *Journal of Cancer Research and Therapeutics*. 2015;11 Suppl 2:C185–C190.

[92] Scott LJ. Lacosamide: A Review in Focal Seizures in Patients with Epilepsy. *Drugs*. 2015;75:2143–2154.

[93] Gruber JJ and Colevas AD. Differentiated thyroid cancer: focus on emerging treatments for radioactive iodine-refractory patients. *The Oncologist*. 2015;20:113–126.

[94] Shen CT, Qiu ZL and Luo QY. Sorafenib in the treatment of radioiodine-refractory differentiated thyroid cancer: a meta-analysis. *Endocrine-Related Cancer*. 2014;21:253–261.

[95] Cooper DS, Doherty GM, Haugen BR, Kloos RT, Lee SL, Mandel SJ, Mazzaferri EL, McIver B, Sherman SI and Tuttle RM. Management guidelines for patients with thyroid nodules and differentiated thyroid cancer. *Thyroid: Official Journal of the American Thyroid Association*. 2006;16:109–142.

[96] McGriff NJ, Csako G, Gourgiotis L, Lori CG, Pucino F and Sarlis NJ. Effects of thyroid hormone suppression therapy on adverse clinical outcomes in thyroid cancer. *Annals of Medicine*. 2002;34:554–564.

[97] Durante C, Haddy N, Baudin E, Leboulleux S, Hartl D, Travagli JP, Caillou B, Ricard M, Lumbroso JD, De Vathaire F and Schlumberger M. Long-term outcome of 444 patients with distant metastases from papillary and follicular thyroid carcinoma:

benefits and limits of radioiodine therapy. *The Journal of Clinical Endocrinology and Metabolism*. 2006;91:2892–2899.

[98] Linskey ME, Andrews DW, Asher AL, Burri SH, Kondziolka D, Robinson PD, Ammirati M, Cobbs CS, Gaspar LE, Loeffler JS, McDermott M, Mehta MP, Mikkelsen T, Olson JJ, Paleologos NA, Patchell RA, Ryken TC and Kalkanis SN. The role of stereotactic radiosurgery in the management of patients with newly diagnosed brain metastases: a systematic review and evidence-based clinical practice guideline. *Journal of Neuro-oncology*. 2010;96:45–68.

[99] Kalkanis SN, Kondziolka D, Gaspar LE, Burri SH, Asher AL, Cobbs CS, Ammirati M, Robinson PD, Andrews DW, Loeffler JS, McDermott M, Mehta MP, Mikkelsen T, Olson JJ, Paleologos NA, Patchell RA, Ryken TC and Linskey ME. The role of surgical resection in the management of newly diagnosed brain metastases: a systematic review and evidence-based clinical practice guideline. *Journal of Neuro-oncology*. 2010;96:33–43.

[100] Droz JP, Schlumberger M, Rougier P, Ghosn M, Gardet P and Parmentier C. Chemotherapy in metastatic nonanaplastic thyroid cancer: experience at the Institut Gustave-Roussy. *Tumori*. 1990;76:480–483.

[101] Ahuja S and Ernst H. Chemotherapy of thyroid carcinoma. *Journal of Endocrinological Investigation*. 1987;10:303–310.

[102] Mazzaferri EL. Management of a solitary thyroid nodule. *The New England Journal of Medicine*. 1993;328:553–559.

[103] Sherman SI. Cytotoxic chemotherapy for differentiated thyroid carcinoma. *Clinical Oncology (Royal College of Radiologists (Great Britain))*. 2010;22:464–468.

[104] Hay ID, Lee RA, Davidge-Pitts C, Reading CC and Charboneau JW. Long-term outcome of ultrasonography-guided percutaneous ethanol ablation of selected "recurrent" neck nodal metastases in 25 patients with TNM stages III or IVA papillary thyroid carcinoma previously treated by surgery and 131I therapy. *Surgery*. 2013;154:1448–1454; discussion 1454–1455.

[105] Guenette JP, Monchik JM and Dupuy DE. Image-guided ablation of postsurgical locoregional recurrence of biopsy-proven well-differentiated thyroid carcinoma. *Journal of Vascular and Interventional Radiology: JVIR*. 2013;24:672–679.

[106] Heilo A, Sigstad E, Fagerlid KH, Haskjold OI, Groholt KK, Berner A, Bjoro T and Jorgensen LH. Efficacy of ultrasonography-guided percutaneous ethanol injection treatment in patients with a limited number of metastatic cervical lymph nodes from papillary thyroid carcinoma. *The Journal of Clinical Endocrinology and Metabolism*. 2011;96:2750–2755.

[107] Park KW, Shin JH, Han BK, Ko EY and Chung JH. Inoperable symptomatic recurrent thyroid cancers: preliminary result of radiofrequency ablation. *Annals of Surgical Oncology*. 2011;18:2564–2568.

[108] Baek JH, Kim YS, Sung JY, Choi H and Lee JH. Locoregional control of metastatic well-differentiated thyroid cancer by ultrasonography-guided radiofrequency ablation. *AJR American Journal of Roentgenology*. 2011;197:W331–W336.

[109] Monchik JM, Donatini G, Iannuccilli J and Dupuy DE. Radiofrequency ablation and percutaneous ethanol injection treatment for recurrent local and distant well-differentiated thyroid carcinoma. *Annals of Surgery*. 2006;244:296–304.

[110] Papini E, Bizzarri G, Bianchini A, Valle D, Misischi I, Guglielmi R, Salvatori M, Solbiati L, Crescenzi A, Pacella CM and Gharib H. Percutaneous ultrasonography-guided laser ablation is effective for treating selected nodal metastases in papillary thyroid cancer. *The Journal of Clinical Endocrinology and Metabolism*. 2013;98:E92–E97.

Chapter 9

Emerging Therapeutic Approaches for the Most Aggressive Epithelial Thyroid Cancers

Alessandro Antonelli, Enke Baldini,
Salvatore Sorrenti, Poupak Fallahi, Paolo Miccoli,
Angelo Filippini and Salvatore Ulisse

Additional information is available at the end of the chapter

http://dx.doi.org/10.5772/64086

Abstract

The majority of epithelial thyroid carcinomas (TC) have a differentiated (DTC) histotype and include the papillary (PTC) and the follicular (FTC) TC which, ensuing dedifferentiation, generate the aggressive poorly differentiated (PDTC) and anaplastic (ATC) TC. Although derived from the same cell type, each TC shows specific histological features, biological behavior, and degree of differentiation because of different genetic alterations. Total thyroidectomy, followed by adjuvant therapy with ^{131}I, is the treatment of choice for most patients affected by DTC. The prognosis of DTC patients is favorable, with 10-year survival rate of nearly 90%. However, one third of them face the morbidity of disease recurrence and TC-related deaths. The worst outcomes are encountered in patients with PDTC and ATC. The latter, in particular, has a mean survival time of few months from the diagnosis, which is not influenced by current anticancer treatments. Following the progress made in the comprehension of the underlying molecular mechanisms deregulated in TC progression, novel therapeutic approaches have come to light. Here, we will attempt to review new targeted therapies, which are currently being exploited in preclinical and clinical studies, with tyrosine kinase inhibitors as well as with emerging inhibitors of mitotic kinases, in PDTC and ATC.

Keywords: thyroid carcinoma, therapy, tyrosine kinase inhibitors, mitotic kinases, aurora kinase inhibitors

1. Introduction

Thyroid cancer (TC) incidence has increased from about 5 new cases per 100,000 persons observed in the early 1990s to 15 new cases per 100,000 persons recorded in 2012 [1]. The reason of such increase resides essentially in the improved diagnostic ability to detect malignancy in small non-palpable thyroid nodules [2, 3]. Data from the Surveillance, Epidemiology, and End Results (SEER) program Cancer Statistics Review indicate that 62,450 new cases of TC are expected to be diagnosed in the US population in 2015 [1]. In addition, 1950 deaths related to TC are estimated to occur [1].

TC represents about 96% of all endocrine malignancies and one of the most frequent cancers in women [1]. Based on histological criteria and clinical behavior, TC are classified as well-differentiated TC (DTC), comprising the papillary (PTC) and follicular (FTC) TC and poorly differentiated TC (PDTC) and undifferentiated or anaplastic (ATC) TC. The PTC accounts for about 86% of all epithelial TC and has a propensity to spread via lymphatic vessels to local lymph nodes [4]. The FTC accounts for approximately 9% of all TC and is characterized by hematogenous spread producing lung and bone metastases [4]. The less differentiated and more aggressive PDTC and ATC, each of which accounts for 1–2% of all TC, develop from the dedifferentiation of DTC, according to the multistep model of thyroid carcinogenesis [4–6]. The latter is supported by the common observation of coexistence of DTC with PDTC or ATC bearing similar genetic alterations [7, 8]. The PDTC, included as a separate entity in the WHO classification of TC in 2004, is defined as a thyroglobulin-producing, non-follicular and non-papillary TC, having an intermediate clinical behavior between DTC and ATC and showing high-grade features such as widely infiltrative growth, necrosis, vascular invasion, and numerous mitotic figures [6, 9]. PDTC may show three different pathological subtypes including the solid, trabecular, and insular architectures [4]. The ATC appears as disseminated fleshy masses with areas of necrosis and hemorrhage. It is composed of undifferentiated cells negative for thyroglobulin and originating three morphological patterns: squamoid cells, pleomorphic giant cells, and spindle cells [4].

Total thyroidectomy followed by adjuvant therapy with ^{131}I is the treatment of choice for most patients affected by DTC [10]. Although the prognosis of these patients is favorable, with 10-year survival rate around 90%, nearly one third of them face the morbidity of disease recurrence and TC-related deaths [10]. The worst outcomes are usually observed in patients with PDTC and ATC, in which the reduced expression of the thyroid specific gene natrium/iodide symporter (NIS) renders ^{131}I treatment less effective [11–13]. In particular, patients affected by ATC have a dismal prognosis with a mean survival time of few months from the diagnosis [12]. These patients present with a rapidly growing thyroid mass and locoregional symptoms, which may include dyspnea, dysphagia, neck pain, hoarseness, and stroke [14]. Outcome of ATC patients is not, or only minimally, influenced by current anticancer treatments, including palliative surgery, when possible, chemotherapy (doxorubicin), and radiotherapy [12, 14]. In the majority of patients, death occurs following tumor airway obstruction [14]. Therefore, the identification of new therapeutic approaches capable of ameliorating the prognosis of PDTC and ATC patients is sorely needed.

2. Molecular alterations underlying thyroid cancer progression

Established risk factors for TC include radiation exposure, family history of TC, lymphocytic thyroiditis, reduced iodine intake, and female gender [15]. These risk factors are thought to induce genetic instability in thyrocytes through still poorly defined direct and indirect mechanisms [15]. Genomic instability, a hallmark of solid tumors including TC, is thought to represent the driving force responsible for acquisition by malignant cells of novel functional capabilities, including self-sufficiency in growth signals, insensitivity to anti-growth signals, evasion of apoptosis, limitless replicative potential, sustained angiogenesis, and tissue invasion and metastasis [16–18]. In fact, the number and the frequency of chromosomal abnormalities observed during TC progression have been shown to increase from DTC to PDTC and ATC [18]. Genomic instability is also sustained by alterations in cell-cycle regulators, frequently encountered in TC [15]. In particular, a deregulated control of the G1/S transition, due either to an increased expression of promoting factors (cyclin D1 and E2F) or to the downregulation or presence of loss-of-function mutations of factors inhibiting the G1/S transition (retinoblastoma, p16INK4A, p21CIP1, p27KIP1, and p53), has been demonstrated in TC [15]. In addition, the aberrant expression of mitotic kinases, such as the polo-like kinase and the three members of the Aurora kinase family (Aurora-A, Aurora-B, and Aurora-C), regulating the G2/M phase transition and several mitotic processes (i.e., centrosome maturation, spindle formation, chromosome segregation, and cytokinesis), is held co-responsible for abnormal cell divisions and the establishment of aneuploid TC cells [19, 20].

The PTC are characterized by mutually exclusive activating somatic mutations of genes encoding proteins involved the MAPK (mitogen-activated protein kinase) signaling pathway [4, 21]. These include rearrangements of the RET (rearranged during transformation) (RET/PTC) and NTRK1 (neurotrophic tyrosine kinase receptor 1) genes and activating point mutations of the three RAS oncogenes (HRAS, KRAS, and NRAS) and BRAF [21]. All together these genetic alterations are held responsible for about 80% of all PTC. In addition, mutations of genes encoding key players of the phosphoinositide 3-kinase (PI3K) pathway, such as PTEN, PIK3CA, and AKT1, have been reported in PTC at lower frequencies [21].

Genetic alterations encountered in FTC include activating point mutations of RAS, present in about 45% of FTC; rearrangement of the paired-box gene 8 (PAX-8) with the peroxisome proliferator-activator receptor-γ (PAX8-PPARγ), observed in 35% of FTC; loss-of-function mutations of the tumor suppressor PTEN gene, encountered in about 10% of FTC; and activating mutations or amplification of the PI3KCA gene, encoding the catalytic subunit of the PI3K, present in about 10% of FTC [22, 23].

In agreement with the multistep model of thyroid carcinogenesis, some of the early genetic events characterizing DTC are also found in PDTC and ATC. In particular, RAS and BRAF gene mutations are found in approximately 35% and 15% of PDTC, respectively [4]. On the contrary, other early genetic alterations such as the rearrangements RET/PTCs and PAX8-PPARγ are very rarely found in PDTC and ATC suggesting that these oncogenes prevent tumor dedifferentiation. Progression of DTC to PDTC and ATC implies, however, tumor acquisition of novel genetic alterations, which are absent or present with low frequency in DTC tissues. Among these are mutations of the tumor suppressor gene p53, thought to be a gatekeeper of TC progression from the indolent DTC to the aggressive PDTC and lethal ATC [24]. In fact, p53 mutations are rarely encountered in DTC (5–9% of cases), while they increase in the PDTC (17–38% of cases) and ATC (67–88% of cases) [15, 25, 26]. A similar trend regards the CTNNB1 gene, encoding the β-catenin, involved in cell adhesion and in the wingless (Wnt) signaling pathway [15]. In particular, CTNNB1 gene mutations are not found in DTC, while they are present in PDTC (25% of cases) and ATC (66% of cases) [27, 28]. Last but not least, the conversion of early-stage TC to more aggressive and invasive malignancies occurs through an epithelial-to-mesenchymal transition (EMT), which implies the loss of cell-cell contacts, remodeling of cytoskeleton, and the acquisition of a migratory phenotype [29, 30]. Reduced expression of E-cadherin and abnormal expression of integrins, Notch, MET, TGFβ, NF-kB, PI3K, TWIST1, matrix metalloproteinases, components of the urokinase plasminogen-activating system, and p21-activated kinase, all of them involved in the EMT, have been identified in TC progression [29–34].

3. Small-molecule inhibitors of protein kinases: a new hope for the treatment of the most aggressive thyroid cancers

As above mentioned, the identification of new therapeutic approaches able to improve the prognosis of PDTC and ATC patients is urgently required. Over the last decade, the advancements made in the comprehension of the molecular mechanisms underlying TC progression gave the opportunity to develop novel therapeutic approaches, based on small molecule inhibitors of tyrosine kinases and mitotic kinases, showing promising results in preclinical and clinical studies (**Table 1**) [19, 35, 36]. In the following paragraphs, the results of these studies will be reviewed.

Kinase inhibitors			
Drug	**Molecular target(s)**	**Status**	**References**
CLM3 and CLM29	RET, EGFR, and VEGFR	Preclinical	[43–47]
Sorafenib (Nexavar)	VEGFR-2, VEGFR-3, c-KIT, PDGFR, RET/PTC, Raf	Phase III	[48–52]
Vandetanib (ZD6474)	VEGFR-2, VEGFR-3, EGFR, and RET	Phase II	[53, 54]
Motesanib (AMG 706)	VEGFR, PDGFR, and c-KIT	Phase II	[55, 56]
Axitinib (AG-013736)	VEGFR, PDGFR-beta	Phase II	[57–61]
Sunitinib (SU011248)	VEGFR, PDGFR, and RET/PTC	Phase II	[62–68]
Cabozantinib (XL184)	VEGFR, C-MET, RET, c-KIT, FLT3, AXL, TRKB, and Tie-2	Phase I	[69–71]
Pazopanib (GW786034)	VEGFR, PDGFR, c-KIT, and Aurora-A kinase	Phase II	[72, 73, 108, 109]
Lenvatinib (E7080)	VEGFR, FGFRs PDGFRa, RET, and c-KIT	Phase II	[74–76]

http://dx.doi.org/10.5772/64086

Kinase inhibitors			
Drug	**Molecular target(s)**	**Status**	**References**
Vemurafenib (PLX4032)	BRAF	Phase II	[80]
CEP-32496	BRAF	Preclinical	[81]
Everolimus (RAD001)	mTORC1	Phase I	[82, 87]
MK-0457 (VX-680)	Aurora kinases	Preclinical	[101]
SNS-314	Aurora kinases	Preclinical	[102]
ZM447439	Aurora kinases	Preclinical	[103]
AZD1152	Aurora-B	Preclinical	[97, 104, 106]
MLN8054	Aurora-A	Preclinical	[105, 107]
MLN8237	Aurora-A	Preclinical	[106, 108]
BI 2536	Polo-like kinase 1	Preclinical	[110–112]
GSK461364A	Polo-like kinase 1	Preclinical	[113]

Table 1. New potential drugs for the treatment of aggressive epithelial thyroid cancer being exploited in preclinical and clinical studies.

3.1. Tyrosine kinase inhibitors

An increased knowledge of the molecular mechanisms involved in cancer has allowed the development of therapeutic agents that target specific pathways involved in the tumor growth

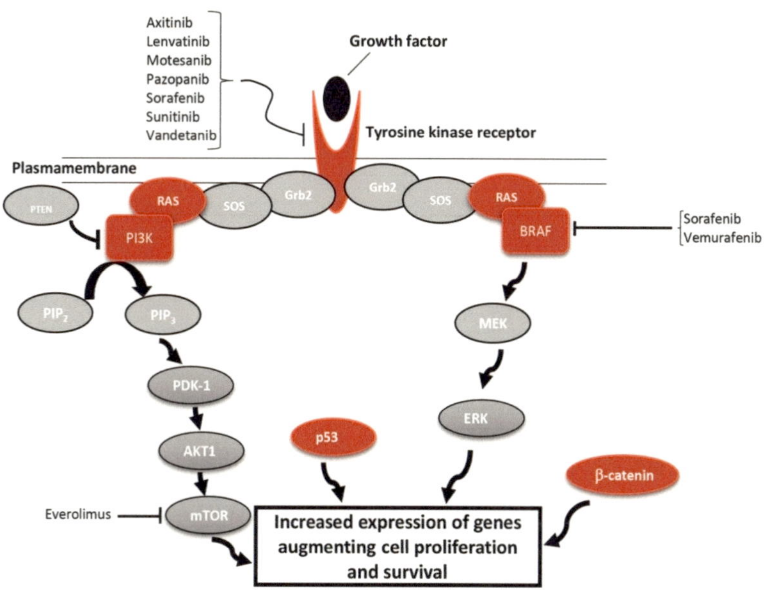

Figure 1. Molecular alterations (in red) involved in thyroid cancer progression and new targeted therapies being exploited in preclinical and clinical studies.

and progression, including RET, BRAF, RAS, epidermal growth factor receptor (EGFR), vascular endothelial growth factor (VEGF) receptor (VEGFR), etc. [37] (**Figure 1** and **Table 1**). Among these, tyrosine kinase inhibitors (TKI) have come out as a new class of anticancer drugs [38]. TKI are small compounds that compete with the ATP-binding sites of the TK catalytic domains, affecting TK-dependent oncogenic pathways [39]. TKI act through the occupation of these sites inhibiting autophosphorylation and activation of TKs and preventing the activation of intracellular signaling cascades. These compounds can be specific to one or several homologous TKs [40]. However, a resistance to TKI treatment could occur when the inhibition of one kinase receptor is compensated by the activation of other TK pathways [41]. This suggests that the best way to approach cancer may be the simultaneous inhibition of multiple activated TKs [42].

3.1.1. RET pathway

The pyrazolo[3, 4-d]pyrimidine (PP) heterocyclic core is one of the most explored chemical templates, with a large spectrum of activity and active against RET. CLM3 and CLM29, pyrazolo[3, 4-d]pyrimidine derivatives with antiangiogenic activity, targeting RET, EGFR, and VEGFR, are capable of impairing the migration of dedifferentiated PTC (DePTC) cells [43–45]. Moreover, CLM3 and CLM29 exert antineoplastic activity in primary ATC cells [43, 46, 47].

3.1.2. Raf kinase pathway

Sorafenib is a bi-aryl urea multi-targeted TKI, with inhibitory activity against VEGFR-2 and 3, c-KIT, PDGFR, RET/PTC, Raf kinases, and the Raf/Mek/Erk pathway, able to induce apoptosis through downregulation of Mcl-1 [48, 49]. Sorafenib has been approved for the treatment of primary kidney cancer and advanced primary liver cancer. After several phase II trials, it has been conducted a multicenter double-blind randomized phase III study (DECISION trial), evaluating sorafenib versus placebo in advanced/metastatic radioactive iodine (RAI)-refractory DTC [50–52]. Patients in treatment with sorafenib showed a median progression-free survival (PFS) significantly longer (10.8 months) compared to those treated with placebo (5.8 months).

3.1.3. VEGF pathway

Vandetanib (ZD6474) is an orally active TKI with a good inhibitory activity on VEGFR-2 and also targeting VEGFR-3, EGFR, and RET kinases [53]. One hundred and forty-five patients with locally advanced/metastatic DTC, 72 of whom receiving vandetanib (300 mg/daily) and 73 placebo, were involved in a double-blind phase II study. Improved PFS were recorded in TKI-treated patients (11.1 months), compared to ones who received placebo (5.9 months), and partial response (PR) and stable disease (SD) were 8% and 57% in the former against 5% and 42% in the second group [54].

Motesanib diphosphate (AMG 706) is an ATP-competitive inhibitor of VEGFR-1, VEGFR-2, VEGFR-3, PDGFR, and KIT. It was studied in several phase I and one phase II trials, where it was given orally 125 mg/day in patients with metastatic TC [55, 56]. The phase II trial was conducted in 184 patients (93 DTC and 91 MTC) for 48 weeks. Among the DTC patients 57 were PTC (61%): PR was obtained in 14% of cases; SD was obtained in 35% for 24 weeks (or longer); serum thyroglobulin diminished with respect to the baseline in 81%; 7 patients (8%) had tumor progression, and median PFS was 40 weeks [56].

Axitinib (AG-013736) is an indazole derivative inhibitor of tyrosine kinase receptors with picomolar potency against VEGFR-1, VEGFR-2, and VEGFR-3 and nanomolar potency against PDGFR-beta [57–59]. In a phase II trial sixty patients with advanced TC (30 PTC, 15 FTC, and 11 MTC) were treated with axitinib (5 mg twice daily): 38% of patients obtained SD for at least 16 weeks, while 30% achieved PR [60]. Median PFS was 72.4 weeks (18.1 months). Fifty-two patients with metastatic or locally advanced MTC or DTC were involved in another phase II trial with axitinib (5 mg twice daily) [61]. The objective response rate (ORR) was 35% (18 PR), and SD was shown in 18 patients for more than 16 weeks. Median PFS was 16 months, and median overall survival was 27 months [61].

Sunitinib (SU011248), a multitarget TKI, inhibits selectively VEGFR-1, VEGFR-2, and VEGFR-3, PDGFR, c-KIT, and RET/PTC subtypes 1 and 3 [62]. It has been approved to treat gastrointestinal stromal tumor and clear-cell renal carcinoma, and it is now investigated in other human cancer types [63]. This TKI strongly inhibits the growth of the PTC-derived TPC1 cell line, bearing RET/PTC rearrangements [64]. However, indications emerged that clinical application of sunitinib should be directed by genotyping, since it inhibits RET/PTC- but not BRAF-mutated cells, as highlighted by another preclinical study in which the different inhibitory mechanisms of this drug against BRAF mutations or RET/PTC rearrangements were evaluated in cell lines or orthotopic TC mouse model [65]. In the largest open-label phase II trial performed to date, 28 patients with aggressive DTC and 7 with MTC were administered with sunitinib (37.5 mg) on continuous basis, showing a complete response (CR) in 3%, PR in 28%, and SD in 46% of cases [66]. Recently, several studies reported the efficacy of the therapy with sunitinib in progressive metastatic DTC patients [67]. Twenty-three patients were enrolled in a single center, nonrandomized, open-label, phase II clinical trial and treated with a starting daily, oral dose of 37.5 mg sunitinib. Six (26%) patients achieved a PR, and 13 (57%) had SD for a clinical benefit rate (PR + SD) of 83%. The overall median PFS was 241 days [68].

The oral multiple receptor kinase inhibitor cabozantinib (XL184) inhibits VEGFR-1, VEGFR-2, VEGFR-3, C-MET, RET, c-KIT, TRKB, AXL, FLT3, and Tie-2 [69, 70]. One phase I trial was recently carried out in a cohort of 15 patients with metastatic DTC who had failed standard radioactive iodine therapy [71]. Patients received cabozantinib with 140 mg free base (the same as 175 mg salt form) daily: PR was shown in 8/15 (53%), while SD in 6/15 (40%) [71].

Another VEGFR-1, VEGFR-2, VEGFR-3, PDGFR, and c-KIT inhibitor is pazopanib (GW786034), approved for the treatment of renal cell carcinoma [72]. In a phase II trial, 37 patients with metastatic, rapidly progressive, and radioiodine-refractory DTC received pazopanib: a PR was achieved in 18 patients (49%) with 800 mg/day orally, but no CR were observed [73]. However, disease progression (PD) or clinical deterioration was ultimately observed in 27 of the 37 patients [73].

Lenvatinib (E7080) is an oral, multitarget TKI of the VEGFR-1, VEGFR-2, and VEGFR-3, FGFRs 1 to 4, PDGFR α, RET, and KIT [74]. After a phase II study, a randomized, double-blind, multicenter phase III study was carried out on lenvatinib (SELECT) in patients with progressive RAI-refractory TC, who randomly received the drug (261 patients, at a daily dose of 24 mg per day in 28-day cycles) or placebo (131 patients) [75, 76]. Median PFS was 18.3 months in the lenvatinib group and 3.6 months in the placebo one ($P < 0.001$). In the lenvatinib group, there were 4 CR and 165 PR, with a response rate of 64.8% *versus* 1.5% in the placebo group ($P < 0.001$).

3.1.4. BRAF inhibitors

BRAF is a serine-threonine kinase that mediates the signal transduction of the MAP/extracellular signal-regulated kinase (ERK) kinase (MEK)-ERK pathway, and it is a critical regulator of normal growth, differentiation, and oncogenic transformation (**Figure 1**). BRAF mutations are associated with lymph node metastases, extrathyroidal extension, tumor size, and multifocality in PTC [77, 78]. In addition, activation of BRAF significantly reduces NIS expression through the induction of robust TGFβ secretion. TGFβ, acting via Smad, was described as a potent repressor of NIS transcription through the functional antagonism of Smads and Pax8, a transcription factor essential for thyroid differentiation [79]. Although this mechanism is MEK-ERK independent, secreted TGFβ cooperates with MEK-ERK signaling in BRAF-induced cell migration, invasion of extracellular matrix, and EMT.

Vemurafenib (PLX4032), an oral analog of PLX 4720, inhibits BRAF and it is already approved for treatment of advanced melanoma. Safety and efficacy of vemurafenib in advanced PTC are currently under study in a phase II trial [80].

Another BRAF inhibitor having multi-kinase binding activity, CEP-32496, showed in vitro selective cellular cytotoxicity for BRAF(V600E) versus wild-type cells. Sustained tumor stasis and regressions were observed with oral administration (30–100 mg/kg twice daily) against $BRAF^{V600E}$ melanoma and colon carcinoma xenografts, with no adverse effect. Thus, it is expected to be effective in the treatment of BRAF-dependent malignancies, among which TC [81].

3.1.5. Mammalian target of rapamycin (mTOR) inhibitors

The mTOR is a serine/threonine kinase that nucleates at least two distinct multi-protein complexes, mTOR complex 1 (mTORC1) and mTOR complex 2 (mTORC2), and acts through the phosphorylation of a number of proteins regulating protein synthesis, metabolism, and cell growth and survival [82, 83]. The mTOR is a major downstream effector of the PI3K/Akt pathway, involved in thyroid carcinogenesis. Activated mTOR is known to control protein synthesis through phosphorylation of the eukaryotic initiation factor 4E (eIF4E) binding protein 1 (4E-BP1) and release of active eIF4E, a key regulator of translation of gene products that participate in regulation of the cell cycle. In aggressive types of PTC and MTC cells, it was seen a strong activation of the mTOR signaling and overexpression of the initial factor eIF4E, whose levels were correlated with tumor aggressiveness [84].

Everolimus (RAD001) is an orally active rapalog (rapamycin analog) that inhibits mTORC1 upon binding FKBP12, a member of the FKBP family of immunophilins [85, 86]. The RAD001-FKBP12 complex interacts with the FKBP12 binding domain of mTOR and blocks the assembly of a functional TORC-1. Everolimus has been approved by FDA for the treatment of patients with advanced renal carcinoma and tested in vivo on MTC [87]. Fury et al. administered everolimus plus cisplatin in 30 patients with advanced solid tumors in a recent phase I study, seven of which had TC (5 DTC, 2 MTC). One patient with PTC completed 14 cycles and achieved SD [82].

3.2. Mitotic kinase inhibitors

The recognition that cell-cycle deregulation represents a hallmark of human cancers has led to the generation of several mitosis-based anticancer therapies [88]. Spindle microtubule-targeting agents (MTA) remain to date the most widely used and reliable antimitotic drugs for the treatment of several human cancers [89, 90]. MTA include microtubule-destabilizing agents, like vinca alkaloids, that inhibit microtubule polymerization and microtubule-stabilizing agents, like taxanes, that stimulate microtubule polymerization [89, 90]. A major limitation in the use of MTAs derives from the side effects observed on the microtubules of quiescent interphasic cells (i.e., neurotoxicity), by disrupting physiological processes such as vesicular trafficking, axonal transport, and cytoskeleton functions. Myeloid toxicity, resulting from the mitotic arrest of bone marrow cells, also occurs. This, along with the tumor cell resistance to MTAs, which appears in ATC, has prompted further research for the identification of new antimitotic drugs nontargeting the spindle microtubules [91].

The three members of the Aurora kinase family, Aurora-A, Aurora-B, and Aurora-C, and the polo-like kinase 1 (PLK1) are serine/threonine kinases playing a major role in the G2/M phase transition and in the regulation of several mitotic processes [19, 92]. Consistent with their role, the expression and activity of the Aurora kinases and PLK1 are low in the G0, G1, and S phases, rise in the late G2, and peak during the M phase [19, 93]. Aurora-A and PLK1 cooperate in the activation of the CDK1/cyclin B complex allowing the transition of the cell from the G2 to the M phase [19]. In addition, both Aurora-A and PLK1 are essential for centrosome maturation and bipolar spindle formation [19, 93]. Aurora-B, along with INCENP, Survivin, and Borealin, is a component of the chromosomal passenger complex (CPC), which localizes on the chromosome arms in prophase, concentrates in the inner centromere region from prometaphase to metaphase, then moves to the central spindle and cortex in anaphase, and remains in the midbody in telophase [19]. The CPC ensures accurate chromosome segregation by regulating chromosome structure, cohesin removal from the chromosomal arms, spindle formation, kinetochore assembly, correction of non-bipolar chromosome-microtubule connections, spindle assembly checkpoint, and cytokinesis [19]. Aurora-C, similarly to Aurora-B, takes part in the CPC, but it is mainly expressed in germ cells during spermatogenesis and oogenesis and in some cancer cell lines [94, 95]. Also PLK1 has been demonstrated to be involved in sister chromatid cohesion and formation of kinetochore-microtubule attachments, mitotic exit, and cytokinesis [93]. Therefore, in view of their important mitotic roles, aberrant expression and/or function of Aurora kinases and PLK1 may lead to abnormal cell divisions with consequent generation of aneuploid cells.

An increased expression of all three Aurora kinases and PLK1 was shown in various cell lines originating from different epithelial TC histotypes, compared to normal thyrocytes, as well as in DTC and ATC tissues, compared to normal matched tissues [19, 20, 88, 96–98]. In addition, a study aimed to evaluate the gene expression profile in ATC, by means of tissue microarray and immunohistochemistry, identified the gene encoding Aurora-A as one of the most frequently and most strongly overexpressed in these tumors [99]. This is consistent with the observation that gain of chromosome 20q, where Aurora-A gene is located (20q13.2), is often encountered in ATC [100]. Based on these findings, the potential therapeutic value of Aurora kinases and PLK1 inhibition on the proliferation and growth of ATC cells has been evaluated in preclinical and clinical studies (**Table 1**).

Concerning the Aurora kinases, the in vitro effects of different small molecule pan-inhibitors, including the MK-0457 (VX-680), the SNS-314 mesylate, and the ZM447439, were investigated on proliferation, apoptosis, cell cycle, ploidy, and anchorage-independent growth of a panel of ATC-derived cell lines [101–103]. All these inhibitors were found to reduce proliferation of ATC cells in a time- and dose-dependent manner and to inhibit colony formation in soft agar. Cytofluorimetric analysis of cell cultures exposed to the Aurora inhibitors revealed an accumulation of tetra- and polyploid cells because of endoreplication events followed by activation of the apoptotic process [101–103]. Treated cells showed mitotic alterations consistent with Aurora kinase inhibition, including major spindle defects, inhibition of histone H3 phosphorylation, and cytokinesis failure [101–103]. Similar effects were obtained with the selective inhibition of either Aurora-A or Aurora-B [97, 104–106]. Suppression of Aurora-B expression by means of RNA interference, or of Aurora-B function by AZD1152, was demonstrated, in vivo and in vitro, to reduce growth and tumorigenicity of different ATC-derived cells [97, 104, 106]. In the same way, selective functional inhibition of Aurora-A by MLN8054 or MLN8237 was shown to inhibit cell proliferation and to induce cell-cycle arrest and apoptosis in a panel of ATC-derived cell lines [105, 106]. In xenograft experiments MLN8054 was found to reduce tumor volume by 86% [105]. Moreover, the combined treatment with MLN8054 and bortezomib, targeting the ubiquitin-proteasome system, showed additive effects on ATC-derived cell proliferation and apoptosis, compared to monotherapy [107]. It is worth to note that pazopanib, a TKI abovementioned, was found to potentiate the cytotoxic effects of paclitaxel in a preclinical study on ATC-derived cell lines in vitro and in vivo [108]. This effect of pazopanib was attributed to an unexpected off-target inhibition of Aurora-A. In fact, similar results were obtained when paclitaxel was combined with the selective Aurora-A inhibitor MLN8237. Remarkably, in the same study the authors showed that the combined administration of pazopanib and paclitaxel achieved a strong and long-lasting regression of lung metastasis in a single ATC patient [108]. However, while pazopanib was shown to have impressive therapeutic activity in patients affected by RAI-refractory PDTC, it was ineffective when tested in a phase II clinical trial on ATC patients [73, 109]. Although several of them had a transient disease regression, no Response Evaluation Criteria in Solid Tumors (RECIST) response was obtained [109].

Regarding PLK1, different studies demonstrated that it could represent a valuable therapeutic target in PDTC and ATC [110–112]. The potential of PLK1 inhibition in cancer treatment was investigated by means of antisense oligonucleotides, small interfering (si) RNA, and small molecule inhibitors targeting either the N-terminal catalytic domain or the C-terminal polo-box (PB) domain, responsible for kinase subcellular localization [113]. In vitro experiments on a panel of ATC-derived cell lines showed that PLK1 inactivation by BI 2536, an ATP-competitive small molecule inhibitor, induced cell arrest in prometaphase with accumulation of cells with 4N DNA content and mitotic spindle aberrations [110]. ATC cells finally died, as evidenced by the increased levels of cleaved caspase-3 and apoptotic nuclear morphology [110]. In agreement with the results of this study, more recently a different PLK1 inhibitor, the GSK461364A, was reported to inhibit cell proliferation and to induce cell death in different PDTC- and ATC-derived cell lines, independent of the nature of their driver mutations [113]. Consistent with PLK1 inhibition, the drug was shown to induce a G2/M arrest, followed by apoptosis. GSK461364A was also effective in vivo, in an allograft model of ATC [113]. Taken together, these data suggest that PLK1 targeting is a promising and effective therapeutic approach against PDTC and ATC [113].

4. Conclusions

In spite of the generally good prognosis of patients affected by thyroid carcinomas, approximately 5% of them will develop metastatic disease not responsive to traditional therapies. New drugs have been developed following the increased knowledge of the molecular alterations occurring in thyroid carcinomas. Tyrosine kinase and mitotic kinase inhibitors are now emerging as new drugs for the therapy of aggressive thyroid cancers, capable of prolonging patients' median progression-free survival. So far, however, no significant improvement has been observed on overall patients' survival. It has also to bear in mind that side effects are common, limiting the dose and time of drug administration. Aims of a future development in this field will be the identification of new, more effective and safe compounds and tailoring of the new targeted therapies in each patient based on tumor-specific genetic background.

Author details

Alessandro Antonelli[1], Enke Baldini[2], Salvatore Sorrenti[2], Poupak Fallahi[1], Paolo Miccoli[1], Angelo Filippini[2] and Salvatore Ulisse[2*]

*Address all correspondence to: salvatore.ulisse@uniroma1.it

1 Department of Clinical and Experimental Medicine, University of Pisa, Pisa, Italy

2 Department of Surgical Sciences, "Sapienza" University of Rome, Rome, Italy

References

[1] Howlader N, Noone AM, Krapcho M, Garshell J, Miller D, Altekruse SF, Kosary CL, Yu M, Ruhl J, Tatalovich Z, Mariotto A, Lewis DR, Chen HS, Feuer EJ, Cronin KA (eds). SEER Cancer Statistics Review, 1975–2012, National Cancer Institute. Bethesda, MD, http://seer.cancer.gov/csr/1975_2012/.

[2] Grodski S, Brown T, Sidhu S, Gill A, Robinson B, Learoyd D, Sywak M, Reeve T, Delbridge L. Increasing incidence of thyroid cancer is due to increased pathologic detection. Surgery 2008;144:1038-1043.

[3] Trimboli P, Ulisse S, Graziano FM, Marzullo A, Ruggieri M, Calvanese A, Piccirilli F, Cavaliere R, Fumarola A, D'Armiento M. Trend in thyroid carcinoma size, age at diagnosis, and histology in a retrospective study of 500 cases diagnosed over 20 years. Thyroid 2006;16:1151-1155.

[4] Nikiforov YE, Biddinger PW, Thompson LDR. Diagnostic Pathology and Molecular Genetics of the Thyroid. Philadelphia, PA: Volters Kluver & Lippincott Williams & Wilkins; 2009. 382 p.

[5] Nikiforov YE, Nikiforova MN. Molecular genetics and diagnosis of thyroid cancer. Nat Rev Endocrinol 2011;7:569-580.

[6] DeLellis RA, Lloyd R, Heitz PU, Heng C, editors. World Health Organization Classification of Tumors, Pathology & Genetics—Tumors of Endocrine Organs. Lyon, France: IARC Press; 2004.

[7] Nikiforov YE. Genetic alterations involved in the transition from well-differentiated to poorly differentiated and anaplastic thyroid carcinomas. Endocr Pathol 2004;15:319-327.

[8] Hunt JL, Tometsko M, LiVolsi VA, Swalsky P, Finkelstein SD, Barnes EL. Molecular evidence of anaplastic transformation in coexisting well-differentiated and anaplastic carcinomas of the thyroid. Am J Surg Pathol 2003;27:1559-1564.

[9] Eloy C, Ferreira L, Salgado C, Soares P, Sobrinho-Simões M. Poorly differentiated and undifferentiated thyroid carcinomas. Turk Patoloji Derg 2015;31:48-59.

[10] American Thyroid Association (ATA) Guidelines Taskforce on Thyroid Nodules and Differentiated Thyroid Cancer, Cooper DS, Doherty GM, Haugen BR, Kloos RT, Lee SL, Mandel SJ, Mazzaferri EL, McIver B, Pacini F, Schlumberger M, Sherman SI, Steward DL, Tuttle RM. Revised American Thyroid Association management guidelines for patients with thyroid nodules and differentiated thyroid cancer. Thyroid 2009;19:1167-1214.

[11] Ibrahimpasic T, Ghossein R, Carlson DL, Nixon I, Palmer FL, Shaha AR, Patel SG, Tuttle RM, Shah JP, Ganly I. Outcomes in patients with poorly differentiated thyroid carcinoma. J Clin Endocrinol Metab 2014;99:1245-1252.

[12] Romesser PB, Sherman EJ, Shaha AR, Lian M, Wong RJ, Sabra M, Rao SS, Fagin JA, Tuttle RM, Lee NY. External beam radiotherapy with or without concurrent chemotherapy in advanced or recurrent non-anaplastic non-medullary thyroid cancer. J Surg Oncol 2014;110:375-382.

[13] Antonelli A, Fallahi P, Ferrari SM, Carpi A, Berti P, Materazzi G, Minuto M, Guastalli M, Miccoli P. Dedifferentiated thyroid cancer: a therapeutic challenge. Biomed Pharmacother 2008;62:559-563.

[14] Keutegen XM, Sadowski SM, Kebebew E. Management of anaplastic thyroid cancer. Gland Surg 2015;4:44-51.

[15] Kondo T, Ezzat S, Asa SL. Pathogenetic mechanisms in thyroid follicular-cell neoplasia. Nat Rev Cancer 2006;6:292-306.

[16] Shahedian B, Shi Y, Zou M, Farid NR. Thyroid carcinoma is characterized by genomic instability: evidence from p53 mutations. Mol Gen Metab 2001;72:155-163.

[17] Wressmann VB, Ghossein RA, Patel SG, Harris CP, Schnaser EA, Shaha AR, et al. Genome-wide appraisal of thyroid cancer progression. Am J Pathol 2002;161:1549-1556.

[18] Hanahan D, Weinberg RA. Hallmarks of cancer: the next generation. Cell 2011;144:646-674.

[19] Baldini E, D'Armiento M, Ulisse S. A new aurora in anaplastic thyroid cancer therapy. Int J Endocrinol 2014;2014:816430.

[20] Ito Y, Miyoshi E, Sasaki N, Kakudo K, Yoshida H, Tomoda C, Uruno T, Takamura Y, Miya A, Kobayashi K, Matsuzuka F, Matsuura N, Kuma K, Miyauchi A. Polo-like kinase 1 overexpression is an early event in the progression of papillary carcinoma. Br J Cancer 2004;90:414-418.

[21] The Cancer Genome Atlas Research Network. Integrated genomic characterization of papillary thyroid carcinoma. Cell 2014;159:676-690.

[22] Omur O, Baran Y. An update on molecular biology of thyroid cancer. Crit Rev Oncol Hematol 2014;90:233-252.

[23] Giordano TJ, Au AY, Kuick R, Thomas DG, Rhodes DR, Wilhelm KG Jr, Vinco M, Misek DE, Sanders D, Zhu Z, Ciampi R, Hanash S, Chinnaiyan A, Clifton-Bligh RJ, Robinson BG, Nikiforov YE, Koenig RJ. Delineation, functional validation, and bioinformatic evaluation of gene expression in thyroid follicular carcinomas with the PAX8-PPARG translocation. Clin Cancer Res 2006;12:1983-1993.

[24] Patel KN, Shaha AR. Poorly differentiated and anaplastic thyroid cancer. Cancer Control 2006;13:119-128.

[25] Ito T, Seyama T, Mizuno T, Tsuyama N, Hayashi T, Hayashi Y, Dohi K, Nakamura N, Akiyama M.Unique association of p53 mutations with undifferentiated but not with differentiated carcinomas of the thyroid gland. Cancer Res 1992;52:1369-1371.

[26] Donghi R, Longoni A, Pilotti S, Michieli P, Della Porta G, Pierotti MA. Gene p53 mutations are restricted to poorly differentiated and undifferentiated carcinomas of the thyroid gland. J Clin Invest 1993;91:1753-1760.

[27] Garcia-Rostan G, Camp RL, Herrero A, Carcangiu ML, Rimm DL, Tallini G. Beta-catenin dysregulation in thyroid neoplasms: down-regulation, aberrant nuclear expression, and CTNNB1 exon 3 mutations are markers for aggressive tumor phenotypes and poor prognosis. Am J Pathol 2001;158:987-996.

[28] Miyake N1, Maeta H, Horie S, Kitamura Y, Nanba E, Kobayashi K, Terada T. Absence of mutations in the beta-catenin and adenomatous polyposis coli genes in papillary and follicular thyroid carcinomas. Pathol Int 2001;51:680-685.

[29] Huber MA, Kraut N, Beug H. Molecular requirements for epithelial-mesenchymal transition during tumor progression. Curr Opin Cell Biol 2005;17:548-558.

[30] Vasko V, Espinosa AV, Scouten W, He H, Auer H, Liyanarachchi S, et al. Gene expression and functional evidence of epithelial-to-mesenchymal transition in papillary thyroid carcinoma invasion. Proc Natl Acad Sci USA 2007;104:2803-2808.

[31] Baldini E, Toller M, Graziano FM, Russo FP, Pepe M, Biordi L, Marchioni E, Curcio F, Ulisse S, Ambesi-Impiombato FS, D'Armiento M.Expression of matrix metalloproteinases and their specific inhibitors (TIMPs) in normal and different human thyroid tumor cell lines. Thyroid 2004;14:881-888.

[32] Ulisse S, Baldini E, Toller M, Marchioni E, Giacomelli L, De Antoni E, Ferretti E, Marzullo A, Graziano FM, Trimboli P, Biordi L, Curcio F, Gulino A, Ambesi-Impiombato FS, D'Armiento M.Differential expression of the components of the plasminogen activating system in human thyroid tumour derived cell lines and papillary carcinomas. Eur J Cancer 2006;42:2631-2638.

[33] Ulisse S, Baldini E, Sorrenti S, Barollo S, Gnessi L, Catania A, Pellizzo MR, Nardi F, Mian C, De Antoni E, D'Armiento M, Frati L.High expression of the urokinase plasminogen activator and its cognate 1 receptor associates with advanced stages and reduced disease-free interval in papillary thyroid carcinoma. J Clin Endocrinol Metab 2011;96:504-508.

[34] Ulisse S, Baldini E, Sorrenti S, Barollo S, Prinzi N, Catania A, Nesca A, Gnessi L, Pelizzo MR, Mian C, De Vito C, Calvanese A, Palermo S, Persechino S, De Antoni E, D'Armiento M. In papillary thyroid carcinoma BRAFV600E is associated with increased expression of the urokinase plasminogen activator and its cognate receptor, but not with disease-free interval. Clin Endocrinol 2012;77:780-786.

[35] Ferrari SM, Fallahi P, Politti U, Materazzi G, Baldini E, Ulisse S, Miccoli P, Antonelli A. Molecular Targeted Therapies of Aggressive Thyroid Cancer. Front Endocrinol 2015;6:176.

[36] Ranganath R, Shah MA, Shah AR. Anaplastic thyroid cancer. Curr Opin Endocrinol Diabetes Obes 2015:22:387-391.

[37] Krause DS, Van Etten RA. Tyrosine kinases as targets for cancer therapy. N Engl J Med 2005;353:172-187.

[38] Fallahi P, Ferrari SM, Vita R, Di Domenicantonio A, Corrado A, Benvenga S, Antonelli A. Thyroid dysfunctions induced by tyrosine kinase inhibitors. Expert Opin Drug Saf 2014;13:723-733.

[39] Tolmachev V, Stone-Elander S, Orlova A. Radiolabelled receptor-tyrosine-kinase targeting drugs for patient stratification and monitoring of therapy response: prospects and pitfalls. Lancet Oncol 2010;11:992-1000.

[40] Sarlis NJ, Benvenga, S. Molecular signaling in thyroid cancer. Cancer Treat Res 2004;122:237-264.

[41] Stommel JM, Kimmelman AC, Ying H, Nabioullin R, Ponugoti AH, Wiedemeyer R, Stegh AH, Bradner JE, Ligon KL, Brennan C, Chin L, DePinho RA. Coactivation of receptor tyrosine kinases affects the response of tumor cells to targeted therapies. Science 2007;318:287-290.

[42] Sherman SI. Lessons learned and questions unanswered from use of multitargeted kinase inhibitors in medullary thyroid cancer. Oral Oncol 2013;49:707-710.

[43] Antonelli A, Bocci G, La Motta C, Ferrari SM, Fallahi P, Fioravanti A, Sartini S, Minuto M, Piaggi S, Corti A, Alì G, Berti P, Fontanini G, Danesi R, Da Settimo F, Miccoli P. Novel pyrazolopyrimidine derivatives as tyrosine kinase inhibitors with antitumoral activity in vitro and in vivo in papillary dedifferentiated thyroid cancer. J Clin Endocrinol Metab 2011;96:E288-E296.

[44] Bocci G, Fioravanti A, La Motta C, Orlandi P, Canu B, Di Desidero T, Mugnaini L, Sartini S, Cosconati S, Frati R, Antonelli A, Berti P, Miccoli P, Da Settimo F, Danesi R. Antiproliferative and proapoptotic activity of CLM3, a novel multiple tyrosine kinase inhibitor, alone and in combination with SN-38 on endothelial and cancer cells. Biochem Pharmacol 2011;81:1309-1316.

[45] Sartini S, Coviello V, Bruno A, La Pietra V, Marinelli L, Simorini F, Taliani S, Salerno S, Marini AM, Fioravanti A, Orlandi P, Antonelli A, Da Settimo F, Novellino E, Bocci G, La Motta C. Structure-based optimization of tyrosine kinase inhibitor CLM3. Design, synthesis, functional evaluation, and molecular modeling studies. J Med Chem 2014;57:1225-1235.

[46] Antonelli A, Bocci G, Fallahi P, La Motta C, Ferrari SM, Mancusi C, Fioravanti A, Di Desidero T, Sartini S, Corti A, Piaggi S, Materazzi G, Spinelli C, Fontanini G, Danesi R, Da Settimo F, Miccoli P. CLM3, a multitarget tyrosine kinase inhibitor with antiangiogenic properties, is active against primary anaplastic thyroid cancer in vitro and in vivo. J Clin Endocrinol Metab 2014;99:E572-E581.

[47] Antonelli A, Bocci G, La Motta C, Ferrari SM, Fallahi P, Ruffilli I, Di Domenicantonio A, Fioravanti A, Sartini S, Minuto M, Piaggi S, Corti A, Alì G, Di Desidero T, Berti P, Fontanini G, Danesi R, Da Settimo F, Miccoli P. CLM94, a novel cyclic amide with anti-VEGFR-2 and antiangiogenic properties, is active against primary anaplastic thyroid cancer in vitro and in vivo. J Clin Endocrinol Metab 2012;97:E528-E536.

[48] Fallahi P, Ferrari SM, Santini F, Corrado A, Materazzi G, Ulisse S, Miccoli P, Antonelli A. Sorafenib and thyroid cancer. BioDrugs 2013;27:615-628.

[49] Ruan M, Liu M, Dong Q, Chen L. Iodide- and glucose-handling gene expression regulated by sorafenib or cabozantinib in papillary thyroid cancer. J Clin Endocrinol Metab 2015;100:1771-1779.

[50] Gupta-Abramson V, Troxel AB, Nellore A, Puttaswamy K, Redlinger M, Ransone K, Mandel SJ, Flaherty KT, Loevner LA, O'Dwyer PJ, Brose MS. Phase II trial of sorafenib in advanced thyroid cancer. J Clin Oncol 2008;26:4714-4719.

[51] Kloos RT, Ringel MD, Knopp MV, Hall NC, King M, Stevens R, Liang J, Wakely PE Jr, Vasko VV, Saji M, Rittenberry J, Wei L, Arbogast D, Collamore M, Wright JJ, Grever M, Shah MH. Phase II trial of sorafenib in metastatic thyroid cancer. J Clin Oncol 2009;27:1675-1684.

[52] Brose MS, Nutting CM, Jarzab B, Elisei R, Siena S, Bastholt L, de la Fouchardiere C, Pacini F, Paschke R, Shong YK, Sherman SI, Smit JW, Chung J, Kappeler C, Peña C, Molnár I, Schlumberger MJ; DECISION investigators. Sorafenib in radioactive iodine-refractory, locally advanced or metastatic differentiated thyroid cancer: a randomised, double-blind, phase 3 trial. Lancet 2014;384:319-328.

[53] Carlomagno F, Vitagliano D, Guida T, Ciardiello F, Tortora G, Vecchio G, Ryan AJ, Fontanini G, Fusco A, Santoro M. ZD6474, an orally available inhibitor of KDR tyrosine kinase activity, efficiently blocks oncogenic RET kinases. Cancer Res 2002;62:7284-7290.

[54] Leboulleux S, Bastholt L, Krause T, de la Fouchardiere C, Tennvall J, Awada A, Gómez JM, Bonichon F, Leenhardt L, Soufflet C, Licour M, Schlumberger MJ. Vandetanib in locally advanced or metastatic differentiated thyroid cancer: a randomised, double-blind, phase 2 trial. Lancet Oncol 2012;13:897-905.

[55] Rosen LS, Kurzrock R, Mulay M, Van Vugt A, Purdom M, Ng C, Silverman J, Koutsoukos A, Sun YN, Bass MB, Xu RY, Polverino A, Wiezorek JS, Chang DD, Benjamin R, Herbst RS. Safety, pharmacokinetics, and efficacy of AMG 706, an oral multikinase inhibitor, in patients with advanced solid tumors. J Clin Oncol 2007;25:2369-2376.

[56] Sherman SI, Wirth LJ, Droz JP, Hofmann M, Bastholt L, Martins RG, Licitra L, Eschenberg MJ, Sun YN, Juan T, Stepan DE, Schlumberger MJ; Motesanib Thyroid Cancer Study Group. Motesanib diphosphate in progressive differentiated thyroid cancer. N Engl J Med 2008;359:31-42.

[57] Kelly RJ, Rixie O. Axitinib—a selective inhibitor of the vascular endothelial growth factor (VEGF) receptor. Target Oncol 2009;4:297-305.

[58] Bagcchi, S. Axitinib: VEGF inhibition in advanced thyroid cancer. Lancet Oncol 2014; 15:e310.

[59] Hu-Lowe D, Hallin M, Feeley R, Zou H, Rewolinski D, Wickman G, Chen E, Kim Y, Riney S, Reed J, Heller D, Simmons B, Kania R, McTigue M, Niesman M, Gregory S, Shalinsky D, Bender S. Characterization of potency and activity of the VEGF/PDGF receptor tyrosine kinase inhibitor AG013736. Proc Am Assoc Cancer Res. 2002;43:A5357.

[60] Cohen EE, Rosen LS, Vokes EE, Kies MS, Forastiere AA, Worden FP, Kane MA, Sherman E, Kim S, Bycott P, Tortorici M, Shalinsky DR, Liau KF, Cohen RB. Axitinib is an active treatment for all histologic subtypes of advanced thyroid cancer: results from a phase II study. J Clin Oncol 2008;26:4708-4713.

[61] Locati LD, Licitra L, Agate L, Ou SH, Boucher A, Jarzab B, Qin S, Kane MA, Wirth LJ, Chen C, Kim S, Ingrosso A, Pithavala YK, Bycott P, Cohen EE. Treatment of advanced thyroid cancer with axitinib: phase 2 study with pharmacokinetic/pharmacodynamic and quality-of-life assessments. Cancer 2014;120:2694-2703.

[62] Rini BI. Sunitinib. Expert Opin Pharmacother 2007;8:2359-2369.

[63] Adams VR, Leggas M. Sunitinib malate for the treatment of metastatic renal cell carcinoma and gastrointestinal stromal tumors. Clin Ther 2007;29:1338-1353.

[64] Kim DW, Jo YS, Jung HS, Chung HK, Song JH, Park KC, Park SH, Hwang JH, Rha SY, Kweon GR, Lee SJ, Jo KW, Shong M. An orally administered multitarget tyrosine kinase inhibitor, SU11248, is a novel potent inhibitor of thyroid oncogenic RET/papillary thyroid cancer kinases. J Clin Endocrinol Metab 2006;91:4070-4076.

[65] Jeong WJ, Mo JH, Park MW, Choi IJ, An SY, Jeon EH, Ahn SH. Sunitinib inhibits papillary thyroid carcinoma with RET/PTC rearrangement but not BRAF mutation. Cancer Biol Ther 2011;12:458-465.

[66] Carr LL, Mankoff DA, Goulart BH, Eaton KD, Capell PT, Kell EM, Bauman JE, Martins RG. Phase II study of daily sunitinib in FDG-PET-positive, iodine-refractory differentiated thyroid cancer and metastatic medullary carcinoma of the thyroid with functional imaging correlation. Clin Cancer Res 2010;16:5260-5268.

[67] Dìez JJ, Iglesias P, Alonso T, Grande E. Activity and safety of sunitinib in patients with advanced radioactive iodine-refractory differentiated thyroid carcinoma in clinical practice. Endocrine 2015;48:582-588.

[68] Bikas A, Kundra P, Desale S, et al. Phase 2 clinical trial of sunitinib as adjunctive treatment in patients with advanced differentiated thyroid cancer. Eur J Endocrinol 2016;174:373-380.

[69] Durante C, Russo D, Verrienti A, Filetti S. XL184 (cabozantinib) for medullary thyroid carcinoma. Expert Opin Investig Drugs 2011;20:407-413.

[70] Cui JJ. Inhibitors targeting hepatocyte growth factor receptor and their potential therapeutic applications. Expert Opin Ther Pat 2007;17:1035-1045.

[71] Cabanillas ME, Brose MS, Ramies DA, Lee Y, Miles D, Sherman SI. Antitumor activity of cabozantinib (XL184) in a cohort of patients (pts) with differentiated thyroid cancer (DTC). (Abstract #5547) ASCO Annual Meeting, Chicago, IL, 2012.

[72] Sternberg CN, Davis ID, Mardiak J, Szczylik C, Lee E, Wagstaff J, Barrios CH, Salman P, Gladkov OA, Kavina A, Zarbá JJ, Chen M, McCann L, Pandite L, Roychowdhury DF, Hawkins RE. Pazopanib in locally advanced or metastatic renal cell carcinoma: results of a randomized phase III trial. J Clin Oncol 2010;28:1061-1068.

[73] Bible KC, Suman VJ, Molina JR, Smallridge RC, Maples WJ, Menefee ME, Rubin J, Sideras K, Morris JC 3rd, McIver B, Burton JK, Webster KP, Bieber C, Traynor AM, Flynn PJ, Goh BC, Tang H, Ivy SP, Erlichman C; Endocrine Malignancies Disease Oriented Group; Mayo Clinic Cancer Center; Mayo Phase 2 Consortium. Efficacy of pazopanib in progressive, radioiodine-refractory, metastatic differentiated thyroid cancers: results of a phase 2 consortium study. Lancet Oncol 2010;11:962-972.

[74] Matsui J, Yamamoto Y, Funahashi Y, Tsuruoka A, Watanabe T, Wakabayashi T, Uenaka T, Asada M. E7080, a novel inhibitor that targets multiple kinases, has potent antitumor activities against stem cell factor producing human small cell lung cancer H146, based on angiogenesis inhibition. Int J Cancer 2008;122:664-671.

[75] Cabanillas ME, Schlumberger M, Jarzab B, Martins RG, Pacini F, Robinson B, McCaffrey JC, Shah MH, Bodenner DL, Topliss D, Andresen C, O'Brien JP, Ren M, Funahashi Y, Allison R, Elisei R, Newbold K, Licitra LF, Sherman SI, Ball DW. A phase 2 trial of lenvatinib (E7080) in advanced, progressive, radioiodine-refractory, differentiated thyroid cancer: a clinical outcomes and biomarker assessment. Cancer 2015;121:2749-2756.

[76] Schlumberger M, Tahara M, Wirth LJ, Robinson B, Brose MS, Elisei R, Habra MA, Newbold K, Shah MH, Hoff AO, Gianoukakis AG, Kiyota N, Taylor MH, Kim SB, Krzyzanowska MK, Dutcus CE, de las Heras B, Zhu J, Sherman SI. Lenvatinib versus placebo in radioiodine-refractory thyroid cancer. N Engl J Med 2015;372:621-630.

[77] Fallahi P, Mazzi V, Vita R, Ferrari SM, Materazzi G, Galleri D, Benvenga S, Miccoli P, Antonelli A. New therapies for dedifferentiated papillary thyroid cancer. Int J Mol Sci 2015;16:6153-6182.

[78] Li C, Lee KC, Schneider EB, Zeiger MA. BRAF V600E mutation and its association with clinicopathological features of papillary thyroid cancer: a meta-analysis. J Clin Endocrinol Metab 2012;97:4559-4570.

[79] Costamagna E, García B, Santisteban P. The functional interaction between the paired domain transcription factor Pax8 and Smad3 is involved in transforming growth factor-beta repression of the sodium/iodide symporter gene. J Biol Chem 2004;279:3439-3446.

[80] Sharma A, Shah SR, Illum H, Dowell J. Vemurafenib: targeted inhibition of mutated BRAF for treatment of advanced melanoma and its potential in other malignancies. Drugs 2012;72:2207-2222.

[81] James J, Ruggeri B, Armstrong RC, Rowbottom MW, Jones-Bolin S, Gunawardane RN, Dobrzanski P, Gardner MF, Zhao H, Cramer MD, Hunter K, Nepomuceno RR, Cheng M, Gitnick D, Yazdanian M, Insko DE, Ator MA, Apuy JL, Faraoni R, Dorsey BD, Williams M, Bhagwat SS, Holladay MW. CEP-32496: a novel orally active BRAF(V600E) inhibitor with selective cellular and in vivo antitumor activity. Mol Cancer Ther 2012;11:930-941.

[82] Fury MG, Sherman E, Haque S, Korte S, Lisa D, Shen R, Wu N, Pfister D. A phase I study of daily everolimus plus low-dose weekly cisplatin for patients with advanced solid tumors. Cancer Chemother Pharmacol 2012;69:591-598.

[83] Kouvaraki MA, Liakou C, Paraschi A, Dimas K, Patsouris E, Tseleni-Balafouta S, Rassidakis GZ, Moraitis D. Activation of mTOR signaling in medullary and aggressive papillary thyroid carcinomas. Surgery 2011;150:1258-1265.

[84] Yeager N, Brewer C, Cai KQ, Xu XX, Di Cristofano A. Mammalian target of rapamycin is the key effector of phosphatidylinositol-3-OH-initiated proliferative signals in the thyroid follicular epithelium. Cancer Res 2008;68:444-449.

[85] de Souza EC, Padrón AS, Braga WM, de Andrade BM, Vaisman M, Nasciutti LE, Ferreira AC, de Carvalho DP. MTOR downregulates iodide uptake in thyrocytes. J Endocrinol 2010;206:113-120.

[86] Kogai T, Sajid-Crockett S, Newmarch LS, Liu YY, Brent GA. Phosphoinositide-3-kinase inhibition induces sodium/iodide symporter expression in rat thyroid cells and human papillary thyroid cancer cells. J Endocrinol 2008;199:243-252.

[87] Faggiano A, Ramundo V, Dicitore A, Castiglioni S, Borghi MO, Severino R, Ferolla P, Crinò L, Abbruzzese A, Sperlongano P, Caraglia M, Ferone D, Hofland L, Colao A, Vitale G. Everolimus is an active agent in medullary thyroid cancer: a clinical and in vitro study. J Cell Mol Med 2012;16:1563-1572.

[88] Ulisse S, Delcros JG, Baldini E, Toller M, Curcio F, Giacomelli L, Prigent C, Ambesi-Impiombato FS, D'Armiento M, Arlot-Bonnemains Y. Expression of Aurora kinases in human thyroid carcinoma cell lines and tissues. Int J Cancer 2006;119:275-282.

[89] K-S Chan, C-G Koh, H-Y Li. Mitosis-targeted anti-cancer therapies: where they stand. Cell Death Dis 2012;3:e411.

[90] Campos SM, Dizon DS. Antimitotic inhibitors. Hematol Oncol Clin North Am 2012;26:607-628.

[91] Jackson JR, Patrick DR, Dar MM, Huang PS. Targeted anti-mitotic therapies: can we improve on tubulin agents? Nat Rev Cancer 2007;7:107–117.

[92] McInnes C, Mezna M, Fischer PM. Progress in the discovery of Polo-like kinase inhibitors. Curr Top Med Chem 2005;5:181–197.

[93] Strebhardt K, Ullrich A. Targeting polo-like kinase 1 for cancer therapy. Nat Rev Cancer 2006;6:321–330.

[94] Gabillard JC, Ulisse S, Baldini E, Sorrenti S, Cremet JY, Coccaro C, Prigent C, D'Armiento M, Arlot-Bonnemains Y. Aurora-C interacts with and phosphorylates the transforming acidic coiled-coil 1 protein. Biochem Biophys Res Co 2011;408:647-653.

[95] Baldini E, Sorrenti S, D'Armiento E, Prinzi N, Guaitoli E, Favoriti P, Gnessi L, Moretti C, Bianchini M, Alessandrini S, Catania A, De Antoni E, Ulisse S. Aurora kinases: new molecular targets in thyroid cancer therapy. Clin Ter 2012;163:e457-462.

[96] Ulisse S, Baldini E, Toller M, Delcros JG, Guého A, Curcio F, De Antoni E, Giacomelli L, Ambesi-Impiombato FS, Bocchini S, D'Armiento M, Arlot-Bonnemains Y. Transforming Acidic Coiled-Coil 3 and Aurora-A interact in human thyrocytes and their expression is deregulated in thyroid cancer tissues. Endocr Relat Cancer 2007;14:827-837.

[97] Sorrentino R, Libertini S, Pallante PL, Troncone G, Palombini L, Bavetsias V, Spalletti-Cernia D, Laccetti P, Linardopoulos S, Chieffi P, Fusco A, Portella G. Aurora B overexpression associates with the thyroid carcinoma undifferentiated phenotype and is required for thyroid carcinoma cell proliferation. J Clin Endocrinol Metab 2005;90:928-935.

[98] Salvatore G, Nappi TC, Salerno P, Jiang Y, Garbi C, Ugolini C, Miccoli P, Basolo F, Castellone MD, Cirafici AM, Melillo RM, Fusco A, Bittner ML, Santoro M. A cell proliferation and chromosomal instability signature in anaplastic thyroid carcinoma. Cancer Res 2007;67:10148-10158.

[99] Wiseman SM1, Masoudi H, Niblock P, Turbin D, Rajput A, Hay J, Bugis S, Filipenko D, Huntsman D, Gilks B. Anaplastic thyroid carcinoma: expression profile of targets for therapy offers new insights for disease treatment. Ann Surg Oncol 2007;14:719-729.

[100] Rodrigues RF, Roque L, Rosa-Santos J, Cid O, Soares J. Chromosomal imbalances associated with anaplastic transformation of follicular thyroid carcinomas. Br J Cancer 2004;90:492-496.

[101] Arlot-Bonnemains Y, Baldini E, Martin B, Delcros JG, Toller M, Curcio F, Ambesi-Impiombato FS, D'Armiento M, Ulisse S. Effects of the Aurora kinase inhibitor VX-680 on anaplastic thyroid cancer-derived cell lines. Endocr Relat Cancer 2008;15:559-568.

[102] Baldini E, Sorrenti S, D'Armiento E, Guaitoli E, Morrone S, D'Andrea V, Gnessi L, Moretti C, Antonelli A, Catania A, De Antoni E, Ulisse S. Effects of the Aurora kinases

pan-inhibitor SNS-314 mesylate on anaplastic thyroid cancer derived cell lines. Clin Ter 2012;163:e307-e313.

[103] Baldini E, Tuccilli C, Prinzi N, Sorrenti S, Antonelli A, Gnessi L, Catania A, Moretti C, Mocini R, Carbotta G, Morrone S, Persechino S, Redler A, De Antoni E, D' Armiento M, Ulisse S. The dual Aurora kinase inhibitor ZM447439 prevents anaplastic thyroid cancer cell growth and tumorigenicity. J Biol Reg Homeost Agents 2013;27:705-715.

[104] Libertini S, Abagnale A, Passaro C, Botta G, Barbato S, Chieffi P, Portella G. AZD1152 negatively affects the growth of anaplastic thyroid carcinoma cells and enhances the effects of oncolytic virus dl922-947. Endocr Relat Cancer, 2011;18:129-141.

[105] Wunderlich A, Fischer M, Schlosshauer T, Ramaswamy A, Greene BH, Brendel C, Doll D, Bartsch D, Hoffmann S. Evaluation of Aurora kinase inhibition as a new therapeutic strategy in anaplastic and poorly differentiated follicular thyroid cancer. Cancer Sci 2011;102:762-768.

[106] Baldini E, Tuccilli C, Prinzi N, Sorrenti S, Antonelli A, Gnessi L, Morrone S, Moretti C, Bononi M, Arlot-Bonnemains Y, D'Armiento M, Ulisse S. Effects of selective inhibitors of Aurora kinases on anaplastic thyroid carcinoma cell lines. Endocr Relat Cancer 2014;21:797-811.

[107] Wunderlich A, Roth S, Ramaswamy A. Combined inhibition of cellular pathways as a future option in fatal anaplastic thyroid cancer. Endocrinie 2012;42:637-646.

[108] Isham CR, Bossou AR, Negron V. Pazopanib enhances paclitaxel-induced mitotic catastrophe in anaplastic thyroid cancer. Sci Transl Med 2013;5:166ra3.

[109] Bible KC, Suman VJ, Menefee ME, Smallridge RC, Molina JR, Maples WJ, Karlin NJ, Traynor AM, Kumar P, Goh BC, Lim WT, Bossou AR, Isham CR, Webster KP, Kukla AK, Bieber C, Burton JK, Harris P, Erlichman C; Mayo Phase 2 Consortium; Mayo Clinic Endocrine Malignances Disease Oriented Group. A multiinstitutional phase 2 trial of pazopanib monotherapy in advanced anaplastic thyroid cancer. J Clin Endocrinol Metab 2012;97:3179-3184.

[110] Nappi TC, Salerno P, Zitzelsberger H, Carlomagno F, Salvatore G, Santoro M. Identification of polo-like kinase 1 as potential therapeutic target in anaplastic thyroid carcinoma. Cancer Res 2009;69:1916-1923.

[111] Zhang XG, Lu XF, Jiao XM, Chen B, Wu JX. PLK1 gene suppresses cell invasion of undifferentiated thyroid carcinoma through the inhibition of CD44v6, MMP-2, and MMP-9. Exp Ther Med 2012;4:1005-1009.

[112] Russo MA, Kang KS, Di Cristofano A. The PKL1 inhibitor GSK461364A is effective in poorly differentiated and anaplastic thyroid carcinoma cells, independent of the nature of their driver mutations. Thyroid 2013;23:1284-1293.

[113] Kumar S, Kim J. PLK-1 targeted inhibitors and their potential against tumorigenesis. BioMed Res Int 2015;2015:705745.

Chapter 10

A Perspective on the Current Medical Approach of Advanced Medullary Thyroid Carcinoma

Ana Valea and Carmen Emanuela Georgescu

Additional information is available at the end of the chapter

http://dx.doi.org/10.5772/63650

Abstract

Medullary thyroid carcinoma (MTC) is a neuroendocrine tumor (NET), which originates in neural crest-derived calcitonin-producing C-cells. It occurs either sporadically or as a result of a germline mutation in the RET proto-oncogene, as in multiple endocrine neoplasia (MEN) syndrome type 2A including its variant familial MTC (FMTC) and type 2B. Currently, the only curative treatment for MTC is surgery, accompanied by lymph node dissection. However, the outcome is largely dependent on disease staging, with lymph node and distant metastases often identified at diagnosis, particularly in sporadic forms. Furthermore, the presence of cervical lymph node invasion at surgery predicts residual disease. The development of new treatments is strongly motivated by: (a) the low surgical cure rate when cervical lymph node metastases are present at the time of initial surgery, with 90% of patients having residual disease, (b) the high prevalence of distant metastases at initial diagnosis (lungs, bones and liver) and (c) the poor outcome in patients receiving cytotoxic chemotherapeutic agents. Herein, we focus on current nonsurgical options and perspectives in the treatment of MTC with emphasis on last year's FDA-approved tyrosine kinase inhibitors (TKIs) and other systemic therapies that need to be considered in the setting of advanced disease.

Keywords: thyroid, medullary thyroid carcinoma, therapy, tyrosine kinase inhibitors, everolimus, somatostatin analogues

1. Introduction

Medullary thyroid carcinoma (MTC) accounts for 1–5% of all thyroid cancers worldwide, with an apparently descending slope in the prevalence of MTC, at least in the USA, which rather can be explained by the marked increase in the relative incidence of papillary thyroid carcinoma over the past decades [1]. As many as 25–30% of cases harbor a germline mutation in the RET proto-oncogene and present as a hereditary syndrome, as in multiple endocrine neoplasia (MEN) syndrome types 2A and 2B [2]. MEN2A, which accounts for 95% of all MEN2 cases, presents with four variants: classical MEN2A, MEN2A with cutaneous lichen amyloidosis (CLA), MEN2A with Hirschsprung's disease (HD) and familial MTC (FMTC, i.e. individuals or families with RET germline mutations and MTC but without pheochromocytoma or primary hyperparathyroidism) [1]. Alternatively, MTC develops as a sporadic form, with a peak of incidence between the 4th and 6th decades of life [3].

A feature of medullary cancer is represented by a variety of hormones or biogenic amines as secretory products of MTC cells including calcitonin and carcinoembryonic antigen (CEA; **Figure 1**) in addition to chromogranin A (CgA), serotonin, neurotensin, adrenocorticotrophic hormone (ACTH), B-melanocyte stimulating hormone (MSHB) or somatostatin. Of note, specifically calcitonin and CEA (unspecific) are validated as sensitive tumor markers for the diagnosis and post-therapeutic follow-up of the disease, and their preoperative serum concentrations are directly related to the C-cell mass [4].

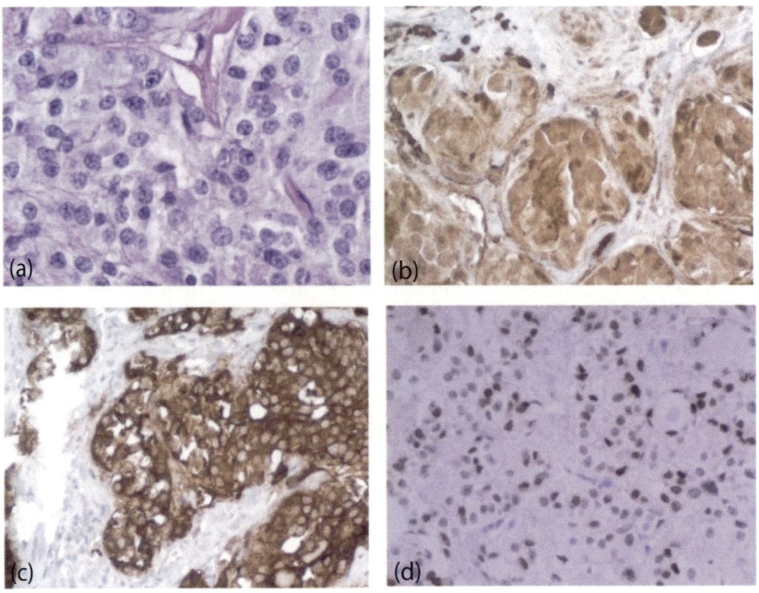

Figure 1. Microscopy of bifocal, bilobar MTC on a thyroidectomy piece in a c.1901G>T codon 634 mutation carrier. (a) H–E 40×; (b) IHC anti-calcitonin 20×; (c) IHC anti-CEA 20×; and (d) IHC anti-TTF 20×. Adapted from Sovrea et al. [5], with permission from the publisher. H–E, haematoxylin–eosin; IHC, immunohistochemistry; CEA, carcinoembryonic antigen; TTF-1, thyroid transcription factor-1.

Early diagnosis of MTC still represents a challenge in clinical practice. About 70% of patients with medullary cancer who present with a palpable thyroid nodule have cervical metastases at initial evaluation; on top of that, 10% have distant metastases [6]. While sporadic forms more often present as a solitary thyroid mass, hereditary syndromes are frequently multicentric and bilateral (**Figure 1**).

On neck ultrasonography, the tumor is typically located in the upper or central parts of the thyroid lobes in correlation with the distribution of C-cells (**Figure 2**). The exhibition of ultrasonographic features of malignancy including hypoechogenicity, irregular margins and intranodular calcifications correlates with tumor aggressiveness and a poor outcome. On the contrary, specific ultrasonographic appearance is lacking, and up to one-third of MTC may appear as non-suspicious on neck ultrasonography [7]. Overall, cost analysis suggests cost-effectiveness of calcitonin screening in patients with nodular goiter [8] and, subsequently, deepening investigations in patients with basal serum calcitonin levels at screening >20 pg/mL is recommended. Use of high-sensitivity immunoassays for measurements of calcitonin or, alternatively, a calcium-stimulation test, is indicated in patients with mildly elevated calcitonin levels.

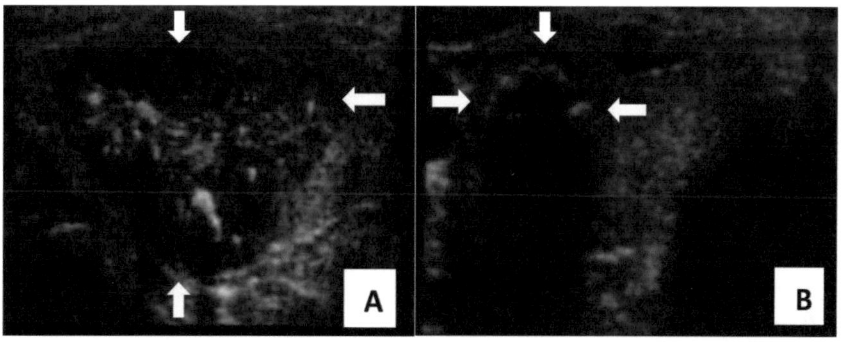

Figure 2. Grey-scale image of medullary thyroid carcinoma (MTC). (A) Cranio-caudal section and (B) transversal section.

Contrast-enhanced computer tomography (CT) scanning of the neck and chest (lymph nodes, lung metastases), contrast-enhanced CT or magnetic resonance imaging (MRI) of the liver, axial MRI and bone scintigraphy should be considered in patients with confirmed, extensive neck disease and signs of regional or distant metastases and in the presence of a serum calcitonin level above 400–500 pg/mL, as these patients almost always harbor systemic disease [9, 10]. Sensitivity of FDG-PET/CT or F-DOPA-PET/CT in detecting MTC metastases appears to be lower compared to other imaging investigations [1].

Recently revised American Thyroid Association (ATA) Guidelines for the management of medullary thyroid carcinoma suggest that fine needle aspiration biopsy (FNAB) should be performed in all thyroid nodules that are 1 cm or greater in size [1]. According to a meta-analysis, FNAB has been shown to have an accuracy of less than 50% in diagnosing MTC in affected subjects; however, diagnostic accuracy of FNAB analysis is significantly improved by measuring calcitonin levels in the FNA washout fluid [11]. In addition, immunohistochemistry analysis with positivity for calcitonin ± CEA and CgA and absence of thyroglobulin (Tg) staining of the FNAB specimen is reassuring [1].

In advanced disease, markedly increased basal CEA in addition to discordantly lower calcitonin, or normal or low levels of both CEA and calcitonin (i.e. nonsecretory MTC) suggests poorly differentiated MTC. Screening for RET mutations is indicated as well, since it has been shown that up to 7% of patients with apparently sporadic MTC have hereditary disease [12].

There is evidence of central and lateral compartment lymph node metastases in 14 and 11% of patients with stage T_1 tumor, whereas an incidence of 86% and 93%, respectively, has been reported in stage T_4 [13]. Ten-year survival rates of 100% for stage I disease, 93% for stage II, 71% for stage III and 21% for stage IV MTC have been reported [14].

2. Conventional treatment strategies of medullary thyroid carcinoma

2.1. Surgery

Thyroidectomy is the only curative treatment for both sporadic and hereditary MTC, accompanied by dissection of cervical lymph node compartments. Patients who carry RET mutations should undergo prophylactic thyroidectomy upon genetic diagnosis, even during childhood but at different ages depending on the risk associated with the specific RET mutation. Radical surgery is rarely possible in advanced regional/distant disease and rather preservation of swallowing, speech and parathyroid function should be attempted [1].

The outcome of surgery is largely dependent on disease staging, with 10-year survival rate of 96% in localized disease but rapidly decreasing to a median survival rate of 3 years after evidence of distant metastases. Normalization of calcitonin (<10 pg/mL) and CEA is only seen in 40% of cases, and approximately 9% of patients who have achieved biochemical cure will later develop recurrent disease [14]. A primary tumor larger than 1 cm diameter in the presence of high preoperative basal calcitonin levels (>20 pg/mL) and CEA concentrations (>10 pg/mL) predicts lymph node metastases in both central and ipsilateral neck compartments [15].

Following surgery, patients undergo levothyroxine replacement therapy in order to maintain serum thyroid stimulating hormone (TSH) levels in the normal range. In patients with unilateral lobectomy in whom MTC was histologically confirmed, completion thyroidectomy is indicated in the presence of elevated postoperative calcitonin or imaging studies indicating residual disease, or patients in whom a positive RET germline mutation was confirmed. In residual MTC, the calcitonin doubling time bears significant prognostic value. Patients whose calcitonin doubling time is 1 year or less have 10-year survival rates of 18%, whereas those with calcitonin doubling time longer than 1 year have a 95% survival rate [16].

According to 2015 ATA guidelines, postoperative care is based upon the dynamics of tumor markers and ultrasonographic findings. Therefore, serum levels of calcitonin and CEA should be measured 3 months after surgery, and if undetectable or within the normal range, every 6–12 months, then yearly. If calcitonin levels are high, yet less than 150 pg/mL, and however, there is no evidence of loco-regional disease on ultrasonography, measurement of serum tumor markers and thyroid ultrasonography every 6 months are strongly recommended.

Should calcitonin levels exceed 150 pg/mL postoperatively, patients should undergo extensive imaging studies to detect persistent disease and/or metastases [1].

2.2. External beam radiation therapy

Adjunctive external beam radiation of the neck or mediastinum could be considered after surgery in MTC patients with high risk for local recurrence (i.e. residual tumor, extra-thyroidal extension, extensive lymph node metastases) or airway obstruction, when repeat surgery is not possible. External beam radiation therapy has been used as a therapeutic method to control local tumor growth in patients with advanced loco-regional disease and implies postoperative delivery of 60–66 Gy over 6 weeks to the thyroid bed, although higher doses may be needed in the presence of important residual disease [1]. Although external radiation therapy positively affects the quality of life [17, 18], it appears not to significantly alter the overall survival rate in patients with lymph node metastases as shown by Martinez et al. [19]. External radiation beam therapy adverse effects include skin erythema, laryngeal edema, mucositis and esophagitis in the early phase. Later on, osteonecrosis, arterial injury, brain or cranial nerve injury are encountered.

Additional indications of external beam radiation therapy are painful bone metastasis, for palliation, or for the prevention of other bone-related complications such as fractures or spinal cord compression. Bone metastases may also benefit from high-dose anti-resorptive therapy (intravenous bisphosphonates or RANK-ligand inhibitor human monoclonal antibody).

2.3. Radioactive iodine

Previous studies certified lack of significant effect of radioactive iodine treatment in patients with MTC, as C-cells do not concentrate iodine. It was hypothesized that radioiodine, concentrated by follicular cells, might induce C-cell apoptosis through a bystander effect, however, not confirmed. In 2013, a controlled multicentre study compared the outcome of 232 patients with local or loco-regional MTC treated only by surgery to 61 matched patients that were also treated with RAI and found no difference in terms of disease-free or disease-specific survival [20]. On the contrary, radioactive iodine therapy should be considered in patients with MTC if the primary tumors or metastases contain MTC mixed with papillary or follicular thyroid carcinoma [1].

2.4. Conventional chemotherapy

Indication of cytotoxic chemotherapy is limited to advanced MTC, when disease control cannot be achieved with other treatments, however, with limited efficacy. Single agent or combination chemotherapeutic regimens generally show low response rates (15–20%), and of short duration (a few months), whereas large clinical trials demonstrating survival benefits are lacking.

According to the National Comprehensive Cancer Network (NCCN), dacarbazine is the drug of choice in patients with disseminated, symptomatic disease [21], in combination to 5-fluorouracil (5FU). Apart from that, dacarbazine has been combined with other cytotoxic agents such as cyclophosphamide, vincristine, streptozotocin and epirubicin, with modest results. Few studies and case reports have focused on the use of capecitabine, a 5FU prodrug that preferentially accumulated in tumors rather than in plasma to inhibit tumor cell proliferation [22], with apparently encouraging effects in stabilizing MTC patients with advanced disease. In a small phase I study, the combination of imatinib with capecitabine and dacarbazine failed to induce an objective response in MTC but four of five patients subjected to the therapeutic regimen maintained stable disease [23]. A combination of capecitabine with temozolomide appears to improve metastatic MTC [24], but experience is limited to isolated case reports.

Alternatively, combination treatment regimens with doxorubicin and another agent (e.g. cisplatin) may be used [1].

3. Molecular targeted therapies in medullary thyroid carcinoma

Systemic therapy is solely reserved for metastatic, unresectable, unstable MTC (i.e. calcitonin doubling time below 2 years) [1] or symptomatic tumor progression that cannot be managed by localized organ therapy [21]. Severe diarrhea that does not respond to symptomatic medication might need systemic therapy.

In contrast to classic cytotoxic chemotherapeutic agents that show weak specificity in discriminating between normal and tumor cells, the use of targeted molecular therapies is advantageous by providing a more narrow and specific therapeutic window and less toxicity. The broader spectrum of targeted therapies in neoplastic disease includes: (a) tyrosine kinases inhibitors (TKIs), (b) anti-sense inhibitors of growth factor receptors and (c) monoclonal antibodies. Tyrosine kinases play key roles in the modulation of growth factors signaling. For instance, RAS activation depends on epidermal growth factor receptor (EGFR), and somatic RAS mutations have been described in patients with MTC in the absence of RET mutations [25]. Apart from the activation by growth factors, protein kinase activation by germline or somatic mutations is a mechanism commonly described in tumor genesis. In fact, about 50% of the patients with sporadic MTC have somatic mutations of RET proto-oncogene, besides patients with MEN2 syndrome, of whom 98% express germline RET mutations [26]. In addition, MTC cells often overexpress vascular endothelial growth factor receptors (VEGFRs). TKI intervenes by blocking the ATP site of the tyrosine kinase receptors to prevent tyrosine kinase activation. They inhibit thyroid tumor cell proliferation, migration and survival and angiogenesis.

3.1. Tyrosine kinase inhibitors

Of all TKIs, the Food and Drug Administration (FDA) recently approved vandetanib and cabozantinib as first-line agents for the treatment of symptomatic or progressive MTC in patients with unresectable or metastatic disease. Both American Thyroid Association (ATA) and National Comprehensive Cancer Network guidelines (NCCN) specifically address the two drugs to patients with advanced MTC [1, 21]. Vandetanib and cabozantinib are multikinase inhibitors, with vandetanib targeting several cell-signaling pathways involved in the pathogenesis of MTC, including receptor tyrosine kinase RET, VEGFR-2 and -3 and EGFR and cabozantinib blocking RET, VEGFR-2 and c-MET [27], without simultaneously over-expressing any of the factors leading to the inhibition of angiogenesis. However, neither drug shows a clear correlation between RET mutational status and efficacy.

3.1.1. Vandetanib

In a trial with a phase II design on 30 adult patients with advanced MTC, of whom 70% had hereditary forms, objective partial response was obtained in 20% of patients while in 53% disease remained stable for 24 weeks during vandetanib 300 mg daily [28]. Vandetanib 100 mg/m^2/d was confirmed as a relatively well-tolerated and effective treatment in children (5–18 years) positive for M918T *RET* germline mutations [29].

In a phase III, randomized, double-blind, placebo-controlled trial (ZETA trial) of 331 patients with unresectable locally advanced (5%) or metastatic (95%) MTC, vandetanib 300 mg once daily resulted in significant prolongation of median progression-free survival to a predicted 30.5 months in the vandetanib group in comparison to 19.3 months in the placebo group [30]. The overall response rate to vandetanib was 44% and was noticed in both patients positive for RET mutations and those without a RET mutation. At the end of the study, 35% of study subjects required dose reductions, and 12% discontinued therapy due to toxicity. A fatal adverse effect was reported in 2.5% of patients.

Tumor markers calcitonin and CEA may fluctuate in patients undergoing therapy with vandetanib, often with an initial drop of the marker levels. A rise in calcitonin levels ≥40% between two follow-ups during the treatment for MTC appears to predict tumor progression early [31].

Vandetanib carries a black box warning for prolongation of the QT interval, *torsades de pointes* and sudden death. During treatment, medications that may prolong the QT interval must be avoided, and patients must undergo regular EKGs and serum electrolyte control. Patients with a history of long QT syndrome, baseline rate-corrected QT >450 ms, or uncorrectable electrolyte abnormalities should be excluded from treatment [32]. Other common adverse effects of vandetanib include diarrhea, nausea, fatigue and abdominal pain. In addition, hypertension, headache, acne and rash were reported. Hypocalcaemia, hepatocytolisis, hypoglycemia, hypertriglyceridemia [33], hypothyroidism and increased creatinine are common laboratory findings. In patients who cannot tolerate recommended dose, there is preliminary evidence that low-dose vandetanib is also efficient [34]; however, further studies are warranted.

Drug resistance to vandetanib has been described. Rare RET mutations V804M and V804L confer resistance to vandetanib as do RAS mutations, identified in 60–80% of RET-negative sporadic MTC cases. Sorafenib could be effective in these particular situations [26]. *In vitro* testing of tumor cell sensitivity to TKI, even in cell cultures prepared from fine needle aspiration specimens [35], has been shown to have a 60% positive predictive value of clinical response in the same patient and a 90% negative predictive value.

3.1.2. *Cabozantinib*

Cabozantinib approval was obtained following a phase III randomized, double-blind, placebo-controlled trial that enrolled 330 patients with progressive, metastatic or locally advanced MTC, in whom median progression-free survival increased significantly from 4.0 months in the placebo group to 11.2 months in the cabozantinib group [36]. The overall response rate was 28%. More than half of patients developed adverse effects such as diarrhea, stomatitis and palmo-plantar erythrodysesthesia. Other adverse effects were similar to those observed for vandetanib (nausea, abdominal pain, fatigue, hypertension). Hepatocytolysis, hyperbilirubinemia, neutropenia and thrombocytopenia were also encountered. Rare but severe adverse effects were gastrointestinal perforation and fistula and hemorrhage, also included on the black box warning. Thromboembolic events, osteonecrosis of the jaw and reversible posterior leukoencephalopathy syndrome were also mentioned. A total of 16% of patients discontinued treatment due to toxicity and 79% required dose reductions; 6% of patients experienced fatal adverse reactions. In view of major adverse effects, patients with a history of diverticulitis, chronic inflammatory gastrointestinal disease, active peptic ulcer, radiation to the neck or mediastinum as well as tumor invasion characteristics that may predispose to fistulas and hemorrhage need to be identified. A systematic review and meta-analysis on small-molecule TKI in patients with thyroid cancer published by Klein Hesselink et al. concluded that vandetanib and cabozantinib resulted in objective responses in 40% (95% CI 34–46%) and 27% (95% CI 22–32%) of patients with advanced MTC [37]. In clinical practice, response to cabozantinib was documented following a failed vandetanib treatment [38].

In conclusion, TKI vandetanib and cabozantinib have demonstrated important rates of disease control at the cost of significant drug toxicity. Still, TKIs are less toxic when compared to conventional cytotoxic agents. Further studies assessing the impact on overall survival for both agents are warranted, as previous studies failed to demonstrate prolonged survival. Head-to-head studies comparing the efficacy of the two drugs in patients with advanced MTC are lacking, therefore selection of one treatment over the other needs evaluation of potential risks and benefits for each patient. Factors that might influence the choice of TKI in patients with MTC are related to patient and drug characteristics, laboratory and cardiologic assessments, past medical history and concomitant medication. Cabozantinib is favored in patients with or at risk for long QT syndrome (baseline QTcF interval >450 ms), patients with uncorrected baseline dyselectrolitemia (hypocalcemia, hypomagnesemia or hypokalemia), patients unable or unwilling to protect from sun exposure or in the case of rapid disease progression. On the contrary, vandetanib should be firstly considered in patients with gastrointestinal comorbidities or tumors invading the trachea, esophagus, or major blood vessels because of the risk of perforation or fistula [39]. Concomitant use of a CYP3A4 inhibitor drug may increase the plasma concentration of cabozantinib, resulting in toxicity, whereas use of a CYP3A4 inducer may decrease the efficacy of vandetanib [32, 39]. Vandetanib may cause weight gain, whereas cabozantinib should be avoided in patients with low body mass index.

Several case reports indicated that both vandetanib and cabozatinib might successfully control ectopic Cushing's syndrome associated to MTC [40].

3.1.3. Sorafenib

Sorafenib, currently approved for the treatment of renal cell and hepatocellular carcinomas, constitutes first-line indication in advanced radioiodine-refractory differentiated thyroid carcinomas (DTCs). Reviewing retrospectively 13 patients with advanced MTC treated with sorafenib 400 mg twice daily, de Castroneves et al. observed stable disease in 10 (83.3%) patients [41]. A systematic review of sorafenib in metastatic thyroid cancer (both DTC and MTC) noticed an overall partial response rate of 22% for MTC patients, with only 6.5% having progressive disease, which suggests a reasonable clinical benefit [42]. However, treatment with sorafenib is associated with considerable toxicity, leading to highest rates of dose reduction or discontinuation [37].

3.1.4. Sunitinib

Sunitinib, available for gastrointestinal stromal tumors (GIST), renal cell carcinomas and pancreatic neuroendocrine tumors (pNET), was investigated in a small phase II study, and a response was objectivized in three of six (50%) patients with metastatic MTC and radiologically evaluable lesions, but more than 10% of treated patients experienced grade 3 or higher toxicities [43]. In a recent meta-analysis, encouraging results were obtained with sunitinib, with a clinical benefit in 43% of patients ($n = 36$) with advanced MTC [37].

3.1.5. Axitinib, motesanib, lenvatinib, ponatinib

Other kinase inhibitors have been investigated, with small trials showing variable results. *Axitinib* is an oral TKI that inhibits VEGFRs, c-KIT and PDGFR-β, approved for the treatment of renal carcinoma. A multicenter, open-label, phase II study examined the efficacy of axitinib in 60 patients with advanced or metastatic thyroid carcinoma of all histological subtypes [44]. Overall, 18% of patients with MTC presented partial response, with median progression-free survival of 18.1 months. Axitinib was relatively well tolerated, with the most common adverse event being hypertension. Another multicenter phase II study aimed at investigating the efficacy and tolerability of *motesanib* in 91 patients with locally advanced or metastatic, progressive or symptomatic MTC. Only two patients (2%) experienced a partial response, and stable disease was achieved in 74 patients (81%), lasting for 24 weeks or longer in 44 (48%) [45].

Ponatinib, a newer multi-kinase inhibitor used in the treatment of chronic myeloid leukemia and acute lymphoblastic leukemia, showed promising results in early trials, but it carries a black box warning due to a high rate of arterial thrombotic events.

A multi-kinase inhibitor targeting VEGFR-1-3, FGFR-1-4, RET, c-KIT and PDGFR-β is *lenvatinib*. Moreover, lenvatinib has been shown to be able to inhibit FGFR-1, thus targeting a pathway involved in resistance to VEGF-pathway inhibitors. In a phase II trial enrolling 59 patients with advanced MTC, an objective response rate was documented in 59%, stable disease was confirmed in 36% and a median progression-free survival of 13.3 months was reported [46].

Neither geftinib nor imatinib induced objective responses in patients with advanced, progressive MTC [37].

The response of individual cases to TKI could be subjected to influence by the expression of RET or RAS mutations in the primary tumor, and Mancikova et al. found that in contrast to RET-positive tumors, RAS-positive tumors express neither PDGFR-β nor MET and poorly express VEGFR-3 [47], thus suggesting that intracellular targets of TKI are expressed according to the presence of RAS mutations, a potentially useful information in the selection of patients receiving treatment with TKI.

Summary

In summary, TKI, specifically vandetanib and cabozantinib, demonstrated a response rate of 27–44% in randomized trials and meta-analyses, to support first-line therapeutic indication in the management of symptomatic or progressive MTC in patients with non-resectable or metastatic disease. Nevertheless, dose-dependent toxicity of these drugs is considerable, including gastrointestinal perforations, fistulas and hemorrhage for cabozantinib and prolongation of the QT interval, *torsades de points* and sudden death for vandetanib. Liver failure, pulmonary arterial hypertension and development of secondary malignancies have been reported. Apparently, regression or stabilization of skeletal metastases related to advanced MTC is weakly influenced by TKI, although cabozantinib may exert some activity against certain types of bone lesions [43]. Overall, the quality of life is markedly affected by TKI with adverse effects reported by 30–60% of patients and serious adverse events occurring in 2% of cases [48]. The evidence for sorafenib and sunitinib in MTC is not as strong, but small studies have demonstrated their efficacy. Other kinase inhibitors have shown variable results.

3.2. Mammalian target of rapamycin (mTOR) inhibitors

There is solid evidence that the PI3K/Akt pathway is extensively involved in cell growth, proliferation and survival of all types of thyroid tumors. The mTOR kinase is a component of the PI3K signaling pathway, and AKT/mTOR activation is demonstrated in DTC and MTC with AKT/mTOR immunostaining present in more than 50% of medullary carcinoma cells [48]. *In vitro* experiments showed oncogenic RET may regulate mTOR activity in patients with MTC. Moreover, low-concentration RET and mTOR inhibitors administered as a combination, to concomitantly target RET and mTOR, acted cooperatively in cell culture experiments [49]. Prospective phase II trials with everolimus, an mTOR inhibitor, in patients with advanced MTC reported promising results. In one small-sized study, stable disease was obtained in five of seven (71%) patients [50]. The most frequent side effects in everolimus trials were fatigue, mucositis and hypertriglyceridemia, but overall the drug was well tolerated. Further investigations are warranted to evaluate the efficacy of everolimus as monotherapy or combined with other targeted agents in patients with advanced MTCs. **Table 1** depicts relevant randomized and non-randomized studies on treatment with TKI and mTOR inhibitors in patients with MTC.

Author	Study design	Drug regimen	Objective partial response (PR)%	Stable disease (SD)%	Common adverse effects
Wells et al., 2010 [28]	Open-label, phase II trial	Vandetanib 300 mg/day	20	53	Diarrhea, rash, fatigue, nausea
Robinson et al., 2010 [34]	Open-label, single-arm trial	Vandetanib 100 mg/day	16	53	Diarrhea, fatigue, rash, constipation, anorexia, back pain, nausea, photosensitivity
Wells et al., 2012 [30]	Randomized, double-blind, placebo-controlled phase III trial	Vandetanib 300 mg/day	45	87	Diarrhea, rash, nausea, hypertension, headache
Chougnet et al., 2015 [51]	Retrospective cohort	Vandetanib 300 mg/day	20	55	Skin toxicity, diarrhea, asthenia
Kurzrock et al., 2011 [38]	Open-label, phase I dose-escalation study	Cabozantinib (maximum-tolerated dose = 175 mg/day)	29	41	Diarrhea, fatigue, decreased appetite, nausea, palmar-plantar erythrodysesthesia (PPE), rash, hepatocytolysis
Elisei et al., 2013 [36]	Randomized, double-blind, placebo-controlled phase III trial	Cabozantinib 140 mg/day	28	47.3 (progression-free at 1 year)	Diarrhea, decreased weight and appetite, PPE, nausea, fatigue
Capdevila et al., 2012 [52]	Retrospective longitudinal study	Sorafenib 2 × 400 mg/day	47	40	PPE, diarrhea, rash, asthenia, anorexia, stomatitis, hypertension, abdominal pain
de Castroneves et al., 2016 [41]	Retrospective, longitudinal study	Sorafenib 2 × 400 mg/day	0	83.3	PPE, weight loss, fatigue
De Souza et al., 2010 [53]	Nonrandomized, open-label, phase II study	Sunitinib 50 mg/day, 4/2 week schedule	35	57	Fatigue, lymphopenia, neutropenia, nausea, diarrhea, mucositis, PPE

Author	Study design	Drug regimen	Objective partial response (PR)%	Stable disease (SD)%	Common adverse effects
Carr et al., 2010 [19]	Non-randomized, open-label, phase II study	Sunitinib 37.5 mg/day	50	71	Fatigue, diarrhea, PPE, neutropenia
Lim et al., 2013 [54]	Non-randomized, open-label, single-arm phase II study	Everolimus 10 mg/day	0	100	Mucositis, anorexia, hepatocytolysis
Schneider et al., 2015 [50]	Non-randomized, open-label, single arm phase II study	Everolimus 10 mg/day	0	71	Mucositis, fatigue, hypertriglyceridemia

Table 1. Randomized and non-randomized studies on tyrosine kinase inhibitors (TKIs) and mammalian target of rapamycin (mTOR) inhibitors in advanced medullary thyroid carcinoma (MTC).

3.3. Somatostatin analogues (SSA)

Medullary thyroid cancers are neuroendocrine tumor (NET) that expresses cell surface somatostatin receptors (SSTRs) in less than 40% of cases; however, these cases may respond favorably to SSA treatment. *Octreotide* and *lanreotide*, the currently available SSA with high affinity for SSTR2 and SSTR5, may be helpful in controlling symptoms in advanced MTC, but they do not appear to significantly affect tumor burden or disease course. Indeed, SSA should be considered in case of flushing and diarrhea, if other drugs are ineffective [55].

3.4. Peptide receptor radiation therapy (PRRT)

There is limited experience with PRRT targeting SSTR2 and cholecystokinin (CCK) receptors A and B, which are expressed by medullary carcinomas, in patients with advanced, metastatic MTC [55]. A phase II trial evaluating systemic ^{90}Y-DOTATOC treatment in selected patients with stage IV MTC showed encouraging response and survival rates: 29% of the 31 study patients experienced reduction of serum calcitonin levels and had a significantly longer median survival from onset of treatment in comparison to non-responders (i.e. 74.5 months vs. 10.8 months); however, 13% of patients developed serious hematological toxicity, and 23% developed nephrotoxicity [56].

One study evaluated CCK-B/gastrin receptor-based PPRT and included eight patients with advanced MTC to whom the radioligand ^{90}Y-DTPT-D-Glu-minigastrin was administered. Of all, two patients developed partial remission and four had stable disease; severe adverse events were encountered, with one patient developing chronic myelogenous leukemia and another patient developing chronic renal failure [57]. Treatment with ^{177}Lu-DOTATATE reached similar results with three of nine patients having partial response and other three presenting stable disease [58]. Current guidelines suggest that PRRT should be taken into account in well-selected cases [1].

3.5. Experimental therapies

A number of other treatments are in the early phases of development. *Pre-targeted radio immunotherapy* with bi-specific monoclonal antibody (BsMAb) and ^{131}I-labeled bivalent hapten has shown positive results in advanced, progressive MTC, but prospective, randomized trials comparing this therapy to other therapies or placebo are needed [1].

Vaccination with autologous dendritic cells pulsed with MTC-specific antigens (CEA or calcitonin) has been attempted, inducing specific immunoreactivity and leading to a clinical response in three of seven patients in one small study [59].

Combination therapy of a TKI (e.g. vandetanib) and a protease inhibitor (bortezomib) appears to induce synergistic effects in cell culture experiments [60], being under evaluation in human trials.

Treatment with *plitidepsin*, an antibiotic that can induce tumor apoptosis, has been used in 16 subjects with unresectable MTC in a phase II trial, with modest clinical benefits and manageable toxicity [61].

The HIV-protease inhibitor *nelfinavir* has been shown to decrease RET expression and induce apoptosis in medullary thyroid cancer cells, but clinical studies are needed to prove its efficacy in treating MTC [62].

Metformin is an anti-diabetic drug that seems to inhibit cancer cell viability through the inhibition of mTOR, an effect that was also observed in MTC cell lines [63]. Metformin is under testing in clinical trials in combination with other agents.

AZD 1480, a JAK 1,2 inhibitor, was shown to block proliferation and tumor growth of RET-activated thyroid cancer cells, supporting its use in advanced MCT; however, further research is needed [64].

Enzastaurin is a protein kinase C inhibitor that has been shown to produce tumor cell apoptosis and suppress tumor-induced angiogenesis. Its value in the treatment of advanced MTC is under investigation.

Epigenetic drugs, that target DNA methylation and acetylation, are regarded with increasing interest. Histone deacetylases regulate gene expression and cell cycle, proliferation and apoptosis. *Histone deacetylase inhibitors* have been shown to suppress proliferation of thyroid cancer cells, but evidence is based on small studies [48]. Combined targeted therapy is also currently under investigation.

3.6. Treatment of hormonally active metastases

Co-secretion of hormones other than calcitonin can often be observed in medullary carcinoma. The prevalence of diarrhea is related to tumor volume. From a pathogenic viewpoint, diarrhea is due to either hypersecretory or increased gastrointestinal motility. Treatment includes anti-motility drugs (loperamide, diphenoxylate/atropine, codeine) and, in selected cases, SSA. When these therapies are insufficient, palliative surgery or chemoembolization may be helpful.

In cases of ectopic CRH or ACTH syndromes associated with unresectable MTC, steroidogenesis inhibitors and ultimately bilateral adrenalectomy should be considered.

4. Conclusions

The treatment of residual or recurrent medullary thyroid carcinoma (MTC) continues to be a challenge. Although surgery remains the mainstay of therapy, it can be curative only in the early stages of the disease. External beam radiotherapy and cytotoxic chemotherapy with dacarbazine and doxorubicin-based regimens may be useful in select patients, but with little or no impact on overall survival. In recent years, there has been significant progress in the treatment of advanced, metastatic MTC. The use of tyrosine kinase inhibitors (TKIs), cabozantinib and vandetanib, as first-line agents for symptomatic metastatic and progressive MTC has significantly improved progression-free survival, showing high rates of partial response and disease stabilization; however, prolonged survival has not been confirmed yet. The search continues for kinase inhibitors that can be used in patients who are unresponsive or develop resistance to existing drugs. Ongoing clinical trials evaluate additional agents that might significantly impact future management of the disease.

Acknowledgements

This work was supported by CNCSIS grant PN-II-ID-PCE-2011-3-0879 and Iuliu Hatieganu University of Medicine and Pharmacy internal grant 4944/20/08/03.2016.

Author details

Ana Valea and Carmen Emanuela Georgescu*

*Address all correspondence to: cgeorgescu@umfcluj.ro

Department of Endocrinology, Iuliu Hațieganu University of Medicine and Pharmacy Cluj-Napoca, Cluj-Napoca, Romania

References

[1] Wells SA Jr, Asa SL, Dralle H, Elisei R, Evans DB, Gagel RF, Lee N, Machens A, Moley JF, Pacini F, Raue F, Frank-Raue K, Robinson B, Rosenthal MS, Santoro M, Schlumberger M, Shah M, Waguespack SG. Revised American Thyroid Association guidelines for the management of medullary thyroid carcinoma. Thyroid. 2015;25(6):567–610. DOI: 10.1089/thy.2014.0335.

[2] Moo-Young TA, Traugott AL, Moley JF. Sporadic and familial medullary thyroid carcinoma: state of the art. Surg Clin North Am. 2009;89(5):1193–204. DOI: 10.1016/j.suc.2009.06.021.

[3] Leboulleux S, Baudin E, Travagli JP, Schlumberger M. Medullary thyroid carcinoma. Clin Endocrinol. 2004;61(3):299–310. DOI: 10.1111/j.1365-2265.2004.02037.

[4] Costante G, Durante C, Francis Z, Schlumberger M, Filetti S. Determination of calcitonin levels in C-cell disease: clinical interest and potential pitfalls. Nat Clin Pract Endocrinol Metab. 2009;5(1):35–44. DOI: 10.1038/ncpendmet1023.

[5] Sovrea AS, Dronca E, Galatâr M, Radian S, Vornicescu C, Georgescu C. Diagnostic correlation between RET proto-oncogene mutation, imaging techniques, biochemical markers and morphological examination in MEN2A syndrome: case report and literature review. Rom J Morphol Embryol. 2014;55(2):389–400.

[6] Moley JF. Medullary thyroid carcinoma: management of lymph node metastases. J Natl Compr Canc Netw. 2010;8(5):549–556.

[7] Trimboli P, Giovanella L, Valabrega S, Andrioli M, Baldelli R, Cremonini N, Rossi F, Guidobaldi L, Barnabei A, Rota F, Paoloni A, Rizza L, Fattorini G, Latini M, Ventura C, Falasca P, Orlandi F, Crescenzi A, D'Ambrosio F, Cantisani V, Romanelli F, Negro R, Saggiorato E, Appetecchia M. Ultrasound features of medullary thyroid carcinoma correlate with cancer aggressiveness: a retrospective multicenter study. J Exp Clin Cancer Res. 2014;33:87. DOI: 10.1186/s13046-014-0087-4.

[8] Mayr B, Brabant G, von zur Mühlen A. Incidental detection of familial medullary thyroid carcinoma by calcitonin screening for nodular thyroid disease. Eur J Endocrinol. 1999;141(3):286–289. DOI: 10.1530/eje.0.1410286.

[9] Machens A, Schneyer U, Holzhausen HJ, Dralle H. Prospects of remission in medullary thyroid carcinoma according to basal calcitonin levels. J Clin Endocrinol Metab. 2005;90(4):2029–2034. DOI: 10.1210/jc.2004-1836.

[10] Machens A, Dralle H. Biomarker-based risk stratification for previously untreated medullary thyroid cancer. J Clin Endocrinol Metab 2010;95(6):2655–2663. DOI: 10.1210/jc.2009-2368.

[11] Trimboli P, Cremonini N, Ceriani L, Saggiorato E, Guidobaldi L, Romanelli F, Ventura C, Laurenti O, Messuti I, Solaroli E, Madaio R, Bongiovanni M, Orlandi F, Crescenzi A,

Valabrega S, Giovanella L. Calcitonin measurement in aspiration needle washout fluids has higher sensitivity than cytology in detecting medullary thyroid cancer: a retrospective multicentre study. Clin Endocrinol. 2014;80(1):135–140. DOI: 10.1111/cen.12234.

[12] Elisei R, Romei C, Cosci B, Agate L, Bottici V, Molinaro E, Sculli M, Miccoli P, Basolo F, Grasso L, Pacini F, Pinchera A. RET genetic screening in patients with medullary thyroid cancer and their relatives: experience with 807 individuals at one center. J Clin Endocrinol Metab. 2007;92(12):4725–4729. DOI: 10.1210/jc.2007-1005.

[13] Machens A, Hinze R, Thomusch O, Dralle H. Pattern of nodal metastasis for primary and reoperative thyroid cancer. World J Surg. 2002;26(1):22–28. DOI: 10.1007/s00268-001-0176-3.

[14] Modigliani E, Cohen R, Campos JM, Conte-Devolx B, Maes B, Boneu A, Schlumberger M, Bigorgne JC, Dumontier P, Leclerc L, Corcuff B, Guilhem I. Prognostic factors for survival and for biochemical cure in medullary thyroid carcinoma: results in 899 patients. Clin Endocrinol. 1998;48(3):265–273. DOI: 10.1046/j.1365-2265.1998.00392.x.

[15] Moley JF, DeBenedetti MK. Patterns of nodal metastases in palpable medullary thyroid carcinoma: recommendations for extent of node dissection. Ann Surg. 1999;229(6):880–887.

[16] Meijer JA, le Cessie S, van den Hout WB, Kievit J, Schoones JW, Romijn JA, Smit JW. Calcitonin and carcinoembryonic antigen doubling times as prognostic factors in medullary thyroid carcinoma: a structured meta-analysis. Clin Endocrinol. 2010;72(4):534–542. DOI: 10.1111/j.1365-2265.2009.03666.x.

[17] Brierley J, Tsang R, Simpson WJ, Gospodarowicz M, Sutcliffe S, Panzarella T. Medullary thyroid cancer: analyses of survival and prognostic factors and the role of radiation therapy in local control. Thyroid. 1996;6(4):305–310.

[18] Schwartz DL, Rana V, Shaw S, Yazbeck C, Ang KK, Morrison WH, Rosenthal DI, Hoff A, Evans DB, Clayman GL, Garden AS, Sherman SI. Postoperative radiotherapy for advanced medullary thyroid cancer-local disease control in the modern era. Head Neck. 2008;30(7):883–888. DOI: 10.1002/hed.20791.

[19] Martinez SR, Beal SH, Chen A, Chen SL, Schneider PD. Adjuvant external beam radiation for medullary thyroid carcinoma. J Surg Oncol. 2010;102(2):175–178. DOI: 10.1002/jso.21557.

[20] Meijer JA, Bakker LE, Valk GD, de Herder WW, de Wilt JH, Netea-Maier RT, Schaper N, Fliers E, Lips P, Plukker JT, Links TP, Smit JA. Radioactive iodine in the treatment of medullary thyroid carcinoma: a controlled multicenter study. Eur J Endocrinol. 2013;168(5):779–786. DOI: 10.1002/jso.21557.

[21] Tuttle RM, Haddad RI, Ball DW, Byrd D, Dickson P, Duh QY, Ehya H, Haymart M, Hoh C, Hunt JP, Iagaru A, Kandeel F, Kopp P, Lamonica DM, Lydiatt WM, McCaffrey J, Moley JF, Parks L, Raeburn CD, Ridge JA, Ringel MD, Scheri RP, Shah JP, Sherman

SI, Sturgeon C, Waguespack SG, Wang TN, Wirth LJ, Hoffmann KG, Hughes M. Thyroid carcinoma, version 2.2014. J Natl Compr Canc Netw. 2014;12(12):1671–1680.

[22] Nakayama Y, Inoue Y, Nagashima N, Katsuki T, Matsumoto K, Kadowaki K, Shibao K, Tsurudome Y, Hirata K, Sako T, Nagata N, Itoh H. Expression levels of thymidine phosphorylase (TP) and dihydropyrimidine dehydrogenase (DPD) in patients with gastrointestinal cancer. Anticancer Res. 2005;25(6A):3755–61.

[23] Halperin DM, Phan AT, Hoff AO, Hoff AO, Aaron M, Yao JC, Hoff PM. A phase I study of imatinib, dacarbazine, and capecitabine in advanced endocrine cancers. BMC Cancer. 2014;14:561. DOI: 10.1186/1471-2407-14-561.

[24] Lacin S, Esin E, Karakas Y, Yalcin S. Metastatic medullary thyroid cancer: a dramatic response to a systemic chemotherapy (temozolomide and capecitabine) regimen. Onco Targets Ther. 2015;8:1039–1042. DOI: 10.2147/OTT.S82906.

[25] Agrawal N, Jiao Y, Sausen M, Leary R, Bettegowda C, Roberts NJ, Bhan S, Ho AS, Khan Z, Bishop J, Westra WH, Wood LD, Hruban RH, Tufano RP, Robinson B, Dralle H, Toledo SP, Toledo RA, Morris LG, Ghossein RA, Fagin JA, Chan TA, Velculescu VE, Vogelstein B, Kinzler KW, Papadopoulos N, Nelkin BD, Ball DW. Exomic sequencing of medullary thyroid cancer reveals dominant and mutually exclusive oncogenic mutations in RET and RAS. J Clin Endocrinol Metab. 2013;98(2):E364–E369. DOI: 10.1210/jc.2012-2703.

[26] Fallahi P, Di Bari F, Ferrari SM, et al. Selective use of vandetanib in the treatment of thyroid cancer. Drug Des Devel Ther. 2015;9:3459–3470. DOI: 10.2147/DDDT.S72495.

[27] Roy S, Narang BK, Rastogi SK, Rawal RK. A novel multiple tyrosine-kinase targeted agent to explore the future perspectives of anti-angiogenic therapy for the treatment of multiple solid tumors: cabozantinib. Anticancer Agents Med Chem. 2015;15(1):37–47. DOI: 10.2174/1871520614666140902153840.

[28] Wells SA Jr, Gosnell JE, Gagel RF, et al. Vandetanib for the treatment of patients with locally advanced or metastatic hereditary medullary thyroid cancer. J Clin Oncol. 2010;28(5):767–772. DOI: 10.1200/JCO.2009.23.6604.

[29] Fox E, Widemann BC, Chuk MK, et al. Vandetanib in children and adolescents with multiple endocrine neoplasia type 2B associated medullary thyroid carcinoma. Clin Cancer Res. 2013;19(15):4239–4248. DOI: 10.1158/1078-0432.CCR-13-0071.

[30] Wells SA Jr, Robinson BG, Gagel RF, Dralle H, Fagin JA, Santoro M, Baudin E, Elisei R, Jarzab B, Vasselli JR, Read J, Langmuir P, Ryan AJ, Schlumberger MJ. Vandetanib in patients with locally advanced or metastatic medullary thyroid cancer: a randomized, double-blind phase II trial. J Clin Oncol. 2012;30(2):134–141. DOI: 10.1200/JCO. 2011.35.5040.

[31] Werner RA, Schmid JS, Muegge DO, Lückerath K, Higuchi T, Hänscheid H, Grelle I, Reiners C, Herrmann K, Buck AK, Lapa C. Prognostic value of serum tumor markers

in medullary thyroid cancer patients undergoing vandetanib treatment. Medicine (Baltimore). 2015;94(45):e2016. DOI: 10.1097/MD.0000000000002016.

[32] Cabanillas ME, Hu MI, Jimenez C. Medullary thyroid cancer in the era of tyrosine kinase inhibitors: to treat or not to treat-and with which drug-those are the questions. J Clin Endocrinol Metab. 2014;99(12):4390–4396. DOI: 10.1210/jc.2014-2811.

[33] Chrisoulidou A, Mandanas S, Margaritidou E, Mathiopoulou L, Boudina M, Georgopoulos K, Pazaitou-Panayiotou K. Treatment compliance and severe adverse events limit the use of tyrosine kinase inhibitors in refractory thyroid cancer. Onco Targets Ther. 2015;8:2435–2442. DOI: 10.2147/OTT.S86322.

[34] Robinson BG, Paz-Ares L, Krebs A, Vasselli J, Haddad R. Vandetanib (100 mg) in patients with locally advanced or metastatic hereditary medullary thyroid cancer. J Clin Endocrinol Metab. 2010;95(6):26642671. DOI: 10.1210/jc.2009-2461.

[35] Antonelli A, Ferrari SM, Fallahi P, Berti P, Materazzi G, Marchetti I, Ugolini C, Basolo F, Miccoli P, Ferrannini E. Evaluation of the sensitivity to chemotherapeutics or thiazolidinediones of primary anaplastic thyroid cancer cells obtained by fine-needle aspiration. Eur J Endocrinol. 2008;159(3):283–291. DOI: 10.1530/EJE-08-0190.

[36] Elisei R, Schlumberger MJ, Müller SP, Schöffski P, Brose MS, Shah MH, Licitra L, Jarzab B, Medvedev V, Kreissl MC, Niederle B, Cohen EE, Wirth LJ, Ali H, Hessel C, Yaron Y, Ball D, Nelkin B, Sherman SI. Cabozantinib in progressive medullary thyroid cancer. J Clin Oncol. 2013;31(29):3639–3646. DOI: 10.1200/JCO.2012.48.4659

[37] Klein Hesselink EN, Steenvoorden D, Kapiteijn E, Corssmit EP, van der Horst-Schrivers AN, Lefrandt JD, Links TP, Dekkers OM. Therapy of endocrine disease: response and toxicity of small-molecule tyrosine kinase inhibitors in patients with thyroid carcinoma: a systematic review and meta-analysis. Eur J Endocrinol. 2015;172(5):R215–R225. DOI: 10.1530/EJE-14-0788.

[38] Kurzrock R, Sherman SI, Ball DW, Forastiere AA, Cohen RB, Mehra R, Pfister DG, Cohen EE, Janisch L, Nauling F, Hong DS, Ng CS, Ye L, Gagel RF, Frye J, Müller T, Ratain MJ, Salgia R. Activity of XL184 (cabozantinib), an oral tyrosine kinase inhibitor, in patients with medullary thyroid cancer. J Clin Oncol. 2011;29(19):2660–2666. DOI: 10.1200/JCO.2010.32.4145.

[39] Weitzman SP, Cabanillas ME. The treatment landscape in thyroid cancer: a focus on cabozantinib. Cancer Manag Res. 2015;7:265–278. DOI: 10.2147/CMAR.S68373.

[40] Baudry C, Paepegaey AC, Groussin L. Reversal of Cushing's syndrome by vandetanib in medullary thyroid carcinoma. N Engl J Med. 2013;369(6):584–586. DOI: 10.1056/NEJMc1301428.

[41] De Castroneves LA, Negrão MV, de Freitas RM, Papadia C, Lima JV Jr, Fukushima JT, Simão EF, Kulcsar MA, Tavares MR, Jorge AA, de Castro G Jr, Hoff PM, Hoff AO.

Sorafenib for the treatment of progressive metastatic medullary thyroid cancer: efficacy and safety analysis. Thyroid. 2016;26(3):414–419. DOI: 10.1089/thy.2015.0334.

[42] Thomas L, Lai SY, Dong W, Feng L, Dadu R, Regone RM, Cabanillas ME. Sorafenib in metastatic thyroid cancer: a systematic review. Oncologist. 2014;19(3):251–258. DOI: 10.1634/theoncologist.2013-0362.

[43] Carr LL, Mankoff DA, Goulart BH, Eaton KD, Capell PT, Kell EM, Bauman JE, Martins RG. Phase II study of daily sunitinib in FDG-PET-positive, iodine-refractory differentiated thyroid cancer and metastatic medullary carcinoma of the thyroid with functional imaging correlation. Clin Cancer Res. 2010;16(21):5260–5268. DOI: 10.1158/1078-0432.CCR-10-0994.

[44] Cohen EE, Rosen LS, Vokes EE, Kies MS, Forastiere AA, Worden FP, Kane MA, Sherman E, Kim S, Bycott P, Tortorici M, Shalinsky DR, Liau KF, Cohen RB. Axitinib is an active treatment for all histologic subtypes of advanced thyroid cancer: results from a phase II study. J Clin Oncol. 2008;26(29):4708–4713. DOI: 10.1200/JCO.2007.15.9566.

[45] Schlumberger M, Elisei R, Bastholt L, Wirth LJ, Martins RG, Locati LD, Jarzab B, Pacini F, Daumerie C, Droz JP, Eschenberg MJ, Sun YN, Juan T, Stepan DE, Sherman SI. Phase II study of safety and efficacy of motesanib in patients with progressive or symptomatic, advanced or metastatic medullary thyroid cancer. J Clin Oncol. 2009;27(23):3794–3801. DOI: 10.1200/JCO.2008.18.7815.

[46] Schlumberger M, Jarzab B, Cabanillas ME, Robinson B, Pacini F, Ball DW, McCaffrey J, Newbold K, Allison R, Martins RG, Licitra LF, Shah MH, Bodenner D, Elisei R, Burmeister L, Funahashi Y, Ren M, O'Brien JP, Sherman SI. A phase II trial of the multitargeted tyrosine kinase inhibitor Lenvatinib (E7080) in advanced medullary thyroid cancer. Clin Cancer Res. 2016;22(1):44–53. DOI: 10.1158/1078-0432.CCR-15-1127.

[47] Mancikova V, Inglada-Pérez L, Curras-Freixes M, de Cubas AA, Gómez Á, Letón R, Kersten I, Leandro-García LJ, Comino-Méndez I, Apellaniz-Ruiz M, Sánchez L, Cascón A, Sastre-Marcos J, García JF, Rodríguez-Antona C, Robledo M. VEGF, VEGFR3, and PDGFRB protein expression is influenced by RAS mutations in medullary thyroid carcinoma. Thyroid. 2014;24(8):1251–1255. DOI: 10.1089/thy.2013.0579.

[48] Links TP, Verbeek HH, Hofstra RM, Plukker JT. Progressive metastatic medullary thyroid carcinoma: first- and second-line strategies. Eur J Endocrinol. 2015;172(6):R241–R251. DOI: 10.1530/EJE-14-0726.

[49] Gild ML, Landa I, Ryder M, Ghossein RA, Knauf JA, Fagin JA. Targeting mTOR in RET mutant medullary and differentiated thyroid cancer cells. Endocr Relat Cancer. 2013;20(5):659–667. DOI: 10.1530/ERC-13-0085.

[50] Schneider TC, de Wit D, Links TP, van Erp NP, van der Hoeven JJ, Gelderblom H, van Wezel T, van Eijk R, Morreau H, Guchelaar HJ, Kapiteijn E. Beneficial effects of the

mTOR inhibitor everolimus in patients with advanced medullary thyroid carcinoma: subgroup results of a phase II trial. Int J Endocrinol. 2015;2015:348124. DOI: 10.1155/2015/348124.

[51] Chougnet CN, Borget I, Leboulleux S, de la Fouchardiere C, Bonichon F, Criniere L, Niccoli P, Bardet S, Schneegans O, Zanetta S, Schvartz C, Drui D, Chauffert B, Rohmer V, Schlumberger M. Vandetanib for the treatment of advanced medullary thyroid cancer outside a clinical trial: results from a French cohort. Thyroid. 2015;25(4):386–391. DOI: 10.1089/thy.2014.0361.

[52] Capdevila J, Iglesias L, Halperin I, Segura A, Martínez-Trufero J, Vaz MÁ, Corral J, Obiols G, Grande E, Grau JJ, Tabernero J. Sorafenib in metastatic thyroid cancer. Endocr Relat Cancer. 2012;19(2):209–216. DOI: 10.1530/ERC-11-0351.

[53] De Souza JA, Busaidy N, Zimrin A, Seiwert TY, Villaflor VM, Poluru KB, Reddy PL, Nam J, Vokes EE, Cohen EE. Phase II trial of sunitinib in medullary thyroid cancer (MTC). J Clin Oncol (Meeting Abstracts). 2010;28:5504.

[54] Lim SM, Chang H, Yoon MJ, Hong YK, Kim H, Chung WY, Park CS, Nam KH, Kang SW, Kim MK, Kim SB, Lee SH, Kim HG, Na II, Kim YS, Choi MY, Kim JG, Park KU, Yun HJ, Kim JH, Cho BC. A multicenter, phase II trial of everolimus in locally advanced or metastatic thyroid cancer of all histologic subtypes. Ann Oncol. 2013;24(12):3089–3094. DOI: 10.1093/annonc/mdt379.

[55] Maxwell JE, Sherman SK, O'Dorisio TM, Howe JR. Medical management of metastatic medullary thyroid cancer. Cancer. 2014;120(21):3287–3301. DOI: 10.1002/cncr.28858.

[56] Iten F, Müller B, Schindler C, Rochlitz C, Oertli D, Mäcke HR, Müller-Brand J, Walter MA. Response to [90yttrium-Dota]-Toc treatment is associated with long-term survival benefit in metastasized medullary thyroid cancer: a phase II clinical trial. Clin Cancer Res. 2007;13(22 Pt 1):6696–6702. DOI: 10.1158/1078-0432.CCR-07-0935.

[57] Behe M, Behr TM. Cholecystokinin-B (Cck-B)/gastrin receptor targeting peptides for staging and therapy of medullary thyroid cancer and other Cck-B receptor expressing malignancies. Semin Nucl Med. 2002;66(6):399–418. DOI: 10.1053/snuc.2002.31028.

[58] Vaisman F, de Castro PH, Lopes FP, Kendler DB, Pessoa CH, Bulzico DA, de Carvalho Leal D, Vilhena B, Vaisman M, Carneiro M, Corbo R. Is there a role for peptide receptor radionuclide therapy in medullary thyroid cancer? Clin Nucl Med. 2015;40(2):123–127. DOI: 10.1097/RLU.0000000000000628.

[59] Schott M, Seissler J, Lettmann M, Fouxon V, Scherbaum WA, Feldkamp J. Immunotherapy for medullary thyroid carcinoma by dendritic cell vaccination. J Clin Endocrinol Metab. 2001;86(10):4965–4969.

[60] Cascone T, Morelli MP, Morgillo F, Kim WY, Rodolico G, Pepe S, Tortora G, Berrino L, Lee HY, Heymach JV, Ciardiello F. Synergistic anti-proliferative and pro-apoptotic activity of combined therapy with bortezomib, a proteasome inhibitor, with anti-

epidermal growth factor receptor (EGFR) drugs in human cancer cells. J Cell Physiol. 2008;217(1):290. DOI: 10.1002/jcp.21444.

[61] Baudin E, Droz JP, Paz-Ares L, van Oosterom AT, Cullell-Young M, Schlumberger M. Phase II study of plitidepsin 3-hour infusion every 2 weeks in patients with unresectable advanced medullary thyroid carcinoma. Am J Clin Oncol. 2010;33(1):83–88. DOI: 10.1097/COC.0b013e31819fdf5e.

[62] Kushchayeva Y, Jensen K, Recupero A, Costello J, Patel A, Klubo-Gwiezdzinska J, Boyle L, Burman K, Vasko V. The HIV protease inhibitor nelfinavir down-regulates RET signaling and induces apoptosis in medullary thyroid cancer cells. J Clin Endocrinol Metab. 2014;99(5):734–745. DOI: 10.1210/jc.2013-3369.

[63] Klubo-Gwiezdzinska J, Jensen K, Costello J, Costello J, Patel A, Hoperia V, Bauer A, Burman KD, Wartofsky L, Vasko V. Metformin inhibits growth and decreases resistance to anoikis in medullary thyroid cancer cells. Endocr Relat Cancer. 2012;19(3):447–456. DOI: 10.1530/ERC-12-0046.

[64] Couto JP, Almeida A, Daly L, Sobrinho-Simões M, Bromberg JF, Soares P. AZD1480 blocks growth and tumorigenesis of RET-activated thyroid cancer cell lines. PLoS One. 2012;7:4686. DOI: 10.1371/journal.pone.0046869.

Chapter 11

Management of Rare Thyroid Malignancies

Moustafa Mourad, David Chan,
Sameep Kadakia and Yadranko Ducic

Additional information is available at the end of the chapter

http://dx.doi.org/10.5772/64141

Abstract

The purpose of this chapter is a focused analysis and review of rare thyroid malignancies including anaplastic thyroid cancer (ATC), medullary thyroid cancer (MTC), primary thyroid lymphoma (PTL), and primary thyroid sarcoma (PTS). The focus will be on the epidemiology, risk factors, workup, and a contemporary review of management of these rare entities.

Keywords: anaplastic thyroid cancer, medullary thyroid cancer, thyroid lymphoma, thyroid sarcoma

1. Introduction

The majority of thyroid neoplasms are well-differentiated lesions that have been extensively studied and reported in the literature with regard to diagnosis and management [1, 2]. While most patients with thyroid malignancy typically fall in to the above-mentioned category, few patients may carry diagnoses of rare thyroid cancers that are not as widely researched. Owing to the dearth of literature on these rare thyroid malignancies, the consensus for management is often unclear and highly debated. As head and neck oncologists should be well versed in the treatment options for these uncommon malignancies, this chapter seeks to coalesce the literature in hopes of providing practitioners with an overview of these challenging pathologies. The chapter will focus on the analysis of anaplastic thyroid cancer (ATC), medullary thyroid cancer (MTC), primary thyroid lymphoma (PTL), and primary thyroid sarcoma (PTS). In the following sections, each of these entities will be discussed beginning with epidemiology and risk factors progressing to work up and management.

2. Anaplastic thyroid cancer

ATC is among the most aggressive and uniformly fatal malignancies afflicting the human species. It is extremely rare, comprising approximately 2–5% of all thyroid malignancies [3–5]. The annual incidence of ATC is one to two cases per million. The majority of patients, greater than 90%, are over the age of 50 [5–7]. Females are more commonly affected than males, with a comparison ratio of approximately 1.5:1 [6, 8]. A large majority of ATC occurs in conjunction with other thyroid cancers and is theorized to be a degeneration of well-differentiated carcinomas [1, 8].

Few patients survive beyond 6 months after initial presentation, with a median survival of 2–12 months [1, 3, 4, 6, 9]. At present, it is reported that more than 50% of patients with ATC have distant metastases [10]. Patients typically present with a rapidly enlarging neck mass, often stating that the neck mass was stable for a significant period of time before the period of rapid growth. Not uncommonly, patients complain of pain, dysphonia, and difficulty breathing as the mass grows and begins to invade the laryngopharyngeal framework [2]. Death from ATC is typically caused by compression of the great vessels, namely the superior vena cava, or asphyxiation from airway compromise [2].

As with any rapidly enlarging neck mass, airway stability is of primary importance and a stable airway should be established even prior to diagnosis if the patient is unstable. In the event the patient has a stable airway, following thorough examination including nasopharyngolaryngoscopy, imaging should be obtained to evaluate the extent and radiographic characteristics of the mass. Computed tomography (CT) is typically the initial imaging study of choice, however, magnetic resonance imaging (MRI) can be obtained to determine the extent of soft tissue and cartilage involvement. Following imaging, tissue diagnosis can be established with fine-needle aspiration (FNA); however, at times a larger tissue sample may be needed to rule out lymphoma [2]. Pathology of ATC typically shows gross macroscopic involvement of surrounding tissue along with areas of florid necrosis. A population of undifferentiated cells is typically seen, along with a heterogeneous population of polygonal, spindle, and giant cells. As cells are poorly differentiated, no thyroglubin production or thyroid hormone receptors are found on further evaluation [1]. After a diagnosis of malignancy is established, practitioners may opt to pursue a fludeoxyglucose (^{18}F-FDG) positron emission tomography (PET) scan or whole body CT scan to evaluate for metastases. Staging of ATC is based on its extension from the thyroid gland and distal metastases. All lesions are considered stage 4; stage 4A for lesions within the thyroid gland without distal spread, stage 4B for lesions that have grown outside the thyroid without distal spread, and stage 4C for any lesion that has distal metastases [11].

The management of ATC poses a number of challenges for the practitioner owing to the advanced nature of the malignancy at diagnosis, short survival time, and often severe functional impairment. Of paramount importance is an understanding of the patient's desires and the goals of care. Treatment options include radiation, surgery, chemotherapy, or a combination. Commonly, patients require tracheostomy and enteral feeding support with a gastrostomy tube [2, 6]. Routine tracheostomy is not advocated and the decision is highly based on the patients desire to undergo a surgical airway procedure in lieu of potential changes in the quality of life [12, 13]. Chemotherapeutic regimens have not been uniformly accepted and as such, there is no standard regimen. In recent studies, however, there have been promising results with newer drug modalities. The combination of carfilzomib, a proteasome inhibitor, and CUDC-101, a histone deacetylase, have been shown to induce apoptosis in anaplastic thyroid cancer cells [14]. Another recent study has shown positive results through the use of doxorubicin nanospheres combined with extracorporeal shock wave therapy [15].

The role of surgery is controversial. In conjunction with the American Thyroid Association, Smallridge et al. report that surgery can be considered with locoregional disease; however, given the lack of survival benefit, they recommend against tumor debulking [16]. Disease extending beyond the thyroid gland has typically represented unresectable disease [17–22].

In a recent study by Brown and Ducic, 16 patients with extrathyroidal ATC were evaluated for long-term survival following complete surgical resection. These patients had stage 4B ATC without evidence of distal metastases, and no disease extension beyond the carotid arteries. Twelve patients required total laryngectomy, four required tracheal resection, and six required cervical esophagectomy. Twelve out of 16 patients also required bilateral complete neck dissection for clinically evident disease. Postoperatively, surgical patients underwent external beam radiation. Of the 16 patients that underwent surgery with adjuvant radiation, 50% had long-term disease free survival ranging from 9 months to 8 years. Six patients died from metastatic disease while one died from a myocardial infarction. Based on their findings, Brown and Ducic believe that specific patients with extrathyroidal ATC that does not extend lateral to the carotid artery and without distal metastases may be suitable surgical candidates for complete resection followed by radiation therapy [23].

Regardless of treatment modality chosen, resectability of locoregional cancer, localized intrathyroidal disease, and absence of distal metastases are associated with a more favorable prognosis [24–26].

Anaplastic thyroid cancer is an aggressive disease with a high mortality rate. Early detection with thoughtful planning involving the patient's family is the cornerstone of managing this challenging malignancy.

3. Primary thyroid sarcoma

PTS is an extremely rare entity with an incidence no higher than 1.5% [27–29]. The rarity of PTS has led to a substantial dearth of literature and the majority of information is based on scattered case reports in the literature, along with several review papers. PTS is a general term for all types of thyroid sarcoma; however, specific entities include angiosarcoma, hemangioendothelioma, fibrosarcoma, leiomyosarcoma, fibrous histiocytoma, and several others.

Patients are typically between the ages of 60 and 80 years and do not possess any other specific risk factors for this entity. Presenting complaints center on a thyroid nodule without any specific signs or symptoms unless they have advanced disease [29]. Diagnosis for PTS is similar to other thyroid nodules, centered on ultrasound imaging followed by FNA. On ultrasound, these lesions have a hypohyperechoic pattern in comparison to normal thyroid tissue. As the pattern is nonspecific, it may raise suspicion for PTS but by no means is pathognomonic [30]. It is important for the practitioner to realize that certain subsets of sarcoma, such as angiosarcoma, can often have similar pathologic findings as other thyroid malignancies. In a study by Bayir et al., it was reported that angiosarcoma can be mistaken as ATC due to similar pathologic findings; however, angiosarcoma tends to bleed more significantly than ATC and often leaves a hematoma at the FNA site [31]. Although treatment is based on surgery with postoperative radiation for advanced disease, there is no standard protocol for treatment given the rare nature of this disease.

In a contemporary review, Surov et al. examined the PTS literature and evaluated the cases of 142 patients with PTS. They reported a slight male preponderance and found that the majority of patients, approximately 70%, did not present with distal metastases at presentation. Patients typically had a painless goiter, and a small subset of patients had dyspnea and dysphagia indicating advanced disease [30]. Of their population, approximately 20% of lesions were angiosarcoma, 15% were malignant hemangioendothelioma, followed by smaller percentages of fibrous histiocytoma, leiomyosarcoma, and fibrosarcoma. Leiomyosarcoma and malignant histiocytoma were reported to be more likely to infiltrate the trachea or esophagus compared to the other subtypes [30].

Fibrosarcoma patients were more likely to present with regional disease while leiomyosarcoma and angiosarcoma patients were more likely to present with distal disease. Patients with distal metastases primarily involved the lung [30]. In their review, 75 patients were treated with surgery as single modality, while 53 had surgery with adjuvant chemo-radiation. One patient had only radiation, two had just chemotherapy, and four had chemo-radiation without surgery. During the follow-up period of 0.5–120 months (median 7 months), 31% of patients were living while the remainder died or were lost to follow-up [30].

As mentioned previously, due to the lack of cohesive literature, there have been no studies reporting the overall 5-year survival or disease free survival of PTS as a group. One study reported a 33% 5-year survival for angiosarcoma of the thyroid and noted that patients present at a late stage [32]. While this statistic may not be applicable to other subtypes of sarcoma, the practitioner must understand that given the possibility of this rare malignancy and its tendency for locally aggressive behavior, any thyroid nodule with suspicious features should be imaged and biopsied in a timely fashion.

4. Primary thyroid lymphoma

PTL comprises 1–5% of all thyroid malignancies with women more commonly affected than men [33, 34]. The disease typically affects individuals between the ages of 50 and 80, and is rarely found in those younger than 40 years of age [35, 36]. Carrying a diagnosis of Hashimoto's thyroiditis is a major risk factor for PTL. Studies by Holm and Kato report a 67–80-fold increased risk of PTL in patients with Hashimoto's thyroiditis [37, 38]. In a 2015 study by Chai et al., 87% of patient with PTL had Hashimoto's [39].

Patients typically present with a painless enlarging neck mass, often in the setting of a known autoimmune thyroiditis. Adenopathy can be associated with the primary complaints as well [40]. Complaints of dysphagia, dyspnea, and hoarseness are uncommon, and signify advanced disease with compressive symptoms or invasion of the recurrent laryngeal nerve [2]. Only an estimated 10% of patients present with constitutional symptoms such as fever, weight loss, and night sweats [5]. Following thorough history and physical examination, thyroid studies can be obtained followed by ultrasound and fine needle aspiration if indicated. FNA by itself may yield inconclusive information and as such, either ultrasound guided FNA or open biopsy is recommended [2, 41, 42].

PLT is a broad term encompassing multiple pathologies. B-cell non-Hodgkin's lymphoma (NHL) is by far the most common cell line in PTL; T-cell lymphoma, plasmacytoma, and Hodgkin's lymphoma have been reported but are exceedingly rare [42, 43]. The three main subtypes of B-cell NHL are mucosal associated lymphoid tissue (MALT) lymphoma, diffuse large B-cell lymphoma (DLBCL), and a mixed variant of DLBCL and MALT [39]. MALT lymphoma is generally of low grade and indolent growth while DLBCL is high grade with aggressive growth. The mixed variant behaves more similarly to DLBCL than MALT [33, 35, 42, 44, 45]. Staging of PTL is based on extension from the thyroid gland. Stage 1 disease is localized to the thyroid gland; stage 2 disease is localized to the thyroid gland but also involves regional lymph nodes; stage 3 disease involves spread to lymph nodes on both sides of the diaphragm; stage 4 disease has spread to distant sites of the body [36].

The management of PTL is primary through chemotherapy and radiation; surgery is reserved for early stage MALT localized to the thyroid gland or for patients suffering from compressive symptoms [5, 46]. The chemotherapeutic regimen commonly utilized, CHOP, consists of cyclophosphamide, hydroxydoxorubicin, vincristine, and prednisone [47, 48].

Chai et al. examined 38 patients with PTL, 92% early stage, treated with a combination of surgery, chemotherapy, radiation, or a combination. Few patients received single modality therapy, while the majority were treated with multimodality therapy. Treatment outcomes were followed from 3 to 156 months with the median follow up being 56 months. They reported a 100% 5-year disease specific survival for MALT lymphoma, 100% for mixed, and 87.5% for DLBCL [39]. This concurs with previous studies reporting a 96–100% 5-year disease specific survival for MALT lymphoma, and shows an improvement in survival compared to the previously reported 71–75% 5-year disease specific survival for DLBCL [35, 36, 49]. Stratifying survival by stage, a surveillance, epidemiology, and end results (SEER) database study by Graff Baker reported 86% 5-year disease-specific survival for stage 1 PTL, 81% for stage 2, and 64% for stages 3 and 4 [36].

As overall prognosis is highly dependent on the subtype of primary thyroid lymphoma and the stage at presentation, the practitioner must have a high suspicion for lymphoma especially in a patient with a history of Hashimoto's presenting with enlarging neck mass. Establishing a diagnosis with sufficient cell volume to perform flow cytometry is crucial in categorizing the subtype of lymphoma and quickly beginning treatment with a multidisciplinary team.

5. Medullary thyroid cancer

MTC is a malignancy that arises from the calcitonin producing parafollicular cells and comprises 3–5% of thyroid malignancies [2, 50]. It is important to note that the parafollicular c-cells also produce carcinoembryonic antigen (CEA), prostaglandin, and serotonin of which excess levels could lead to symptoms [10]. Males and females are equally affected, typically over the age of 50 [51, 52].

The majority of MTC, approximately 75%, occurs in a sporadic fashion and generally are unilateral and unifocal [50, 52]. The remaining MTC is derived from an autosomal dominant hereditary pattern associated with the *RET* proto-oncogene. Hereditary MTC is more likely to be multifocal and bilateral in nature [53–59]. Thirty percent of MTC affects patients younger than 50 and can have a familial inheritance pattern including the association with multiple endocrine neoplasia (MEN) syndromes. MTC in MEN2A is associated with pheochromocytoma and hyperparathyroidism, while MTC associated with MEN2B is associated with mucosal neuromas, Marfanoid habitus, or pheochromocytoma [53, 54, 60, 61].

Patients commonly present with a painless thyroid nodule that can be accompanied by palpable cervical adenopathy [50]. Pain, dyspnea, and dysphagia are worrisome symptoms that can indicate invasion of local structures or compression from mass effect [2]. Symptoms of serotonin production can also be present such as diarrhea or flushing [50]. Initial regional spread can be found in the central neck, lateral neck, or superior mediastinum. Fifty percent of MTC patients have distal metastases on diagnosis, typically involving the mediastinum, liver, bone, or lung [62].

Diagnosis is based on ultrasound, fine needle aspiration, and appropriate testing of serum markers. FNA of MTC shows infiltrating neoplastic cells with marked heterogeneity. Occasionally, amyloid deposits resulting from polymerized calcitonin will be found, strongly indicative of MTC [63]. Following FNA diagnosis of MTC, patients should have calcitonin and CEA levels evaluated, as they are both diagnostic and important for surveillance [2]. Calcitonin strongly correlates with tumor volume and progression while CEA is a predictor of survival. Often, the doubling of calcitonin can be followed to determine the rate of tumor progression. A doubling time of greater than 6 months is associated with a 5-year survival of 92% while a doubling time less than 6 months is associated with a 5-year survival of 25% [64, 65]. CT imaging of the neck and mediastinum can be pursued to evaluate for radiographic evidence of spread. As the uptake of fluorodeoxyglucose is low in MTC, PET scanning is not routinely recommended. However, the use of other radionuclide tracers such as ^{18}F-DOPA can be useful, as ^{18}F-DOPA has been reported to have a sensitivity of 81%, much greater than FDG for metastatic disease [66]. To evaluate for metastases, CT of the chest, abdomen, and head is recommended along with MRI of the liver and brain due to the increased accuracy [50].

Prior to undertaking treatment, the patient should also be evaluated for *RET* mutations and a thorough screening for MEN syndrome should be completed. Genetic testing is becoming more common with these patients and their families as early detection and treatment of family members may lead to favorable prognoses. The workup of MEN syndrome includes evaluation of hyperparathyroidism by checking calcium and parathyroid hormone levels. More importantly, patients should have a 24-h urine screen for catecholamines and metanephrines along with an abdominal MRI to evaluate for the presence of a pheochromocytoma. An undiagnosed or poorly managed pheochromocytoma could result in an intraoperative catastrophe leading to a significant increase in mortality [2, 50].

Initial treatment of MTC is total thyroidectomy and bilateral central neck dissection. Family members with MEN2B or MEN 2C are recommended to have a prophylactic total thyroidectomy [2, 50]. If the patient has positive central neck adenopathy or palpable lateral neck disease, a neck dissection of levels two through six should be performed along with dissection of the superior mediastinal lymph nodes on the ipsilateral side or bilaterally if indicated. If the primary MTC lesion is greater than 1 cm, there can be a greater than 50% chance of occult metastases to the ipsilateral neck and a lateral neck dissection should be performed in that scenario as well [67–69]. As MTC is from parafollicular cells, it does not respond to radioactive iodine therapy [70]. Following surgery, patients should be followed with serial calcitonin and CEA levels to evaluate for recurrence or persistent disease [69]. External beam radiation can be considered for resections with positive margins or unresectable tumor [2]. Serum calcitonin greater than 150 pg/ml signifies residual or metastatic disease [64, 71].

Advanced MTC can be potentially treated with surgery and postoperative radiation, but often patients with extensive local disease or distal metastases are not surgical candidates. Chemotherapy in MTC, often times involving a combination of doxorubicin, dacarbazine, or cisplatin, is indicated only in rapidly progressive metastatic disease, but the response rates have not been reported higher than 20% [72–75]. Currently, molecular therapies targeting kinases of VEGFR2 and *REF* are in clinical trials but reserved for a very specific subset of patients given the adverse risk profile [76]. The overall prognosis of MTC is related to disease stage. Ten-year survival for all MTC is 61–75%; however, the presence of cervical adenopathy decreases survival to 45% [70].

MTC can be an aggressive malignancy with limited treatment options. Early intervention and close surveillance with imaging and serum markers are vital. As this malignancy has the possibility of being associated with concomitant endocrine maladies and familial inheritance, a thorough assessment of the patient and family alike can allow for safe treatment and the prevention of disease progression.

6. Conclusion

Anaplastic thyroid cancer, primary thyroid lymphoma, primary thyroid sarcoma, and medullary thyroid cancer are all extremely rare malignancies that make up a small portion of all thyroid malignancies. The literature available for guiding management is often limited as the small number of cases precludes adequate investigation in clinical trials. Although these rare malignancies are not frequently encountered, they have the potential of being aggressive with poor outcomes if not managed in a timely fashion. Patients with any of the above malignancies should be encouraged to be vigilant in the care and follow up of these conditions. Practitioners should make every attempt to rapidly establish a diagnosis for thyroid nodules and initiate treatment in an expedited fashion while keeping the patients and their families closely involved in the decision making process.

Author details

Moustafa Mourad[1], David Chan[1], Sameep Kadakia[2] and Yadranko Ducic[1*]

*Address all correspondence to: yducic@sbcglobal.net

1 Department of Head and Neck Surgery, Otolaryngology and Facial Plastic Surgery Associates, Dallas-Fort Worth, TX, USA

2 Department of Head and Neck Surgery, New York Eye and Ear Infirmary of Mount Sinai, New York, NY, USA

References

[1] LiVolsi VA, Merino M. Pathology of Thyroid Tumors. Philadelphia: Saunders; 1987.

[2] Lai S, Mandel S, Weber R. Management of thyroid neoplasms. In Flint P, editor. Cummings Otolaryngology, 6th ed.; 2015. p. 1901–1928 [Chapter 123].

[3] Nel CJ, Van heerden JA, Goellner JR, et al. Anaplastic carcinoma of the thyroid: a clinicopathologic study of 82 cases. Mayo Clin Proc. 1985;60(1):51–58.

[4] Nagaiah G, Hossain A, Mooney CJ, Parmentier J, Remick SC. Anaplastic thyroid cancer: a review of epidemiology, pathogenesis, and treatment. J Oncol. 2011;2011:542358.

[5] Green LD, Mack L, Pasieka JL. Anaplastic thyroid cancer and primary thyroid lymphoma: a review of these rare thyroid malignancies. J Surg Oncol. 2006;94:725–736.

[6] Neff RL, Farrar WB, Kloos RT, Burman KD. Anaplastic thyroid cancer. Endocrinol Metab Clin North Am. 2008;37(2):525–538, xi.

[7] Chiacchio S, Lorenzoni A, Boni G, Rubello D, Elisei R, Mariani G. Anaplastic thyroid cancer: prevalence, diagnosis and treatment. Minerva Endocrinol. 2008;33(4):341–357.

[8] Kapp DS, Livolsi VA, Sanders MM. Anaplastic carcinoma following well-differentiated thyroid cancer: etiological considerations. Yale J Biol Med. 1982;55(5–6):521–528.

[9] Are C, Shaha AR. Anaplastic thyroid carcinoma: biology, pathogenesis, prognostic factors, and treatment approaches. Ann Surg Oncol. 2006;13(4):453–464.

[10] Demeter JG, De Jong SA, Lawrence AM, Paloyan E. Anaplastic thyroid carcinoma: risk factors and outcome. Surgery. 1991;110(6):956–961.

[11] American Joint Committee on Cancer. How is thyroid cancer staged? (2015). http://www.cancer.org/cancer/thyroidcancer/detailedguide/thyroid-cancer-staging.

[12] Kebebew E, Greenspan FS, Clark OH, Woeber KA, Mcmillan A. Anaplastic thyroid carcinoma. Treatment outcome and prognostic factors. Cancer. 2005;103(7):1330–1335.

[13] Shaha AR. Airway management in anaplastic thyroid carcinoma. Laryngoscope. 2008;118(7):1195–1198.

[14] Zhang L, Boufraqech M, Lake R, Kebebew E. Carfilzomib potentiates CUDC-101-induced apoptosis in anaplastic thyroid cancer. Oncotarget. 2016;7(13)16517–16528.

[15] Marano F, Argenziano M, Frairia R, et al. Doxorubicin-loaded nanobubbles combined with extracorporeal shock waves: basis for a new drug delivery tool in anaplastic thyroid cancer. Thyroid. 2016;26(5):705–716.

[16] Smallridge RC, Ain KB, Asa SL, et al. American Thyroid Association guidelines for management of patients with anaplastic thyroid cancer. Thyroid. 2012;22(11):1104–1139.

[17] Mciver B, Hay ID, Giuffrida DF, et al. Anaplastic thyroid carcinoma: a 50-year experience at a single institution. Surgery. 2001;130(6):1028–1034.

[18] Venkatesh YS, Ordonez NG, Schultz PN, Hickey RC, Goepfert H, Samaan NA. Anaplastic carcinoma of the thyroid. A clinicopathologic study of 121 cases. Cancer. 1990;66(2):321–330.

[19] Haigh PI. Anaplastic thyroid carcinoma. Curr Treat Options Oncol. 2000;1(4):353–357.

[20] Grant CS, Thompson G. Anaplastic thyroid carcinoma: hope on the horizon?. Surgery. 2011;150(6):1220–1221.

[21] Passler C, Scheuba C, Prager G, et al. Anaplastic (undifferentiated) thyroid carcinoma (ATC). A retrospective analysis. Langenbecks Arch Surg. 1999;384(3):284–293.

[22] Cobin RH, Gharib H, Bergman DA, et al. AACE/AAES medical/surgical guidelines for clinical practice: management of thyroid carcinoma. American Association of Clinical Endocrinologists. American College of Endocrinology. Endocr Pract. 2001;7(3):202–220.

[23] Brown RF, Ducic Y. Aggressive surgical resection of anaplastic thyroid carcinoma may provide long-term survival in selected patients. Otolaryngol Head Neck Surg. 2013;148(4):564–571.

[24] Voutilainen PE, Multanen M, Haapiainen RK, Leppäniemi AK, Sivula AH. Anaplastic thyroid carcinoma survival. World J Surg. 1999;23(9):975–978.

[25] Tan RK, Finley RK, Driscoll D, Bakamjian V, Hicks WL, Shedd DP. Anaplastic carcinoma of the thyroid: a 24-year experience. Head Neck. 1995;17(1):41–47.

[26] Hundahl SA, Fleming ID, Fremgen AM, Menck HR. A National Cancer Data Base report on 53,856 cases of thyroid carcinoma treated in the U.S., 1985–1995 [see comments]. Cancer. 1998;83(12):2638–2648.

[27] Buła G, Waler J, Niemiec A, Trompeta J, Steplewska K, Gawrychowski J. Unusual malignant thyroid tumours—a clinical study of 20 cases. Acta Chir Belg. 2008;108(6): 702–707.

[28] Thompson LD, Wenig BM, Adair CF, Shmookler BM, Heffess CS. Primary smooth muscle tumors of the thyroid gland. Cancer. 1997;79(3):579–587.

[29] Surov A, Holzhausen HJ, Machens A, Dralle H. Imaging findings of thyroidal sarcoma. Clin Imaging. 2014;38(6):826–830.

[30] Surov A, Gottschling S, Wienke A, Meyer HJ, Spielmann RP, Dralle H. Primary thyroid sarcoma: a systematic review. Anticancer Res. 2015;35(10):5185–5191.

[31] Bayır Ö, Yılmazer D, Ersoy R, et al. An extremely rare case of thyroid malignancy from the non-Alpine region: angiosarcoma. Int J Surg Case Rep. 2015;19:92–96.

[32] Kalitova P, Plzak J, Kodet R, Astl J. Angiosarcoma of the thyroid. Eur Arch Otorhinolaryngol. 2009;266(6):903–905.

[33] Widder S, Pasieka JL. Primary thyroid lymphomas. Curr Treat Options Oncol. 2004;5(4):307–313.

[34] Ansell SM, Grant CS, Habermann TM. Primary thyroid lymphoma. Semin Oncol. 1999;26(3):316–323.

[35] Derringer GA, Thompson LD, Frommelt RA, Bijwaard KE, Heffess CS, Abbondanzo SL. Malignant lymphoma of the thyroid gland: a clinicopathologic study of 108 cases. Am J Surg Pathol. 2000;24(5):623–639.

[36] Graff-baker A, Roman SA, Thomas DC, Udelsman R, Sosa JA. Prognosis of primary thyroid lymphoma: demographic, clinical, and pathologic predictors of survival in 1,408 cases. Surgery. 2009;146(6):1105–1115.

[37] Holm LE, Blomgren H, Löwhagen T. Cancer risks in patients with chronic lymphocytic thyroiditis. N Engl J Med. 1985;312(10):601–604.

[38] Kato I, Tajima K, Suchi T, et al. Chronic thyroiditis as a risk factor of B-cell lymphoma in the thyroid gland. Jpn J Cancer Res. 1985;76(11):1085–1090.

[39] Chai YJ, Hong JH, Koo DH, et al. Clinicopathological characteristics and treatment outcomes of 38 cases of primary thyroid lymphoma: a multicenter study. Ann Surg Treat Res. 2015;89(6):295–299.

[40] Kumar R, Khosla D, Kumar N, et al. Survival and failure outcomes in primary thyroid lymphomas: a single centre experience of combined modality approach. J Thyroid Res. 2013;2013:269034.

[41] Matsuda M, Sone H, Koyama H, Ishiguro S. Fine-needle aspiration cytology of malignant lymphoma of the thyroid. Diagn Cytopathol. 1987;3(3):244–249.

[42] Alzouebi M, Goepel JR, Horsman JM, Hancock BW. Primary thyroid lymphoma: the 40 year experience of a UK lymphoma treatment centre. Int J Oncol. 2012;40(6):2075–2080.

[43] Salhany KE, Pietra GG. Extranodal lymphoid disorders. Am J Clin Pathol. 1993;99(4): 472–485.

[44] Tsang RW, Gospodarowicz MK, Pintilie M, et al. Localized mucosa-associated lymphoid tissue lymphoma treated with radiation therapy has excellent clinical outcome. J Clin Oncol. 2003;21(22):4157–4164.

[45] Thieblemont C, Mayer A, Dumontet C, et al. Primary thyroid lymphoma is a heterogeneous disease. J Clin Endocrinol Metab. 2002;87(1):105–111.

[46] Sakorafas GH, Kokkoris P, Farley DR. Primary thyroid lymphoma (correction of lympoma): diagnostic and therapeutic dilemmas. Surg Oncol. 2010;19(4):e124–e129.

[47] Devine RM, Edis AJ, Banks PM. Primary lymphoma of the thyroid: a review of the Mayo Clinic experience through 1978. World J Surg. 1981;5(1):33–38.

[48] Rasbach DA, Mondschein MS, Harris NL, Kaufman DS, Wang CA. Malignant lymphoma of the thyroid gland: a clinical and pathologic study of twenty cases. Surgery. 1985;98(6):1166–1170.

[49] Oh SY, Kim WS, Kim JS, et al. Primary thyroid marginal zone B-cell lymphoma of the mucosa-associated lymphoid tissue type: clinical manifestation and outcome of a rare disease – consortium for improving survival of lymphoma study. Acta Haematol. 2012;127(2):100–104.

[50] Hadoux J, Pacini F, Tuttle RM, Schlumberger M. Management of advanced medullary thyroid cancer. Lancet Diabetes Endocrinol. 2016;4(1):64–71.

[51] Hazard JB. The C cells (parafollicular cells) of the thyroid gland and medullary thyroid carcinoma. A review. Am J Pathol. 1977;88(1):213–250.

[52] Chong GC, Beahrs OH, Sizemore GW, Woolner LH. Medullary carcinoma of the thyroid gland. Cancer. 1975;35(3):695–704.

[53] Delellis RA. Multiple endocrine neoplasia syndromes revisited. Clinical, morphologic, and molecular features. Lab Invest. 1995;72(5):494–505.

[54] Raue F, Frank-raue K, Grauer A. Multiple endocrine neoplasia type 2. Clinical features and screening. Endocrinol Metab Clin North Am. 1994;23(1):137–156.

[55] Wells SA, Asa SL, Dralle H, et al. Revised American Thyroid Association guidelines for the management of medullary thyroid carcinoma. Thyroid. 2015;25(6):567–610.

[56] Elisei R, Cosci B, Romei C, et al. Prognostic significance of somatic RET oncogene mutations in sporadic medullary thyroid cancer: a 10-year follow-up study. J Clin Endocrinol Metab. 2008;93(3):682–687.

[57] Moura MM, Cavaco BM, Pinto AE, Leite V. High prevalence of RAS mutations in RET-negative sporadic medullary thyroid carcinomas. J Clin Endocrinol Metab. 2011;96(5):E863–E868.

[58] Boichard A, Croux L, Al Ghuzlan A, et al. Somatic RAS mutations occur in a large proportion of sporadic RET-negative medullary thyroid carcinomas and extend to a previously unidentified exon. J Clin Endocrinol Metab. 2012;97(10):E2031–E2035.

[59] Agrawal N, Jiao Y, Sausen M, et al. Exomic sequencing of medullary thyroid cancer reveals dominant and mutually exclusive oncogenic mutations in RET and RAS. J Clin Endocrinol Metab. 2013;98(2):E364–E369.

[60] Moley JF. Medullary thyroid cancer. Surg Clin North Am. 1995;75(3):405–420.

[61] Goodfellow PJ, Wells SA. RET gene and its implications for cancer. J Natl Cancer Inst. 1995;87(20):1515–1523.

[62] Ellenhorn JD, Shah JP, Brennan MF. Impact of therapeutic regional lymph node dissection for medullary carcinoma of the thyroid gland. Surgery. 1993;114(6):1078–1081.

[63] Stepanas AV, Samaan NA, Hill CS, Hickey RC. Medullary thyroid carcinoma: importance of serial serum calcitonin measurement. Cancer. 1979;43(3):825–837.

[64] Laure Giraudet A, Al Ghulzan A, Aupérin A, et al. Progression of medullary thyroid carcinoma: assessment with calcitonin and carcinoembryonic antigen doubling times. Eur J Endocrinol. 2008;158(2):239–246.

[65] Barbet J, Campion L, Kraeber-bodéré F, Chatal JF. Prognostic impact of serum calcitonin and carcinoembryonic antigen doubling-times in patients with medullary thyroid carcinoma. J Clin Endocrinol Metab. 2005;90(11):6077–6084.

[66] Beheshti M, Pöcher S, Vali R, et al. The value of ^{18}F-DOPA PET-CT in patients with medullary thyroid carcinoma: comparison with ^{18}F-FDG PET-CT. Eur Radiol. 2009;19(6):1425–1434.

[67] Sherman SI, Angelos P, Ball DW, et al. Thyroid carcinoma. J Natl Compr Cancer Netw. 2007;5(6):568–621.

[68] Block MA. Surgical treatment of medullary carcinoma of the thyroid. Otolaryngol Clin North Am. 1990;23(3):453–473.

[69] Donovan D, Gagel RF. Medullary Thyroid Carcinoma and Multiple Endoscine Neoplasia Syndromes, 2nd ed., Philadelphia: Lippincott-Raven; 1997.

[70] Saad MF, Ordonez NG, Rashid RK, et al. Medullary carcinoma of the thyroid. A study of the clinical features and prognostic factors in 161 patients. Medicine (Baltimore). 1984;63(6):319–342.

[71] Machens A, Schneyer U, Holzhausen HJ, Dralle H. Prospects of remission in medullary thyroid carcinoma according to basal calcitonin level. J Clin Endocrinol Metab. 2005;90(4):2029–2034.

[72] Shimaoka K, Schoenfeld DA, Dewys WD, Creech RH, Deconti R. A randomized trial of doxorubicin versus doxorubicin plus cisplatin in patients with advanced thyroid carcinoma. Cancer. 1985;56(9):2155–2160.

[73] Williams SD, Birch R, Einhorn LH. Phase II evaluation of doxorubicin plus cisplatin in advanced thyroid cancer: a Southeastern Cancer Study Group Trial. Cancer Treat Rep. 1986;70(3):405–407.

[74] Nocera M, Baudin E, Pellegriti G, Cailleux AF, Mechelany-corone C, Schlumberger M. Treatment of advanced medullary thyroid cancer with an alternating combination of doxorubicin-streptozocin and 5 FU-dacarbazine. Groupe d'Etude des Tumeurs à Calcitonine (GETC). Br J Cancer. 2000;83(6):715–718.

[75] Schlumberger M, Abdelmoumene N, Delisle MJ, Couette JE. Treatment of advanced medullary thyroid cancer with an alternating combination of 5 FU-streptozocin and 5 FU-dacarbazine. The Groupe d'Etude des Tumeurs a Calcitonine (GETC). Br J Cancer. 1995;71(2):363–365.

[76] Dunna NR, Kandula V, Girdhar A, et al. High affinity pharmacological profiling of dual inhibitors targeting RET and VEGFR2 in inhibition of kinase and angiogeneis events in medullary thyroid carcinoma. Asian Pac J Cancer Prev. 2015;16(16):7089–7095.

Chapter 12

Radiation Dosimetry in Thyroid Cancer Patients

Lebriz Uslu Beşli and Mustafa Demir

Additional information is available at the end of the chapter

http://dx.doi.org/10.5772/64087

Abstract

Radioactive iodine is utilized commonly for ablation of remnant thyroid tissue after thyroidectomy and treatment of persistent disease and metastases in differentiated thyroid cancer patients. As it involves ionizing radiation, it is important to ensure that the patients receive optimum amount of radiation to destruct the target tissue while keeping the radiation-related side effects to minimum. In clinical practice, standard activity doses are preferred for thyroid cancer patients, assuming that biokinetics are similar in all patients. Lately, many clinicians offered to individualise the radioactive iodine therapy by calculating the optimal amount of radioactivity using patient dosimetry. Radiation dosimetry is used to calculate the minimum effective and maximum tolerated absorbed dose for a successful radioactive iodine therapy. This approach enables to administer increased amount of therapeutic activity while minimizing the related side effects. This chapter presents some of the basic principles of patient dosimetry and radioiodine biokinetics following radioactive iodine administration in differentiated thyroid cancer patients.

Following radioactive iodine therapy, radiation protection measures are necessary to protect the public from ionizing radiation after discharge of the patient from hospital. Radiation exposure to patients, family members and caregivers and attempts to decrease the exposure during therapy are also going to be discussed.

Keywords: radiation dosimetry, radiation exposure, dose rate, radioiodine therapy

1. Introduction

Radioactive iodine is an important component in treatment approach of differentiated thyroid carcinoma patients. Following thyroidectomy, radioactive iodine is used for remnant tissue ablation and to destroy residual tumor foci or metastatic disease. Traditionally a fixed dose of

3700–7400 MBq (100–200 mCi) of radioiodine was recommended for treatment of residual disease [1]. However, concerns related with ionizing radiation led to a significant decrease in the administered dose recommended in the recent thyroid cancer management guidelines [2].

The optimum I-131 activity is controversial as the radioiodine biokinetics is different in each patient. Therefore, radiation dosimetry is preferred especially in the subgroup of patients, where selection of biologically effective dose is more crucial, such as patients with metastatic disease, especially with lung metastases or with comorbidities such as chronic kidney disease, as well as in pediatric and elderly population.

This chapter aims to present the basic principles of radiation dosimetry and common dosimetric methods, as well as main dosimetric approaches for radiation dose selection for thyroid carcinoma patients. Also, concerns about radiation exposure to patients, family members, and caregivers and attempts to decrease the exposure during therapy are discussed.

2. Basic principles of radiation dosimetry

Radiation dosimetry is a general term implying the approach for (1) calculation of the minimum amount of radiation activity necessary for successful treatment of a patient (i.e., therapeutic dose) for treatment planning using radionuclides or external beam radiotherapy, (2) assessment of the radiation dose received by a specific organ or tissue of a patient to ensure that radiation dose received by the patient would not exceed the tolerable limits of certain organs or tissues, (3) determining the total radiation dose received by patients, health care workers, or family members of patients to maintain radiation safety of individuals, (4) measurement of the instantaneous and cumulative radiation dose in the environment where ionizing radiation sources are used to ensure radiation safety of the workers and public, and (5) calculation of the total amount of dose received by the fetus, in case the mother is exposed to ionizing radiation during pregnancy. Radiation dosimetry for treatment planning of thyroid cancer patients involves calculating the minimum amount of I-131 activity to be given to the patient to ensure successful remnant thyroid tissue ablation or treatment of persistent disease and metastases, as well as measuring the radiation dose received by critical or dose-limiting organs to calculate the maximal safe dosage of I-131 that can be given to the patient.

There are two main approaches to determine the amount of I-131 to be given to the thyroid cancer patients after thyroidectomy operation: empirical fixed amount approach, and dosimetrically calculated amount approach. Empirical fixed amount approach is more widely used, as it is a more simple and convenient method. However, it lacks the ability to accurately incorporate the individual biological and physical features of patients, such as radioiodine uptake, release, and residual functioning volume of thyroid tissue. On the other hand, current individual dosimetric approaches are both demanding and inconvenient to calculate the exact uptake and kinetics for each patient. However, it is especially crucial in the subgroup of thyroid cancer patients, who require higher amount of radioiodine due to the presence of metastases or relapsing disease.

The tissue damage caused by ionizing radiation is dependent on many factors, such as the type of radiation emitted, its amount and energy, its biokinetics in the body, including its uptake and clearance in various organs, and the physical arrangement and location of organs emitting radiation. Therefore, unlike external radiation sources, the doses received from internal radiation sources used in nuclear medicine cannot be calculated exactly; rather several formulas and assumptions are used to predict the radiation dose applied to the body.

2.1. Internal radiation dosimetry

The main aim of internal radiation dosimetry is to calculate the *absorbed dose*, which is defined as the mean energy imparted to matter per unit mass by ionizing radiation. Absorbed dose (D) is calculated using the following formula:

$$\boldsymbol{D} = \frac{d\varepsilon}{dm} \tag{1}$$

where $d\varepsilon$ is the mean energy imparted by ionizing radiation and dm is the matter of mass.

In SI system, the unit for absorbed dose is joules per kilogram (J/kg) or ergs per gram (erg/g). The special units for absorbed dose are gray (Gy) and rad:

$$1\ \text{J/kg} = 1\ \text{Gy} = 100\ \text{rad} = 10^4\ \text{erg/g}$$

The term *equivalent dose* is derived from the absorbed dose to refer the different biological effects of different types of ionizing radiation. It is calculated by multiplying the absorbed dose by a radiation weighting factor (w_R), which is dependent on the type and energy of radiation. The formula for the equivalent dose (H) is therefore:

$$\boldsymbol{H} = \boldsymbol{D} \times \boldsymbol{w}_R \tag{2}$$

The unit for equivalent dose is the same as absorbed dose, as the radiation weighting factor does not have a unit. However, special unit names are also defined for equivalent dose, which are *sievert* (Sv) and *rem*. Radiation weighting factor is dependent on the type of radiation. According to the International Commission on Radiological Protection (ICRP), alpha particles have radiation weighting factor of 20, whereas the factor for beta minus, beta plus (positron), gamma rays, and X-rays are 1:

$$1\ \text{Sv} = 100\ \text{rem}$$

Absorbed dose for a certain organ or tissue can be calculated when the energy absorbed per unit mass is identified. Several authors have established similar equations to calculate the absorbed dose, which are known as the Marinelli method [3], Quimby method, Medical

Internal Radiation Dose (MIRD) method [4], and International Commission on Radiological Protection (ICRP) method. For the scope of our chapter, only MIRD method is going to be explained in details, as it is the most commonly used method for radiation dosimetry calculations in nuclear medicine.

A generic equation for the absorbed dose (D) in an organ or tissue has been established as [5, 6]:

$$D = \frac{k\tilde{A}\sum_i n_i E_i \phi_i}{m} \tag{3}$$

where k is the proportionality constant, $\tilde{A}$ is the cumulated activity (μCi-h or MBq-s), n_i is the number of particles with energy E_i emitted per nuclear transition, E_i is the energy per particle (MeV), ϕ_i is the fraction of energy absorbed in the target, and m is the mass of the target region (g or kg).

Source	**Target**	**S-value**
Bladder	Bladder	1.2×10^{-3}
Stomach	Stomach	9.7×10^{-4}
Kidney	Kidney	1.5×10^{-3}
Kidney	Adrenal gland	3.2×10^{-5}
Kidney	Spleen	2.4×10^{-5}
Thyroid gland	Thyroid gland	2.2×10^{-2}
Thyroid gland	Whole body	9.5×10^{-6}
Thyroid gland	Lungs	2.9×10^{-6}
Thyroid gland	Bone marrow	2.4×10^{-6}

Table 1. Some S-factors for I-131.

2.2. Medical internal radiation dose (MIRD) method

MIRD method was established by the Society of Nuclear Medicine to assist radiation dose estimation to various organs using a simplified calculation method. Instead of using numerous variables, MIRD method has shortened the absorbed dose equation by using the "S-factor" for all the absorption parameters, which includes types and energy of radiation emitted, size and shape of the target organ and other related organs, and energy fraction of each emission absorbed in the target organ from radiation that originated in the source organ. S-factor is ascertained for common radiopharmaceuticals, including I-131. S-factors for I-131 and Tc-99m are given in **Tables 1** and **2**. Equation for the S-factor would be:

$$S = \frac{k\sum_i n_i E_i \Phi_i}{m} \tag{4}$$

where k is the proportionality constant (=2.13), n_i is the number of particles with energy E_i emitted per nuclear transition, E_i is the energy per particle (MeV), Φ_i is the fraction of energy absorbed in the target, and m is the mass of the target region (g or kg).

Source	Target	S-value
Liver	Liver	4.6×10^{-7}
Liver	Kidneys	3.9×10^{-6}
Liver	Whole body	2.2×10^{-6}
Liver	Bone marrow	1.6×10^{-6}
Liver	Spleen	9.2×10^{-7}
Spleen	Spleen	3.3×10^{-4}
Spleen	Pancreas	1.9×10^{-5}
Spleen	Stomach	1.0×10^{-5}
Spleen	Whole body	2.2×10^{-6}
Spleen	Bone marrow	1.7×10^{-6}
Spleen	Liver	9.8×10^{-7}
Bone marrow	Bone marrow	3.1×10^{-5}
Bone marrow	Whole body	2.2×10^{-6}
Bone marrow	Liver	9.2×10^{-7}

Table 2. Some S-factors for Tc-99m.

Finally, MIRD equation is as follows:

$$D_t = \sum_s \tilde{A}_s S(t \rightarrow s) \tag{5}$$

$$\tilde{A} = A_0 \times \tau \tag{6}$$

where $\tilde{A}_s$ is the cumulated activity in the source organ, t is the target organ, s is the source organ, A_0 is the initial activity given, and τ is the residence time.

For the MIRD equation, various body phantoms, which represent human body and enable accurate measurement of absorbed fractions, organ masses, and relationship of organs, were established to determine the cumulated activity. Either external probes, such as thyroid uptake device, or time-activity curves obtained from scintigraphic imaging are used to calculate the cumulative activity. Using MIRD equation, the calculation of radiation dose of patients after radiopharmaceutical application is possible, but MIRD equation is not suitable for establishment of radiation dose received by radiation workers and family members.

Following the establishment of MIRD phantom, various other phantoms were introduced representing human body more realistically, such as female and male phantoms, pregnant female phantom [7], family phantoms including pediatric phantom series [8], and bone and marrow phantom [9]. The data obtained using these phantoms are inserted in special software programs dedicated for internal dose calculations, such as MIRDOSE [10] and OLINDA/EXM 1.0 [11].

The recent development in computer and anatomical imaging technologies led to the creation of more realistic voxel phantoms, which include three-dimensional digital images of internal organs and hybrid phantoms enabling a realistic and rapid modeling of human body **(Figure 1)** [12, 13].

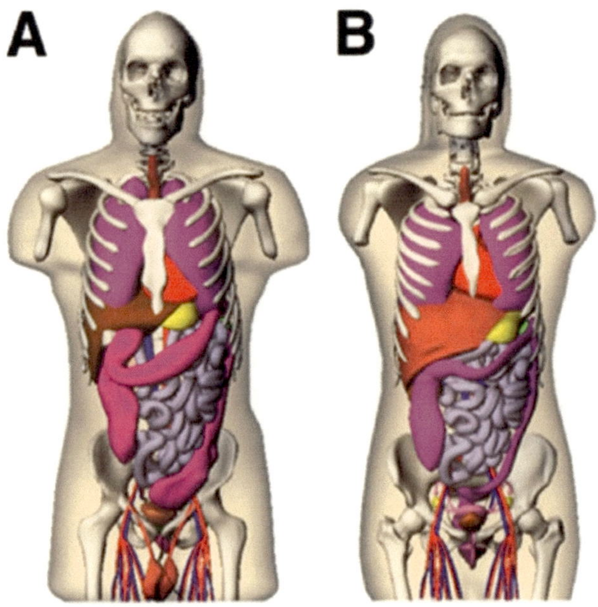

Figure 1. Adult male (A) and adult female (B) phantom by Segars [13]. There are also different age-specific phantoms for dose evaluation in pediatric patients.

3. Dosimetric approaches for thyroid carcinoma

There are two main dosimetric approaches for administration of radioiodine for the treatment of thyroid carcinoma: bone marrow-based approach, which aims to limit the radiation dose to be within safe limits for bone marrow, and lesion-based approach, which aims to give at least the minimum amount of radiation dose to destroy the lesions.

3.1. Bone marrow-based dosimetric approach

Bone marrow depression is one of the most important complications of radioiodine therapy as bone marrow is susceptible to ionizing radiation. Bone marrow-based dosimetry aims to calculate the maximum amount of radiation that bone marrow can tolerate for radioiodine treatment. This method was first developed by Benua et al. and it allows estimating the radiation dose received by the hematopoietic system from each unit (GBq or mCi) of I-131 activity given to the patient [14]. The procedure involves an initial administration of a tracer activity of I-131 to the patient, followed by serial blood sampling and whole-body activity measurement for at least 4 days to follow the clearance of radioiodine from the body. Although the name of this approach is bone marrow based, the calculations involve whole blood compartment, not only the bone marrow. In the study by Benua et al., the group of patients that received a whole blood dose of more than 200 cGy showed serious complications related to ionizing radiation, whereas the group of patients that received less than 200 cGy to the blood did not have serious side effects. Therefore, 2 Gy limit was proposed to be the safety limit for bone marrow.

I-131 has both gamma (γ) and beta minus (β) radiation; so both radiation types are included in radiation dose calculations. I-131 activity to be administered to the patient is calculated as combined absorbed doses for gamma and beta radiation and is within safety limits for bone marrow, which is accepted as 2 Gy:

$$A_{administered}\left(MBq\right)=\frac{2\ Gy}{D_{\beta}\left(Gy/MBq\right)+D_{\gamma}\left(Gy/MBq\right)} \tag{7}$$

According to the original Benua protocol, a standard tracer I-131 activity was given to the patient before the therapy and measurement of serial blood samples in a gamma counter is performed for the detection of β-radiation dose (D_{β}), whereas radiation dose for γ-radiation (D_{γ}) is calculated either by serial measurement of the whole body of the patient using a gamma probe or by measurement of the periodic urine collection.

After the introduction of the Benua protocol, several studies were performed with different modifications to the original protocol, such as using gamma camera instead of gamma probe [15], using geometric mean of the body activity counts instead of anterior measurement, delaying the onset of whole body counting to 2 hours, and elimination of urine collection. EANM Dosimetry Committee has also published a detailed guideline providing most recent recommendations on how to perform blood- and bone marrow–based dosimetry in thyroid cancer patients [16].

Further studies revealed that serious bone marrow toxicity is avoided in radiation doses of less than 3 Gy; so 3 Gy is accepted today as bone marrow safety limit and it is used generally for treatment of thyroid carcinoma patients with multiple metastases. Bone marrow dosimetry is not recommended for patients with extended bone metastases, as blood-based absorbed dose calculation could underestimate the absorbed dose to bone marrow [16]. Also, in the presence of multiple pulmonary micrometastasis, lung would be the critical organ instead of bone marrow, therefore, bone marrow dosimetry would not be appropriate in those patients.

3.2. Lesion-based dosimetric approach

Bone marrow-based dosimetry aims to give the maximum safe amount of I-131, ignoring the absorbed dose in the tumor, which may end up with giving a higher amount of radioiodine than the actual therapeutic amount. Lesion-based dosimetric approach aims to calculate the therapeutic amount of radioiodine that provides the minimum necessary radiation dose to the residual thyroid tissue and metastatic foci. For lesion-based dosimetry, uptake and clearance of I-131 from residual thyroid tissue and all metastatic foci are needed to be calculated.

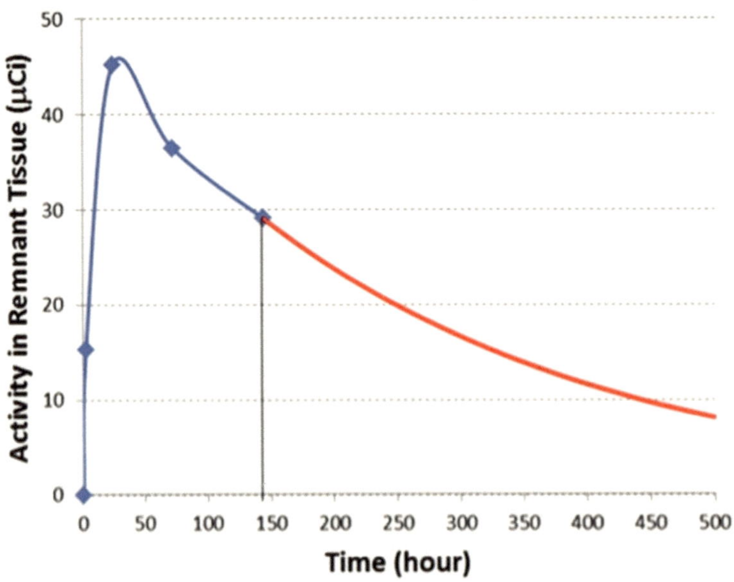

Figure 2. Time-activity curve obtained from series of scintigraphic images of a thyroid cancer patient. Series of whole body scintigraphy with empty bladder and rectum were acquired at different time points following tracer radioiodine administration.

The lesion-based dosimetric approach was first described by Maxon et al. in 1983 in a study with 76 thyroid carcinoma patients. Clinical response was detected in the group of patients that received minimum 300 Gy radiation dose to residual thyroid tissue and 80 Gy to metastatic foci, whereas less values were found to be inadequate for treatment [17].

The equation for assessment of lesion dose is as follows [18]:

$$\boldsymbol{Dose}(\boldsymbol{cGy}) = 0.63 \times \boldsymbol{C}_0(\boldsymbol{\mu Ci}/\boldsymbol{g}) \times \boldsymbol{T}_{1/2\ \boldsymbol{lesion}}(\boldsymbol{h}) \tag{8}$$

where C_0 is the initial concentration of I-131 in the lesion and $T_{1/2\ \text{lesion}}$ is the effective half-life of the lesion activity.

To obtain the initial concentration of I-131 in the lesion, either serial whole body scintigraphic imaging or radioiodine uptake test are performed after the administration of an initial tracer I-131 activity. Using scintigraphic images, region of interest is drawn around the residual thyroid tissue and all metastatic foci and time-activity curves are obtained to calculate the initial activity and the effective half-life **(Figure 2)**. Measurements were performed at the 2nd, 6th, 24th, 48th, 72nd, and 96th hours following radioiodine administration and additional measurements are performed if the excretion is delayed. Also, the lesion mass is calculated either using the gamma camera images or using radiological imaging tools, such as computerized tomography (CT) or ultrasonography (USG).

Selection of optimum administered dose is challenging in the presence of chronic renal failure, as delayed excretion of radioiodine in these patients lead to increased radiation exposure of the whole body including the critical dose limiting organs such as bone marrow. Dosimetry is therefore recommended for these patients to refrain from radiation-related side effects and to limit the exposure of the healthcare providers [19, 20].

3.3. Dosimetry using I-124

Traditionally, dosimetric methods for thyroid carcinoma involve use of low dose of I-131. However, concerns about the stunning effect of I-131 limit its usage and lead to search for alternative radionuclides, such as I-123 or I-124. I-123 is a cyclotron product with a half-life of 13 h. Being a pure gamma emitter, it is more favorable for diagnostic imaging but its supply is limited. I-124 is also produced in a cyclotron, but it has a longer half-life of 4.18 days and it is a positron emitter, which makes the isotope a promising tool for imaging of the residual disease using PET/CT, for detection of patients who would benefit from radioiodine therapy and for dosimetry of lesions especially for patients who require higher amount of radioiodine [21].

I-124 PET-based dosimetry protocol involves serial PET/CT imaging starting 2–4 h after oral administration of I-124 until 72–96 h. There are also simplified protocols proposed involving imaging only at the 24th and 96th hours for lesion dosimetry [22]. Data obtained from I-124 PET/CT image can also be used to simplify the blood dose protocol, reducing the number of blood sampling [23].

I-124 PET/CT was reported to provide a better assessment of lesion dosimetry in thyroid cancer patients as it enables to determine the concentration of radionuclide in the lesion, providing higher spatial resolution and imaging sensitivity than images acquired using gamma cameras [24, 25]. Also, it allows estimating the lesion absorbed dose per administered I-131 activity for each radioiodine positive tumor foci [24]. In a study investigating the relationship between the absorbed radiation dose detected by I-124 PET and lesion response after I-131 administration, similar response rates were found for thyroid remnant tissue compared to the historical data of Maxon et al., who used planar I-131 scintigraphy to detect absorbed radiation dose [23]. It was shown that I-124 PET/CT lesion dosimetry could be used as a prognostic tool to predict lesion-based I-131 response [26]. Moreover, I-124 PET was found to be promising for detection of radioiodine avidity of the remnant thyroid tissue and metastatic foci [27, 28]. However, high false negative rate of I-124 PET/CT was also reported in patients who had received rhTSH stimulation [29].

4. Radiation safety

Increased usage of radiation in science, technology, and medicine led to a need for establishment of an international organization to provide recommendations on radiation protection. International Commission on Radiological Protection (ICRP, former name "International X-ray and Radium Protection Committee") is an international, nongovernmental organization that was founded in 1928 in Sweden to provide recommendations and guidance on radiation protection.

4.1. Biological effects of radiation

Biological effects of radiation can be divided into two categories: deterministic effects and stochastic effects.

Tissue/organ	Effects	Equivalent dose for single exposure (Sv)	Equivalent dose rate for prolonged exposure (Sv/year)
Testis	Temporary infertility	0.15	0.4
	Permanent infertility	>3.5	2.0
Ovaries	Permanent infertility	>2.5	>0.2
Lens of the eye	Detectable opacities	>0.5	>0.1
	Cataract	>2.0	>0.15
Bone marrow	Impairment of blood cell production	>0.5	>0.4

Table 3. Threshold for deterministic for different tissues and organs by ICRP [30].

Deterministic effects can be seen in medium to high radiation doses. The effects related with radiation are seen only above a certain threshold, when there is loss of tissue function and the damage will increase with the absorbed dose. Bone marrow, testis, and lens of the eye are the most sensitive tissues for radiation; therefore, deterministic effects such as pancytopenia, infertility, and cataract are first seen in those tissues. Although skin is not one of the most sensitive organs for radiation, erythema is another common deterministic effect, which occurs due to accidental skin contamination. Doses of radionuclides used for nuclear medicine imaging procedures are below the threshold for deterministic effects. During radionuclide therapy, including I-131 therapy for thyroid cancer, doses are selected that exceed the deterministic threshold only for the thyroid tissue, preserving the other tissues. ICRP has published recommendations including the thresholds for deterministic effects of different tissues and organs **(Table 3)** [30].

Stochastic effects can be seen in low level of exposure, there is not a certain threshold for the effects and the severity is not dependent on the absorbed dose. The name stochastic is given to refer that the effects can be seen by chance and the proportion of the population that are effected can be predicted statistically but the exact persons that will be affected cannot be foreseen. Stochastic effects occur when radiation does not kill the cell but modifies its DNA. Radiation-related cancers and hereditary disorders are examples for stochastic effects of radiation.

4.2. Practical dosimetry

Despite many advantages of radiation dosimetry, it is difficult to be performed for all thyroid carcinoma patients undergoing radioiodine therapy. Some information, on the other hand, obtained from dosimetry principles can guide clinicians in treatment planning of patients. Retention of radioiodine can be easily determined using a standard uptake probe and if high radioiodine retention is detected, prescribed radioiodine dose could be decreased to ensure safety [31]. On the contrary, if radioiodine retention is low, then prescribed dose of I-131 could be increased to optimize the efficacy. Bone marrow is the dose-limiting organ for radioiodine therapy, as the bone marrow depression is one of the most important complications of the therapy. Radiation to blood and to bone marrow is correlated with body retention. Also, increased serum thyroxine concentration in the blood in the absence of thyroid hormone medication can be used as an indicator of increased blood radiation and reduction of prescribed activity could be taken into consideration. Thyroid carcinomas, which are at least 1 cm in diameter but are not visible on scintigraphic image, usually cannot be eliminated with a usual therapeutic I-131 dose of 3700–7400 MBq (100–200 mCi); therefore, either dose increase or dosimetric approaches should be considered for those patients [31]. Presence of radiation-related side effects after the first radioiodine therapy, such as bone marrow toxicity, sialadenitis, and lacrimal gland dysfunction, should be assessed prior further therapy planning to avoid cumulative radiation toxicity.

4.3. Radiation-related risks in thyroid cancer patients

The risk of radioiodine-related secondary cancer in thyroid cancer patients is controversial. There are several long-term follow-up studies investigating the secondary malignancies in thyroid cancer patients and only a very low associated risk of malignancy could be found. Therefore, recent thyroid cancer management guidelines do not recommend any specific screening after radioiodine administration in thyroid cancer patients [2]. The risk of secondary cancers is dose related and generally seen in patients who receive cumulative I-131 activity of more than 22,200 MBq (600 mCi) and there is no direct evidence of increased risk in patients who have received 1110–3700 MBq (30–100 mCi) radioiodine in a single session [32]. In a meta-analysis including 16,502 patients from two distinct multicenter studies, overall risk of secondary cancer was shown to be increased by 1.2 (95% CI: 1.04–1.36; $p < 0.01$) [33]. The most significant risk increase was reported to be in leukemias, with a relative risk of 2.5 (95% CI: 1.13–5.53; $p < 0.024$) [33]. Other cancers reported to have increased risk are bone and soft tissue cancers, breast cancer, colorectal cancer, salivary gland tumors, and kidney cancer [32, 34, 35].

There are also several other studies that show increased risk of secondary malignancies in thyroid cancer patients, that is not associated with radioiodine administration [36, 37].

4.4. Radiation safety precautions for family members and public

Three of basic elements of radiation safety are distance, shielding, and time. Distance is the most important and simple way to ensure radiation safety. For point sources, the intensity of radiation is inversely related with the square of distance (inverse square law). For nonpoint sources, such as the patients, this law is not as accurate as in point sources, but still the exposure decreases as the distance in between increases. Shielding is another important parameter to ensure radiation safety. During radioiodine therapy, protection against beta and gamma radiation of I-131 is necessary. Beta radiation can be absorbed in a few centimeters of wood and they cannot penetrate out of patient body. Gamma rays are absorbed by atoms with heavy nuclei, such as lead. Reducing the exposure time reduces the cumulative dose proportionally. So the shorter time patients spend with their family, the smaller the radiation dose the family members receive.

ICRP and International Atomic Energy Agency (IAEA) recommend a dose limit of 1 mSv/year to the general public and 5 mSv/year to family members and caregivers of patients who have received radionuclide therapy **(Table 4)** [30, 38]. According to the European Atomic Energy Community (EURATOM), patients are allowed to be discharged after a radiation dose rate limit of 20 μSv/h at 1 m is achieved. After discharge, patients are advised to take further precautions at home.

Organ or tissue	Radiation worker (mSv/year)	Public (mSv/year)
Whole body	20	1
Gonads	50	5
Bone marrow	50	5
Bone	500	50
Skin	500	50
Thyroid gland	500	50
Extremities	500	75

Table 4. Dose limits to radiation workers and public recommended by ICRP.

Patients undergoing radioiodine therapy for thyroid cancer treatment and ablation are hospitalized in radionuclide therapy units to ensure proper shielding and waste control. Special precautions are taken in design of the patient rooms: The walls are lead lined to limit the gamma ray exposure of the health care workers and other patients. Also, lead lined tanks are used to store the waste of patients for decay to limit the release of I-131 to public sewage system. After discharge, patients are advised to maximize their distance from pregnant women and children, sleep in separate beds, to avoid spending extended time in public places, and to

http://dx.doi.org/10.5772/64087

limit travel for some time depending on the amount of radioiodine given [39, 40]. Also, several attempts are being discussed to decrease the radiation-related side effects of the patient, such as increased amount of daily water intake, frequent urination to decrease the absorbed dose to kidneys and bladder, and chewing-gum stimulation to decrease the absorbed dose to salivary glands [41]. Pregnancy is contra-indicated for radioiodine administration and according to ICRP female patients are advised to refrain from pregnancy for at least 4 months following radioiodine administration. Also, breast-feeding is not allowed after radioiodine administration.

Author details

Lebriz Uslu Beşli and Mustafa Demir*

*Address all correspondence to: demirm@istanbul.edu.tr

Department of Nuclear Medicine, Istanbul University Cerrahpaşa Medical Faculty, Istanbul, Turkey

References

[1] Cooper DS, Doherty GM, Haugen BR, Kloos RT, Lee SL, Mandel SJ, et al. Revised American Thyroid Association management guidelines for patients with thyroid nodules and differentiated thyroid cancer. Thyroid: Official Journal of the American Thyroid Association. 2009;19:1167–1214. doi: 10.1089/thy.2009.0110.

[2] Haugen BR, Alexander EK, Bible KC, Doherty GM, Mandel SJ, Nikiforov YE, et al. 2015 American Thyroid Association management guidelines for adult patients with thyroid nodules and differentiated thyroid cancer: The American Thyroid Association Guidelines Task Force on Thyroid Nodules and Differentiated Thyroid Cancer. Thyroid: Official Journal of the American Thyroid Association. 2016;26:1–133. doi: 10.1089/thy.2015.0020.

[3] Marinelli LD, Quimby EH, Hine GJ. Dosage determination with radioactive isotopes; biological considerations and practical applications. Nucleonics. 1948;2:44–49.

[4] Zanzonico PB. Internal radionuclide radiation dosimetry: a review of basic concepts and recent developments. Journal of Nuclear Medicine: Official Publication, Society of Nuclear Medicine. 2000;41:297–308.

[5] Toohey RE, Stabin MG, Watson EE. The AAPM/RSNA physics tutorial for residents: internal radiation dosimetry: principles and applications. Radiographics: A Review Publication of the Radiological Society of North America, Inc. 2000;20:533–546; quiz 1–2. doi: 10.1148/radiographics.20.2.g00mc33533.

[6] Stabin MG. Dosimetric and radiobiologic considerations. In: Ell PJ, Gambhir SS, editors. Nuclear Medicine in Clinical Diagnosis and Treatment. 3rd edition. Churchill Livingstone, New York; 2004. Pp 363–373.

[7] Stabin MG. Mathematical models and specific absorbed fractions of photon energy in the nonpregnant adult females and at the end of each trimester of pregnancy. Oak Ridge, TN: Oak Ridge National Laboratory; 1995.

[8] Cristy M. Development of mathematical pediatric phantoms for internal dose calculations: designs, limitations, and prospects. In: Watson EE, Stelson A, Coffey J, Cloutier R, editors. Proceedings of the Third International Radiopharmaceutical Dosimetry Symposium (FDA 81–8166). Oak Ridge, TN: Oak Ridge Associated Universities; 1981. Pp. 496–517.

[9] Eckerman K. Aspects of the dosimetry of radionuclides in the skeleton with particular emphasis on the active marrow. In: Stelson A, Watson E, editors. Proceedings of the Fourth International Radiopharmaceutical Dosimetry Symposium (CONF-851113). Oak Ridge, TN: Oak Ridge Associated Universities; 1986. Pp. 514–534.

[10] Stabin MG. MIRDOSE: personal computer software for internal dose assessment in nuclear medicine. Journal of Nuclear Medicine: Official Publication, Society of Nuclear Medicine. 1996;37:538–546.

[11] Stabin MG, Sparks RB, Crowe E. OLINDA/EXM: the second-generation personal computer software for internal dose assessment in nuclear medicine. Journal of Nuclear Medicine: Official Publication, Society of Nuclear Medicine. 2005;46:1023–1027.

[12] Zaidi H, Xu XG. Computational anthropomorphic models of the human anatomy: the path to realistic Monte Carlo modeling in radiological sciences. Annual Review of Biomedical Engineering. 2007;9:471–500. doi:10.1146/annurev.bioeng.9.060906.151934.

[13] Stabin MG, Emmons MA, Segars WP, Fernald MJ. Realistic reference adult and paediatric phantom series for internal and external dosimetry. Radiation Protection Dosimetry. 2012;149:56–59. doi:10.1093/rpd/ncr383.

[14] Benua RS, Cicale NR, Sonenberg M, Rawson RW. The relation of radioiodine dosimetry to results and complications in the treatment of metastatic thyroid cancer. The American Journal of Roentgenology, Radium Therapy, and Nuclear Medicine. 1962;87:171–182.

[15] Wahl RL, Kroll S, Zasadny KR. Patient-specific whole-body dosimetry: principles and a simplified method for clinical implementation. Journal of Nuclear Medicine: Official Publication, Society of Nuclear Medicine. 1998;39:14s–20s.

[16] Lassmann M, Hanscheid H, Chiesa C, Hindorf C, Flux G, Luster M. EANM Dosimetry Committee series on standard operational procedures for pre-therapeutic dosimetry I: blood and bone marrow dosimetry in differentiated thyroid cancer therapy. European

Journal of Nuclear Medicine and Molecular Imaging. 2008;35:1405–1412. doi:10.1007/s00259-008-0761-x.

[17] Maxon HR, Thomas SR, Hertzberg VS, Kereiakes JG, Chen IW, Sperling MI, et al. Relation between effective radiation dose and outcome of radioiodine therapy for thyroid cancer. The New England Journal of Medicine. 1983;309:937–941. doi:10.1056/nejm198310203091601.

[18] Atkins FB, Van Nostrand D, Wartofsky L. Dosimetrically-determined prescribed activity of radioiodine for the treatment of metastatic thyroid carcinoma. In: Wartofsky L, Van Nostrand D, editors. Thyroid Cancer: A Comprehensive Guide to Clinical Management. 2nd edition. Humana Press, Totowa, New Jersey; 2006. Pp. 433–446.

[19] Alevizaki C, Molfetas M, Samartzis A, Vlassopoulou B, Vassilopoulos C, Rondogianni P, et al. Iodine 131 treatment for differentiated thyroid carcinoma in patients with end stage renal failure: dosimetric, radiation safety, and practical considerations. Hormones (Athens, Greece). 2006;5:276–287.

[20] Yeyin N, Cavdar I, Uslu L, Abuqbeitah M, Demir M. Effects of hemodialysis on iodine-131 biokinetics in thyroid carcinoma patients with end-stage chronic renal failure. Nuclear Medicine Communications. 2016;37:283–287. doi: 10.1097/mnm.0000000000000439.

[21] Lassmann M, Reiners C, Luster M. Dosimetry and thyroid cancer: the individual dosage of radioiodine. Endocrine-Related Cancer. 2010;17:R161–R172. doi: 10.1677/erc-10-0071.

[22] Jentzen W, Freudenberg L, Eising EG, Sonnenschein W, Knust J, Bockisch A. Optimized ^{124}I PET dosimetry protocol for radioiodine therapy of differentiated thyroid cancer. Journal of Nuclear Medicine: Official Publication, Society of Nuclear Medicine. 2008;49:1017–1023. doi: 10.2967/jnumed.107.047159.

[23] Jentzen W, Bockisch A, Ruhlmann M. Assessment of simplified blood dose protocols for the estimation of the maximum tolerable activity in thyroid cancer patients undergoing radioiodine therapy using 124I. Journal of Nuclear Medicine: Official Publication, Society of Nuclear Medicine. 2015;56:832–838. doi: 10.2967/jnumed.114.153031.

[24] Freudenberg LS, Jentzen W, Stahl A, Bockisch A, Rosenbaum-Krumme SJ. Clinical applications of 124I-PET/CT in patients with differentiated thyroid cancer. European Journal of Nuclear Medicine and Molecular Imaging. 2011;38(Suppl 1):S48–S56. doi: 10.1007/s00259-011-1773-5.

[25] Chen MK, Cheng DW. What is the role of dosimetry in patients with advanced thyroid cancer? Current Opinion in Oncology. 2015;27:33–37. doi: 10.1097/cco.0000000000000145.

[26] Wierts R, Brans B, Havekes B, Kemerink G, Halders S, Schaper N, et al. Dose–response relationship in differentiated thyroid cancer patients undergoing radioiodine treatment

assessed by means of ^{124}I PET/CT. Journal of Nuclear Medicine: Official Publication, Society of Nuclear Medicine. 2016. doi: 10.2967/jnumed.115.168799.

[27] Pettinato C, Spezi E, Nanni C, Grassetto G, Monari F, Allegri V, et al. Pretherapeutic dosimetry in patients affected by metastatic thyroid cancer using ^{124}I PET/CT sequential scans for ^{131}I treatment planning. Clinical Nuclear Medicine. 2014;39:e367-74. doi: 10.1097/rlu.0000000000000490.

[28] Pettinato C, Monari F, Nanni C, Allegri V, Marcatili S, Civollani S, et al. Usefulness of ^{124}I PET/CT imaging to predict absorbed doses in patients affected by metastatic thyroid cancer and treated with ^{131}I. The Quarterly Journal of Nuclear Medicine and Molecular Imaging: Official Publication of the Italian Association of Nuclear Medicine (AIMN) [and] the International Association of Radiopharmacology (IAR), [and] Section of the Society of Radiopharmaceutical Chemistry and Biology. 2012;56:509–514.

[29] Kist JW, de Keizer B, van der Vlies M, Brouwers AH, Huysmans DA, van der Zant FM, et al. 124I PET/CT to predict the outcome of blind 131I treatment in patients with biochemical recurrence of differentiated thyroid cancer: Results of a multicenter diagnostic cohort study (THYROPET). J Nucl Med. 2016;57(5):701–7.

[30] International Commission on Radiological Protection. 1990 Recommendations of the International Commission on Radiological Protection. Annals of the ICRP. ICRP Publication 60 ed. Oxford: Pergamon Press; 1991. Pp. 1–201.

[31] Sisson JC. Practical dosimetry of 131I in patients with thyroid carcinoma. Cancer Biotherapy & Radiopharmaceuticals. 2002;17:101–105. doi: 10.1089/10849780252824118.

[32] Rubino C, de Vathaire F, Dottorini ME, Hall P, Schvartz C, Couette JE, et al. Second primary malignancies in thyroid cancer patients. British Journal of Cancer. 2003;89:1638–1644. doi: 10.1038/sj.bjc.6601319.

[33] Sawka AM, Thabane L, Parlea L, Ibrahim-Zada I, Tsang RW, Brierley JD, et al. Second primary malignancy risk after radioactive iodine treatment for thyroid cancer: a systematic review and meta-analysis. Thyroid: Official Journal of the American Thyroid Association. 2009;19:451–457. doi: 10.1089/thy.2008.0392.

[34] Brown AP, Chen J, Hitchcock YJ, Szabo A, Shrieve DC, Tward JD. The risk of second primary malignancies up to three decades after the treatment of differentiated thyroid cancer. The Journal of Clinical Endocrinology and Metabolism. 2008;93:504–515. doi: 10.1210/jc.2007-1154.

[35] Chen AY, Levy L, Goepfert H, Brown BW, Spitz MR, Vassilopoulou-Sellin R. The development of breast carcinoma in women with thyroid carcinoma. Cancer. 2001;92:225–231.

[36] Berthe E, Henry-Amar M, Michels JJ, Rame JP, Berthet P, Babin E, et al. Risk of second primary cancer following differentiated thyroid cancer. European Journal of Nuclear Medicine and Molecular Imaging. 2004;31:685–691. doi: 10.1007/s00259-003-1448-y.

[37] Sandeep TC, Strachan MW, Reynolds RM, Brewster DH, Scelo G, Pukkala E, et al. Second primary cancers in thyroid cancer patients: a multinational record linkage study. The Journal of Clinical Endocrinology and Metabolism. 2006;91:1819–1825. doi: 10.1210/jc.2005-2009.

[38] International Atomic Energy Agency. Radiological Protection for Medical Exposure to Ionizing Radiation. Vienna: IAEA; 2002.

[39] Sisson JC, Freitas J, McDougall IR, Dauer LT, Hurley JR, Brierley JD, et al. Radiation safety in the treatment of patients with thyroid diseases by radioiodine ^{131}I: practice recommendations of the American Thyroid Association. Thyroid: Official Journal of the American Thyroid Association. 2011;21:335–346. doi: 10.1089/thy.2010.0403.

[40] Barrington SF, Kettle AG, O'Doherty MJ, Wells CP, Somer EJ, Coakley AJ. Radiation dose rates from patients receiving iodine-131 therapy for carcinoma of the thyroid. European Journal of Nuclear Medicine. 1996;23:123–130.

[41] Jentzen W, Richter M, Nagarajah J, Poeppel TD, Brandau W, Dawes C, et al. Chewing-gum stimulation did not reduce the absorbed dose to salivary glands during radioiodine treatment of thyroid cancer as inferred from pre-therapy (124)I PET/CT imaging. EJNMMI Physics. 2014;1:100. doi: 10.1186/s40658-014-0100-1.

Chapter 13

Thyroid Cancer in Children and Adolescents

Eman Marie, Mahnaz Kousha and Reza Vali

Additional information is available at the end of the chapter

http://dx.doi.org/10.5772/64190

Abstract

Thyroid cancer is the most common endocrine malignancy in children and adolescents. Although the basis of the thyroid cancer management in children is the same as those of the adults, thyroid cancer may behave different in pediatric population than adults. Unlike adults, children usually present with more advanced disease and the risk of recurrence and metastases are higher. However, the prognosis and survival of pediatric thyroid cancer is better than those of adults. This chapter will review the frequency, epidemiology, and clinical behavior of pediatric thyroid cancer with emphasis on the appropriate management in nuclear medicine.

Keywords: thyroid cancer, iodine scan, thyroid, thyroglobulin, ultrasound, children, adolescents

1. Introduction

Thyroid cancer is the most common endocrine malignancy; in 2014, it affected >60,000 people in North America [1]. Only approximately 2% of thyroid cancer has been reported to occur in children and adolescents [2]. The most frequent type of thyroid cancer is the differentiated type, mainly papillary (90–95%) and to a lesser extent follicular (~5%) [3–5]. Conventionally, thyroid cancers in both adult and pediatric patients are managed by total or near-total thyroidectomy, with resection of the affected regional lymph nodes, followed by ablation of the thyroid remnant and associated metastases using ^{131}I. The patients then receive subsequent treatment involving thyroid-stimulating hormone (TSH) suppression with levothyroxine [6, 7]. Accurate staging (to avoid overtreatment) and the choice of surveillance methods are important in children. On one hand, the risk of recurrence and regional lymph node involvement are higher in children. On the other hand, because of the long lifespan of these patients and their susceptibility to treatment side effects, the risk of long-term complications associated with therapy (e.g., high doses of radioiodine) is higher than those of adults [8, 9]. In this chapter, the management of thyroid cancer in children is discussed, with the focus on nuclear medicine therapies.

2. Epidemiology

In general, the risk of thyroid cancers has increased globally over the last decades [3, 10]. Unlike many other cancers, thyroid cancer is rare in early childhood; the incidence increases during adolescence and early adult life and will reach a plateau at age approximately 40 years with little subsequent changes at older ages [11]. Thyroid cancer is the eighth most common cancer diagnosed in patients aged 15–19 years, and is the second most common cancer among adolescent girls [12, 13]. Many other cancers are rare in early childhood and are common in older people; some (usually those with immature tumor cells such as retinoblastoma or neuroblastoma) are more common in early childhood and are rare in adults [11]. Thyroid nodules are more common in teenagers than in younger children [14]; however, the risk of malignancy is greater when a nodule in diagnosed in children aged <10 years [15].

3. Risk factors

Age, sex, family history of thyroid disease, and radiation exposure are among the risk factors affecting the frequency of thyroid cancers in children. Generally, differentiated thyroid cancer (DTC) is more common in adolescent girls [2]. The sex distribution of thyroid carcinoma differs between adults and children. In adults, thyroid cancer is four times more common in women than in men. In the pediatric population, the incidence of thyroid cancer is only slightly higher in younger girls before puberty as compared with boys (female-to-male ratio, 1.5:1). The risk of thyroid cancer then increases rapidly and reaches a peak during puberty in teenage girls (female-to-male ratio, 3:1 to 14:1) [16–18]. Although it has not yet been confirmed, sex hormones may play a major role in the rapid increase in the incidence of thyroid cancer in female individuals during puberty [19].

The higher frequency of thyroid cancers after radiotherapy involving the neck has been confirmed in patients who were treated with external radiation for conditions such as tinea capitis, chronic tonsillitis, acne, and thymus hyperplasia [20, 21], and in children years after the Chernobyl incident [22, 23]. Analysis of the age of individuals at the time of radiation exposure showed that younger children had the highest risk of thyroid carcinoma after the Chernobyl incident [24].

4. Presentation

An asymptomatic neck mass (located in either the thyroid bed or elsewhere in the neck as an enlarged lymph node) is usually the first clinical presentation of thyroid cancer in children [25].

The possibility of malignancy increases if the mass is firm, nonmobile with associated lymphadenopathy, and/or there is vocal cord paralysis [25]. At presentation, the tumor size is often greater in children than in adults [26, 27]. The frequency of regional lymph node involvement is also higher in children relative to adults. More than half of the patients (60–90%) will have regional lymph node involvement either at diagnosis or on follow-up [8, 25, 27].

Lung metastasis is the most common site of distant metastases [28, 29]. Presentation with lung symptoms is very rare. Lung metastasis is more commonly seen in patients with extracapsular invasion, bilateral tumors, and in patients aged <7 years at diagnosis [30, 31]. In our experience, we found ≤20% of pulmonary metastases either at presentation or in follow-up studies [32]; all of them had a thyroglobulin (Tg) level of >10 ng/mL. In contrast to adults, pulmonary metastases in children are usually miliary and rarely nodular [30, 31]. Metastases to the lungs are functional in 95% of the cases. Metastases to the bone or central nervous system are very rare [28, 29, 33]. Thyroid function tests are usually normal in pediatric patients with DTC at presentation [25].

5. Management

The management of children with DTC should be undertaken by a medical team with appropriate experience and skills. The treatment of thyroid cancer in adult patients has been studied in detail by several investigators, and general guidelines exist. Pediatric oncologists have attempted to extrapolate from these guidelines, but there are insufficient data to answer many questions regarding children. Patients with thyroid cancer require the assistance of a diversified group of healthcare providers during literally every step of their care, from the time of diagnosis to the extended period of follow-up. The American Thyroid association (ATA) 2015 guidelines endeavor to summarize, in a practical way, the optimal management of patients with thyroid cancer; they detail how the fabric of their care is carefully woven by a group of providers with specialized skills, each of whom adds a unique component regarding the patient's overall care [34]. Without this broad multidisciplinary approach, gaps may occur at every turn in management, which may pose serious obstacles in achieving the best long-term results for the patients.

Generally, after a comprehensive analysis of patient history and physical examination, further investigation using high-resolution ultrasound (US) is recommended for the diagnosis of solid thyroid nodules, and to check for extrathyroid extension of the disease and regional neck lymph node involvement (**Figure 1**). This is frequently followed by fine needle aspiration (FNA) of the nodule, usually under the guidance of US [35, 36]. According to the pediatric-specific ATA guidelines recommendations, the US characteristics and clinical context, rather than size alone, should be used to determine if nodules warrant FNA [34]. Moreover, in children it is recommended that all FNAs are performed under US guidance [34]. Evaluation of regional lymph node involvement is important because children with evidence of palpable cervical lymph node disease at diagnosis are more likely to have multifocal disease (89 vs. 16%), an increased risk of pulmonary metastasis (20 vs. 0%), and an increased risk of persistent

(30 vs. 0%) and/or recurrent (53 vs. 0%) disease (**Figures 2** and **3**), as compared with children without gross nodal disease [37, 38].

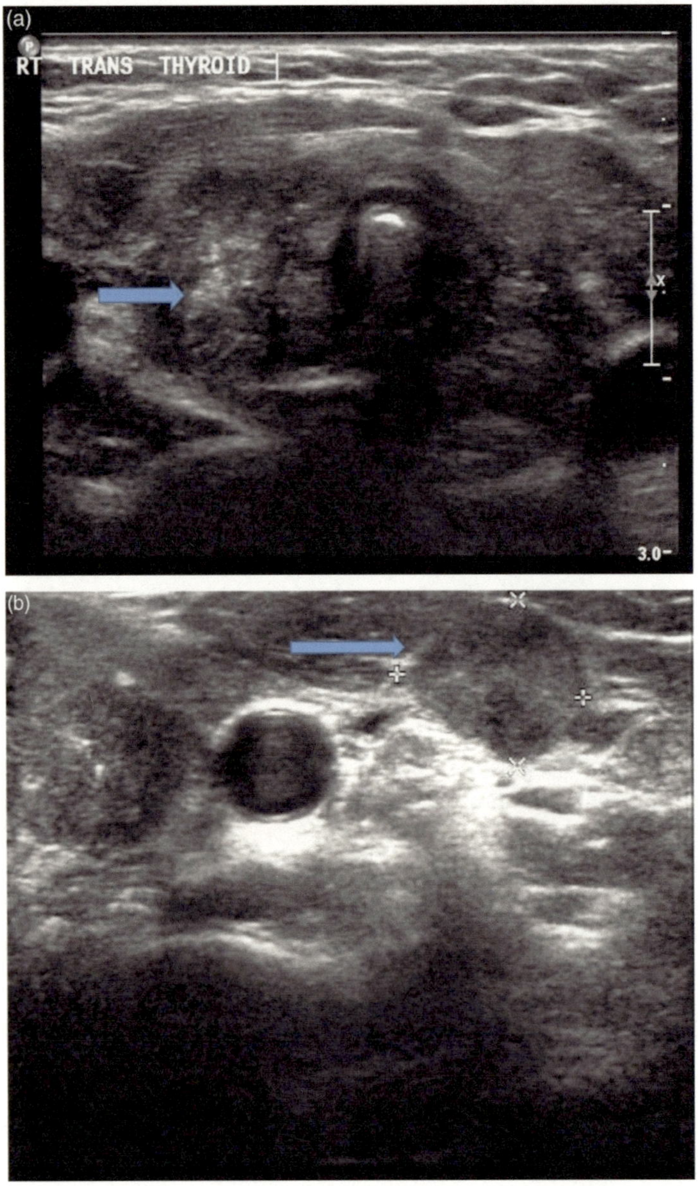

Figure 1. Ultrasound in a 10-year old boy with history of large posterior fossa brain tumour and panhypopituitarism, on thyroid replacement treatment: the patient presented with bilateral vocal cord weakness and stridor. Thyroid gland was enlarged with heterogeneous parenchyma and small foci of calcification (arrow in a). There were enlarged cervical lymph nodes with lost central echogenic hilum and increased short-to-long axis ratio (S/L) >0.5 (b) which is suggestive of malignant infiltration, one of them showed in (b) (arrow). Papillary thyroid cancer was proved on histopathology with neck lymph nodes involvement.

http://dx.doi.org/10.5772/64190

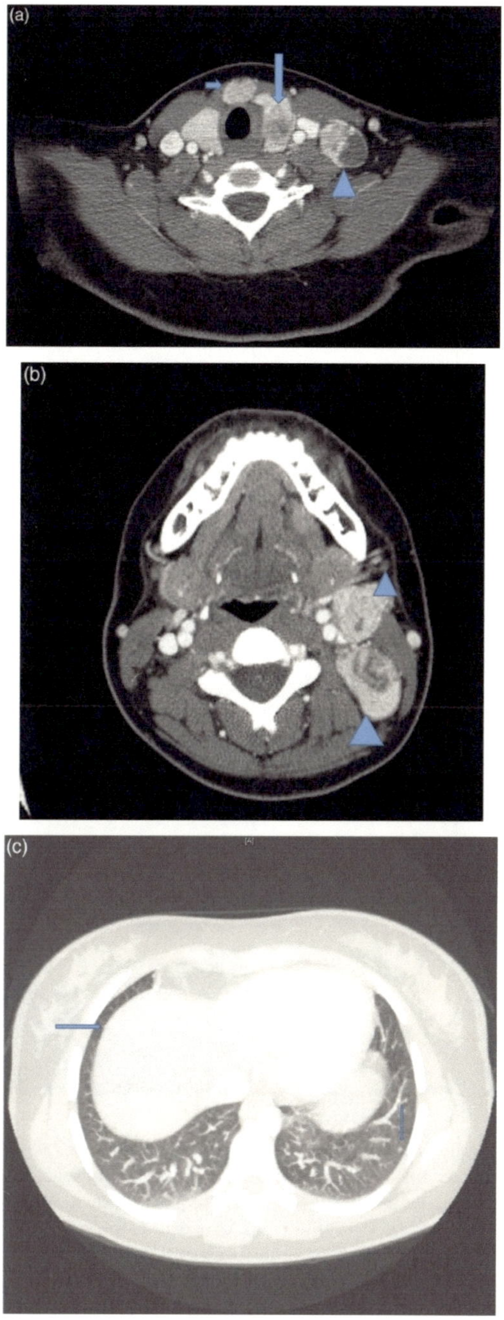

Figure 2. Fifteen-year old girl referred to the clinic for a neck mass. Axial enhanced CT image (a and b) shows a heterogeneous nodule in the left thyroid lobe (big arrow) with enhancing large cystic nodal lymph nodes (arrowheads) in the left levels IIa, IIb, and IV in addition to level VI or Delphian nodes (small arrow). Papillary thyroid carcinoma with lymph nodes involvement was proven on histopathology. CT scan was suggestive for lung metastases (c) with small nodules in both lungs (arrows).

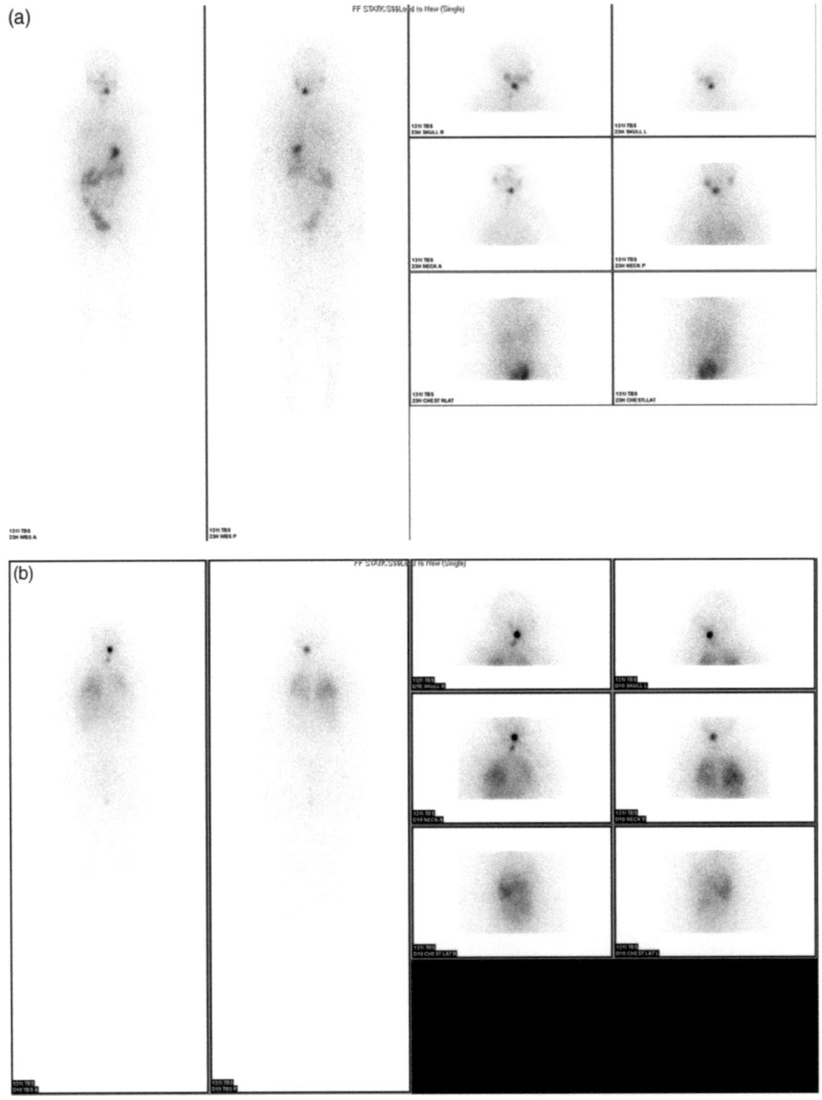

Figure 3. Status postoperative (total thyroidectomy) in the same patient presented in **Figure 2**. Diagnostic whole-body iodine scan after 2 mCi I-123 (a) demonstrated mild residual thyroid activity with a focus in the left submandibular region that might represent lymph node metastatic lesion. There was suspicion of lung metastases on chest CT scan (please see **Figure 2c**). The patient was treated with 145 mCi. On posttherapy scan (b) 7 and 10 days after a therapeutic dose of radioiodine, bilateral chest activity with no definite focus was noted due to pulmonary metastatic.

According to the ATA guidelines for pediatrics, children with papillary thyroid cancer can be divided into low, intermediate, or high risk, based on the clinical presentation, tumor size, and evidence of regional invasion and metastasis [34]. Low-risk patients are those with a cancer confined to the thyroid with no regional lymph nodes involvement or with incidental micro-metastasis to a small number of central neck lymph nodes. If the patient has extensive central lymph nodes involvement (level VI; pretracheal, paratracheal, prelaryngeal/Delphian lymph

http://dx.doi.org/10.5772/64190

nodes), or minimal lymph nodes involvement in the rest of the neck, the patient is categorized as intermediate risk. Locally invasive disease (in the thyroid) or extensive neck lymph nodes involvement (other than region VI), or distant metastases will put the patient into the high-risk group [34]. Similar to adults, the cornerstone of the therapy is based on surgery, radioiodine ablation/therapy, and thyroid hormone replacement/suppression therapy.

6. Surgery

Except under special conditions, it is recommended that more comprehensive thyroid surgery is performed in pediatric patients; this is because of the higher incidence of bilateral and multifocal disease (30 and 65%, respectively) [39–41]. Thyroid lobectomy alone may be sufficient for small unifocal cancers (<1 cm), with no capsular invasion or lymph node involvement, without a prior history of radiotherapy or a family history of thyroid cancer [34]. In comparison with lobectomy, total thyroidectomy has a lower risk of recurrent/persistent disease and subsequent second surgical procedures [34, 40, 42, 43]. Central neck dissection is recommended for patients with evidence of gross extrathyroidal invasion and/or locoregional metastasis on preoperative staging or during surgery [34]. If there is no evidence of gross extrathyroidal invasion and/or locoregional metastasis, prophylactic central neck dissection may be routinely performed [34]. The decision is made based on tumor focality and size, and the experience of the surgeon [34]. Prophylactic lateral neck dissection (levels III, IV, anterior V, and II) is not recommended routinely, unless there is histopathological proof of lateral neck lymph node involvement [34].

7. Radioactive iodine (^{131}I) ablation and therapy

Typically, there is remnant thyroid tissue after a total or near-total thyroidectomy, mainly because of the presence of normal thyroid tissue around the nerves or Berry's ligament. Because multifocal papillary cancer is relatively common in children, most authors recommend radioiodine ablation therapy in younger patients [25, 44]. Ablation therapy presumably not only destroys normal residual thyroid tissue but also possible micrometastases [45]. Moreover, follow-up Tg measurement is easier after radioiodine ablation therapy [46, 47]. In other words, if a patient receives radioiodine ablation therapy and the Tg level reaches an undetectable level, a subsequent rise in Tg level is highly suspicious of recurrence. In contrast, a rise in Tg level in a patient who did not receive ablation therapy may be the result of tumor recurrence or the regrowth of normal thyroid tissue [48, 49]. In the majority of cases, a single radioiodine treatment is sufficient for ablation. However, in some cases more than one treatment is required for complete ablation. It has not been proven in the pediatric population if the response to the first ablation therapy has any prognostic value.

Radioiodine can be provided in liquid and capsule forms. Although selection of the type of administration depends on patient preference, the capsule form is usually preferred to ensure that the activity is fully delivered to the stomach. In some cases, an antiemetic medication is also required before administration of the radioiodine. If it is not clear that the patient can tolerate the capsule form, an empty gelatin capsule can be tried before the actual radioiodine capsule. ^{131}I is also used for the treatment of known or suspected viable malignant disease in patients with DTC to destroy or control the disease. The dose of radioiodine for therapy mainly depends on the presence or absence of metastases, and the organs involved. The diagnostic and therapeutic role of radioiodine must be individualized to each patient through collaboration between the patient's endocrinologist/referring physician and the nuclear medicine physician [50]. Tumor radioiodine avidity and sensitivity to radioiodine can vary significantly between children with DTC, and even in the same patient over time [50, 51]. The selected dose of radioiodine for therapy depends on many factors including the presence or absence of metastases, and intermediate-/high-risk or low-risk patients. There are formulas for the estimation of relative pediatric doses [51]. In general, it is suggested that the ^{131}I doses should not exceed 200 mCi (7400 MBq) for each patient with a total cumulative dose limited to 1000 mCi (37,000 MBq). The absorbed dose to the red marrow should not exceed 200 cGy, and 48-hour whole-body retention should not reach 120 mCi (4440 MBq) to minimize the risk of secondary acute myelogenous leukemia (AML). The 48-hour whole-body retention of activity should be limited to 80 mCi (2960 MBq) in the setting of pulmonary metastases, to minimize the risk of pulmonary fibrosis [50, 51]. In certain cases, especially with pulmonary metastases, formal dosimetry should be performed in children with avid pulmonary metastases [50, 51]. Dosimetry before ^{131}I therapy can also be considered in small children and in patients with a limited bone marrow reserve [34]. If there is a need to repeat the ^{131}I therapy, an interval of ≥12 months is suggested to minimize the risk of secondary AML [50].

In many European and Asian countries, the patient is admitted 2 or 3 days after radioiodine ablation/therapy to minimize radiation exposure to the public. In North America, however, many centers allow the patients to go home after a therapeutic dose of radioiodine [52]. In our center, patients receiving therapeutic radioiodine doses of >30 mCi (1.1 GBq) up to and including 200 mCi (7.4 GBq) can be managed on an outpatient basis, provided that the estimate of radiation exposure to the general public falls within regulatory limits. According to our institutional protocol, an adult family member who is considered to be the primary caregiver is exempt from the 1 mSv public dose limit; however, dose exposure should not exceed 5 mSv for the course of the treatment [53]. Our pediatric patients would prefer to be isolated in their homes rather than be confined in the hospital when medical care is not required. To achieve this, the patient and family must be willing to temporarily modify their lifestyles and comply with the instructions provided (**Table 1**). **Table 2** is an example of a questionnaire for an outpatient therapy with ^{131}I in our institution. Exclusion criteria include patients requiring medical care during the course of the constrained period, any socio-economical factor that would inhibit compliance, and the inability of the primary caregiver or the patient to follow the radiation safety instructions. In a recent study, despite poor compliance with the radiation safety recommendations for patients treated with 100 mCi (3.7 GBq), caregivers received a low measured radiation exposure [54]. In this study, excessive radiation exposure was only seen when the caregivers stayed close to the patient for more than 5.8 hours during the first 3 days after radioiodine treatment [54].

http://dx.doi.org/10.5772/64190

Patients receiving therapeutic radioiodine doses of greater than 30 mCi (1.1 GBq) up to and including 200 mCi (7.4 GBq) can be managed on an outpatient basis provided that the estimate of radiation exposure to the general public fall within regulatory limits.

Procedure

1. The treating physician will conduct an assessment to determine suitability for outpatient treatment. The decision will be based on the patient's or family's response to a questionnaire regarding family members, circumstances and the assurance of compliance with the radiation safety instructions. See **Table 2**.

2. The treating physician will discuss the patient's suitability for this protocol with the radiation safety officer (RSO) or trained designate. In the case of noncompliance with the restrictions given, an estimate of the maximal dose to an individual in the patient's environment should be estimated and taken into account in the decision process.

3. The patient and family will be provided with appropriate written and oral information and instruction about the requirements for treatment. The RSO will verify that the patient and family understand what is required of them and that they are willing to comply with the requirements.

4. Approval for outpatient management of radioiodine therapy must be obtained from the RSO prior to scheduling the therapy.

5. An effort should be made to reduce doses to family members to levels that are as low as reasonably achievable (ALARA) with economic and social factors being taken into account. Dose reductions may require a detailed assessment of family activities to determine where modification in lifestyle can best be made to reduce doses without unnecessary restrictions. One example of a modification would be to have the patient spend the "isolation" period with a compliant grandparent, away from other siblings or a pregnant parent.

6. A primary caregiver will be identified. Since this person will likely receive a higher radiation dose during the course of the patient's treatment, a dose calculation for this person will be made based on activity and occupancy factors during constrained activity for 3 days.

7. On the day of treatment, the RSO (or trained designate) and treating physician will reassess the patient's compliance and give the written and oral precautions for radiation safety. The patient and/or parent will sign two copies of the instructions. One copy will be given to the patient and the other will be retained for the departmental patient record.

8. The therapy dose will be administered and the patient will be discharged.

Table 1. The instructions to assess the patient for outpatient iodine therapy.

Patient Name: _____

MRN# _____

Referring Physician:

_____

1. Confirmation that the patient is not pregnant (≥12 years). Date of negative pregnancy test: _____

2. Is the patient breast feeding? Yes No

3. List the age and relationship of all other household members.

   Who will be the primary caregiver?

   _____

4. Will there be any young children (<10 yrs) or pregnant women at home Yes No
when the patient returns after treatment?
5. How will the patient travel home? _____ How long will it take? _____
Who will accompany the patient?
_____
6. Is the patient scheduled for any other medical tests, procedures, travel or Yes No
vacation 4 weeks prior or 2 weeks after dosing?
7. What is the parent's occupation and specific job duties?
8. Can the patient remain home for the recommended time? Yes/No
(Not applicable for patients receiving less than 30 mCi of I-131) N/A
9. Does the patient require any special medical care or living assistance? Yes No
10. Will patient have use of private bathroom for the next 3 days? Yes No
11. Is the patient incontinent or have any urinary bladder control problems? Yes No
12. Will the patient have a private bedroom for the next 7 days? Yes No
Where is the location of bedroom and adjoining rooms? _____
13. Can the patient maintain at least 10-foot distance from others? Yes No
14. Is the patient capable of following the radiation safety instructions? Yes No
15. Are there any other issues that would prevent the patient from being able to Yes No
Comply with the radiation safety instructions?
Explain:
_____
_____
Individual completing Questionnaire:
_____ Date:
_____
Title: _____

Table 2. A sample questionnaire for outpatient treatment with iodine 131.

8. Radioiodine side effects

The side effects of the radioiodine treatment are similar to those of adult patients and include: radiation thyroiditis (usually in patients with a large thyroid remnant) given sufficient ^{131}I to deliver about 500 Gy (50,000 cGy) [55]; acute and/or chronic parotiditis or submandibular gland sialadenitis (in up to one-third of patients, usually when a large amount of ^{131}I activity was administered to a patient with a small thyroid remnant) [56]; conjunctivitis and nasolacrimal drainage system obstruction [57, 58], radiation sickness (with a high dose); acute tumor edema or hemorrhage; transient vocal cord or facial nerve palsy [59]; transient amenorrhea or menstrual irregularities [60]; and reduced sperm counts (usually transient) [61]. Infertility is rare but may occur after an accumulated high dose of radiation [62]. The majority of these complications are transient and do not require any specific treatment. However, there are two important side effects that are life threatening, namely, secondary leukemia and pulmonary fibrosis [63]; both relate to the cumulative dose of radioiodine. Unfortunately, there is no definite cutoff regarding the safe dose of ^{131}I that can be used to avoid these important complications; the usefulness of the therapy should be assessed prior to each administration, especially where multiple treatments in a single patient are needed, or in patients with pulmonary metastases.

9. Follow-up (surveillance)

Recurrence of DTC in children may be seen years after the initial therapy. Thus, long-term follow-up including periodic physical examinations and evaluation involving Tg measurement and neck US are necessary [1]. In recommendation 16 of the ATA 2105 guidelines, postoperative staging is usually performed within 12 weeks after surgery to identify the patients who will benefit from further treatment. In our center, we evaluate the patients 6 weeks after the surgery. Although low-risk patients may be followed up with only TSH-suppressed Tg, for intermediate- and high-risk patients TSH-stimulated Tg evaluation and a diagnostic whole-body iodine scan are typically recommended to determine if there is evidence of persistent and/or recurrent disease [34]. We suggest to evaluate the low-risk patients with Tg measurement and neck US [32]. The measurement of Tg, either "on T4" (basal Tg level) or "off T4" (stimulated Tg level), is the cornerstone of postoperative surveillance programs [2]. Tg is only produced by thyroid cells (normal thyroid cells and differentiated thyroid carcinomas). Consequently, the level of Tg should be undetectable if all thyroid tissues have been destroyed by surgery and radioiodine ablation therapy. However, Tg measurement is not reliable when there is anti-Tg antibody (TgAb) present in the serum. Tg and TgAb levels should be simultaneously measured using the same laboratory and assay technique [47]. Recommendation 23 of the ATA 2015 guidelines stresses that Tg is a sensitive tumor marker in the evaluation, treatment, and long-term follow-up of pediatric DTC, even in children not previously treated with ^{131}I [47]. The trend in serial Tg and/or TgAb levels is probably more representative of disease status than any single measurement [47]. US is a noninvasive and sensitive method for the evaluation of locoregional lymph node involvement [32]. US is superior in sensitivity to a diagnostic whole-body iodine scan for the detection of involved neck lymph nodes, and it does not require levothyroxine withdrawal. However, the accurate interpretation of US scans in DTC can be complicated by the high frequency of large inflammatory neck lymph nodes in children [4]. According to the ATA guidelines, neck US should be performed at ≥6 months after the initial surgery, and then at 6- to 12-month intervals for intermediate- and high-risk patients, and at annual intervals for low-risk patients [47]. Follow-up beyond 5 years should be individualized based on the risk of recurrence [47].

A whole-body scan using ^{123}I or ^{131}I allows localization of local recurrences or distant metastases, and helps in the decision concerning subsequent radioiodine therapy [5]. Our institutional Protocol for ^{131}I-whole-body scan is summarized in **Table 3**. Routine evaluation using a diagnostic whole-body iodine scan is not recommended. ^{123}I is preferred to ^{131}I for diagnostic imaging. A whole-body iodine scan may be useful in children with known iodine-avid metastases (based on a prior post-therapy scan) at 1–2 years after therapy to evaluate the response to previous ^{131}I treatment [47]. According to the ATA guidelines, a repeat radioiodine scan is not recommended unless recurrent disease is suspected clinically, based on physical examination, US, or rising LT4 levels. In our experience, a radioiodine scan was useful when the Tg level was >10 ng/mL (for the evaluation of lung metastasis), when the results of Tg measurement and ultrasound was incongruent, or when anti-TgAb was positive (Tg can be falsely increased or reduced in the presence of a high anti-TgAb level) [34].

Indications

Follow-up imaging of patients post-thyroidectomy for thyroid cancer.

Follow-up imaging of patients receiving ^{131}I therapy for ablation post-thyroidectomy.

Contraindications

Patient who had a recent (24–48 hours) nuclear medicine scan performed.

The patient must not have had intravenous iodinated contrast agents for at least 1 month. Check with the nuclear medicine (NM) physician.

No recent administration of potassium perchlorate.

Patient preparation

- If the patient is taking thyroid medication, check with the referring physician if the patient can stop taking it for a minimum of 3 weeks prior to this procedure. Note this information on the requisition.
  - Synthroid should be stopped for 4–6 weeks
  - Cytomel 2 weeks
  - PTU 4 days
  - Tapazole 1 week
  - Methimazole 1 week
- Stop cough syrup, multivitamins for 48 hours before the test.
- Ensure other blood work has been done prior to radiopharmaceutical administration. Patients must have a minimum TSH level of 30–40 mIU/L, and all females who have commenced menstruating must have a documented negative bHCG prior to dosing.
- The patient should be NPO for approximately 2 hours before and 1 hour after receiving the dose by mouth to enhance the absorption of the ^{131}I.
- The patient should be encouraged to drink plenty of fluids for the next 24 hours to facilitate soft tissue clearance and to flush saliva from the mouth.

Radiopharmaceutical: ^{131}NaI

Dose: Based on BSA (body surface area) with a maximum dose of 4 mCi (148 MBq)

Dose administration

- This product is given **orally** in either capsule or liquid forms.
- Please inform the responsible NM Physician of the patient's arrival prior to dose administration.

http://dx.doi.org/10.5772/64190

- Please make sure to go over the radiation safety guidelines with the patient and parents to ensure compliance. The guidelines should be followed for **2** days if it is a **diagnostic** ^{131}I TBS (i.e., patient can return to school, etc. the day following whole-body scan). If the patient is getting a **therapeutic** ^{131}I dose, guidelines will be followed for **7** days. Ensure patient/parents are given the instruction sheet to take with them after dose administration and explain how to page the technologist on call if required.
- Pre- and Postdose counting must be done for all patients having an uptake and scan. Please refer to the ^{131}I Thyroid Uptake-Probe Method protocol
- For liquid ^{131}I, administer the dose directly into the patient's mouth. Have a small cup of water handy to use for rinsing the residual dose from the syringe into the patient's mouth—several rinses with the water may be necessary to ensure total dose delivery.
- Patients who are able to swallow a capsule should do so with at least one cup of water.
- Instruct the patient to remain NPO for one more hour and to return for imaging in 48 hours.

Acquisition

Images are done 48 hours following diagnostic dose administration.

- Images post-^{131}I therapy for ablation is performed 7–10 days postadministration.
- Using the high-energy collimator, first acquire an anterior and posterior whole-body pass with the head straight.
- Imaging should be done with a scan speed of 15 min/m using a 256 × 1024 matrix.
- Statics will also need to be done of the RLAT and LLAT skull using a 256 matrix and acquisition time of 10 min/view.
- A 10-minute anterior chest view may also be required but check with the NM physician.
- Patients receiving a diagnostic ^{131}I dose (4 mCi or less) will need to have an uptake performed at 48 hours as well.
- Have all images and uptake value checked by the NM physician. In most instances, the NM physician will want to speak to the patient before he leaves the department.

Table 3. Institutional protocol for ^{131}I-whole-body scans. Please note that there are some variations among different institutes for the protocol including the radiation safety precaution.

10. Prognosis

Despite the occurrence of extensive disease at clinical presentation, a higher risk of locoregional lymph node involvement, and a higher risk of recurrence, children are much less likely to die from thyroid cancer (≤2% long-term cause-specific mortality) than are adults [64], and the overall prognosis is better in pediatric DTC [7, 26]. In a study by Minsk et al., the 5- and 10-year survival rates were 99.3 and 98.5%, respectively [65]. Usually, the prognosis is worse in patients aged <10 years [66]. The prevalence of sodium-iodide transporter expression in pediatric DTC metastases is greater than in adults [67, 68]. This is probably one of the reasons for better prognosis and a superior response to radioiodine therapy in children relative to adults, although the risk of lymph node involvement is higher in pediatric DTC [67, 68].

11. Conclusion

Although the basis of thyroid cancer management in pediatric population is similar to that of adults, because of longer lifespan and susceptibility of children, the risk of therapy side effects may be higher in comparison to that of adults. Therefore, any treatment in these age groups should be individualized considering the risk and benefit of the therapy in that patient.

Acknowledgements

The authors would like to thank Dr. Amer Shammas, Dr. Martin Charron, and Susan McQuattie for sharing the institutional protocol.

Author details

Eman Marie, Mahnaz Kousha and Reza Vali*

*Address all correspondence to: reza.vali@sickkids.ca

Division of Nuclear Medicine, Diagnostic Imaging Department, The Hospital for Sick Children, University of Toronto, Toronto, Canada

References

[1] The Survival, Epidemiology, and End Result Program: SEER stats fact sheet: thyroid cancer. National Cancer Institute (2014). http://seer.cancer.gov/statfacts/html/thyro.html

[2] Hogan AR, Zhuge Y, Perez EA, Koniaris LG, Lew JI, Sola JE (2009) Pediatric thyroid carcinoma: incidence and outcomes in 1753 patients. The Journal of Surgical Research 156 (1):167–172. doi:10.1016/j.jss.2009.03.098

[3] Davies L, Welch HG (2006) Increasing incidence of thyroid cancer in the United States, 1973-2002. JAMA: The Journal of the American Medical Association 295 (18):2164–2167. doi:10.1001/jama.295.18.2164

[4] Hundahl SA, Fleming ID, Fremgen AM, Menck HR (1998) A National Cancer Data Base report on 53,856 cases of thyroid carcinoma treated in the U.S., 1985-1995 [see commetns]. Cancer 83 (12):2638–2648

[5] Harach HR, Williams ED (1995) Childhood thyroid cancer in England and Wales. British Journal of Cancer 72 (3):777–783

[6] Jones MK (2002) Management of papillary and follicular thyroid cancer. Journal of the Royal Society of Medicine 95 (7):325–326

[7] Mazzaferri EL, Massoll N (2002) Management of papillary and follicular (differentiated) thyroid cancer: new paradigms using recombinant human thyrotropin. Endocrine-Related Cancer 9 (4):227–247

[8] Parisi MT, Mankoff D (2007) Differentiated pediatric thyroid cancer: correlates with adult disease, controversies in treatment. Seminars in Nuclear Medicine 37 (5):340–356. doi:10.1053/j.semnuclmed.2007.05.001

[9] Vaisman F, Corbo R, Vaisman M (2011) Thyroid carcinoma in children and adolescents-systematic review of the literature. Journal of Thyroid Research (2011):845362. doi: 10.4061/2011/845362.

[10] Siegel R, Ma J, Zou Z, Jemal A (2014) Cancer statistics, 2014. CA: A Cancer Journal for Clinicians 64 (1):9–29. doi:10.3322/caac.21208

[11] Williams D (2015) Thyroid growth and cancer. European Thyroid Journal 4 (3):164–173. doi:10.1159/000437263

[12] Siegel DA, King J, Tai E, Buchanan N, Ajani UA, Li J (2014) Cancer incidence rates and trends among children and adolescents in the United States, 2001–2009. Pediatrics 134 (4):e945–955. doi:10.1542/peds.2013-3926

[13] Ward E, DeSantis C, Robbins A, Kohler B, Jemal A (2014) Childhood and adolescent cancer statistics, 2014. CA: A Cancer Journal for Clinicians 64 (2):83–103. doi:10.3322/caac.21219

[14] Josefson J, Zimmerman D (2008) Thyroid nodules and cancers in children. Pediatric Endocrinology Reviews: PER 6 (1):14–23

[15] Yip FW, Reeve TS, Poole AG, Delbridge L (1994) Thyroid nodules in childhood and adolescence. The Australian and New Zealand Journal of Surgery 64 (10):676–678

[16] dos Santos Silva I, Swerdlow AJ (1993) Thyroid cancer epidemiology in England and Wales: time trends and geographical distribution. British Journal of Cancer 67 (2):330–340

[17] Farahati J, Bucsky P, Parlowsky T, Mader U, Reiners C (1997) Characteristics of differentiated thyroid carcinoma in children and adolescents with respect to age, gender, and histology. Cancer 80 (11):2156–2162

[18] Henderson BE, Ross RK, Pike MC, Casagrande JT (1982) Endogenous hormones as a major factor in human cancer. Cancer Research 42 (8):3232–3239

[19] Rapkin L, Pashankar FD (2012) Management of thyroid carcinoma in children and young adults. Journal of Pediatric Hematology/Oncology 34 (Suppl 2):S39–46. doi: 10.1097/MPH.0b013e31824e37a6

[20] Catelinois O, Verger P, Colonna M, Rogel A, Hemon D, Tirmarche M (2004) Projecting the time trend of thyroid cancers: its impact on assessment of radiation-induced cancer risks. Health Physics 87 (6):606–614

[21] Ron E, Lubin JH, Shore RE, Mabuchi K, Modan B, Pottern LM, Schneider AB, Tucker MA, Boice JD, Jr. (1995) Thyroid cancer after exposure to external radiation: a pooled analysis of seven studies. Radiation Research 141 (3):259–277

[22] Mahoney MC, Lawvere S, Falkner KL, Averkin YI, Ostapenko VA, Michalek AM, Moysich KB, McCarthy PL (2004) Thyroid cancer incidence trends in Belarus: examining the impact of Chernobyl. International Journal of Epidemiology 33 (5):1025–1033. doi:10.1093/ije/dyh201

[23] Parfitt T (2004) Chernobyl's legacy. 20 years after the power station exploded, new cases of thyroid cancer are still rising, say experts. Lancet 363 (9420):1534

[24] Williams D (2002) Cancer after nuclear fallout: lessons from the Chernobyl accident. Nature Reviews Cancer 2 (7):543–549. doi:10.1038/nrc845

[25] Jarzab B, Handkiewicz-Junak D, Wloch J (2005) Juvenile differentiated thyroid carcinoma and the role of radioiodine in its treatment: a qualitative review. Endocrine-Related Cancer 12 (4):773–803. doi:10.1677/erc.1.00880

[26] Mazzaferri EL, Kloos RT (2001) Clinical review 128: Current approaches to primary therapy for papillary and follicular thyroid cancer. The Journal of Clinical Endocrinology and Metabolism 86 (4):1447–1463. doi:10.1210/jcem.86.4.7407

[27] Zimmerman D, Hay ID, Gough IR, Goellner JR, Ryan JJ, Grant CS, McConahey WM (1988) Papillary thyroid carcinoma in children and adults: long-term follow-up of 1039 patients conservatively treated at one institution during three decades. Surgery 104 (6): 1157–1166

[28] Newman KD, Black T, Heller G, Azizkhan RG, Holcomb GW, 3rd, Sklar C, Vlamis V, Haase GM, La Quaglia MP (1998) Differentiated thyroid cancer: determinants of disease progression in patients <21 years of age at diagnosis: a report from the Surgical Discipline Committee of the Children's Cancer Group. Annals of Surgery 227 (4):533–541

[29] Schlumberger M, De Vathaire F, Travagli JP, Vassal G, Lemerle J, Parmentier C, Tubiana M (1987) Differentiated thyroid carcinoma in childhood: long term follow-up of 72 patients. The Journal of Clinical Endocrinology and Metabolism 65 (6):1088–1094. doi: 10.1210/jcem-65-6-1088

[30] Luster M, Lassmann M, Freudenberg LS, Reiners C (2007) Thyroid cancer in childhood: management strategy, including dosimetry and long-term results. Hormones 6 (4):269–278

[31] Mitsutake N, Knauf JA, Mitsutake S, Mesa C, Jr., Zhang L, Fagin JA (2005) Conditional BRAFV600E expression induces DNA synthesis, apoptosis, dedifferentiation, and chromosomal instability in thyroid PCCL3 cells. Cancer Research 65 (6):2465–2473. doi: 10.1158/0008-5472.CAN-04-3314

[32] Vali R, Rachmiel M, Hamilton J, El Zein M, Wasserman J, Costantini DL, Charron M, Daneman A (2015) The role of ultrasound in the follow-up of children with differentiated thyroid cancer. Pediatric Radiology 45 (7):1039–1045. doi:10.1007/s00247-014-3261-0

[33] Hay ID (1987) Brain metastases from papillary thyroid carcinoma. Archives of Internal Medicine 147 (3):607, 611

[34] Francis GL, Waguespack SG, Bauer AJ, Angelos P, Benvenga S, Cerutti JM, Dinauer CA, Hamilton J, Hay ID, Luster M, Parisi MT, Rachmiel M, Thompson GB, Yamashita S, American Thyroid Association Guidelines Task F (2015) Management guidelines for children with thyroid nodules and differentiated thyroid cancer. Thyroid: Official Journal of the American Thyroid Association 25 (7):716–759. doi:10.1089/thy.2014.0460

[35] Corrias A, Einaudi S, Chiorboli E, Weber G, Crino A, Andreo M, Cesaretti G, de Sanctis L, Messina MF, Segni M, Cicchetti M, Vigone M, Pasquino AM, Spera S, de Luca F, Mussa GC, Bona G (2001) Accuracy of fine needle aspiration biopsy of thyroid nodules in detecting malignancy in childhood: comparison with conventional clinical, laboratory, and imaging approaches. The Journal of Clinical Endocrinology and Metabolism 86 (10):4644–4648. doi:10.1210/jcem.86.10.7950

[36] Ogilvie JB, Piatigorsky EJ, Clark OH (2006) Current status of fine needle aspiration for thyroid nodules. Advances in Surgery 40:223–238

[37] Borson-Chazot F, Causeret S, Lifante JC, Augros M, Berger N, Peix JL (2004) Predictive factors for recurrence from a series of 74 children and adolescents with differentiated thyroid cancer. World Journal of Surgery 28 (11):1088–1092. doi:10.1007/s00268-004-7630-y

[38] Wada N, Sugino K, Mimura T, Nagahama M, Kitagawa W, Shibuya H, Ohkuwa K, Nakayama H, Hirakawa S, Yukawa N, Rino Y, Masuda M, Ito K (2009) Treatment strategy of papillary thyroid carcinoma in children and adolescents: clinical significance of the initial nodal manifestation. Annals of Surgical Oncology 16 (12):3442–3449. doi:10.1245/s10434-009-0673-4

[39] Grigsby PW, Gal-or A, Michalski JM, Doherty GM (2002) Childhood and adolescent thyroid carcinoma. Cancer 95 (4):724–729. doi:10.1002/cncr.10725

[40] Handkiewicz-Junak D, Wloch J, Roskosz J, Krajewska J, Kropinska A, Pomorski L, Kukulska A, Prokurat A, Wygoda Z, Jarzab B (2007) Total thyroidectomy and adjuvant

radioiodine treatment independently decrease locoregional recurrence risk in childhood and adolescent differentiated thyroid cancer. Journal of Nuclear Medicine: Official Publication, Society of Nuclear Medicine 48 (6):879–888. doi:10.2967/jnumed.106.035535

[41] Welch Dinauer CA, Tuttle RM, Robie DK, McClellan DR, Svec RL, Adair C, Francis GL (1998) Clinical features associated with metastasis and recurrence of differentiated thyroid cancer in children, adolescents and young adults. Clinical Endocrinology 49 (5):619–628

[42] Hay ID, Gonzalez-Losada T, Reinalda MS, Honetschlager JA, Richards ML, Thompson GB (2010) Long-term outcome in 215 children and adolescents with papillary thyroid cancer treated during 1940 through 2008. World Journal of Surgery 34 (6):1192–1202. doi:10.1007/s00268-009-0364-0

[43] Machens A, Lorenz K, Nguyen Thanh P, Brauckhoff M, Dralle H (2010) Papillary thyroid cancer in children and adolescents does not differ in growth pattern and metastatic behavior. The Journal of Pediatrics 157 (4):648–652. doi:10.1016/j.jpeds.2010.04.026

[44] American Thyroid Association Guidelines Taskforce on Thyroid N, Differentiated Thyroid C, Cooper DS, Doherty GM, Haugen BR, Kloos RT, Lee SL, Mandel SJ, Mazzaferri EL, McIver B, Pacini F, Schlumberger M, Sherman SI, Steward DL, Tuttle RM (2009) Revised American Thyroid Association management guidelines for patients with thyroid nodules and differentiated thyroid cancer. Thyroid: Official Journal of the American Thyroid Association 19 (11):1167–1214. doi:10.1089/thy.2009.0110

[45] Pacini F, Elisei R, Capezzone M, Miccoli P, Molinaro E, Basolo F, Agate L, Bottici V, Raffaelli M, Pinchera A (2001) Contralateral papillary thyroid cancer is frequent at completion thyroidectomy with no difference in low- and high-risk patients. Thyroid: Official Journal of the American Thyroid Association 11 (9):877–881. doi:10.1089/105072501316973145

[46] Miccoli P, Antonelli A, Spinelli C, Ferdeghini M, Fallahi P, Baschieri L (1998) Completion total thyroidectomy in children with thyroid cancer secondary to the Chernobyl accident. Archives of Surgery 133 (1):89–93

[47] Baloch Z, Carayon P, Conte-Devolx B, Demers LM, Feldt-Rasmussen U, Henry JF, LiVosli VA, Niccoli-Sire P, John R, Ruf J, Smyth PP, Spencer CA, Stockigt JR, Guidelines Committee NAoCB (2003) Laboratory medicine practice guidelines. Laboratory support for the diagnosis and monitoring of thyroid disease. Thyroid: Official Journal of the American Thyroid Association 13 (1):3–126. doi:10.1089/105072503321086962

[48] Durante C, Montesano T, Torlontano M, Attard M, Monzani F, Tumino S, Costante G, Meringolo D, Bruno R, Trulli F, Massa M, Maniglia A, D'Apollo R, Giacomelli L, Ronga G, Filetti S, Group PTCS (2013) Papillary thyroid cancer: time course of recurrences

during postsurgery surveillance. The Journal of Clinical Endocrinology and Metabolism 98 (2):636–642. doi:10.1210/jc.2012-3401

[49] Han JM, Kim WB, Yim JH, Kim WG, Kim TY, Ryu JS, Gong G, Sung TY, Yoon JH, Hong SJ, Kim EY, Shong YK (2012) Long-term clinical outcome of differentiated thyroid cancer patients with undetectable stimulated thyroglobulin level one year after initial treatment. Thyroid: Official Journal of the American Thyroid Association 22 (8):784–790. doi:10.1089/thy.2011.0322

[50] Maxon HR, 3rd, Smith HS (1990) Radioiodine-131 in the diagnosis and treatment of metastatic well differentiated thyroid cancer. Endocrinology and Metabolism Clinics of North America 19 (3):685–718

[51] Robbins J (1994) Treatment of thyroid cancer in childhood. National Institutes of Health, Bethesda, MD

[52] Willegaignon J, Sapienza M, Ono C, Watanabe T, Guimaraes MI, Gutterres R, Marechal MH, Buchpiguel C (2011) Outpatient radioiodine therapy for thyroid cancer: a safe nuclear medicine procedure. Clinical Nuclear Medicine 36 (6):440–445. doi:10.1097/RLU.0b013e3182184fa0

[53] Caldwell CB, Ehrlich LE (1999) Outpatient treatment of thyroid cancer using high doses of iodine 131. Canadian Association of Radiologists Journal 50 (5):331–336

[54] Gabriel S, Farman-Ara B, Bourrelly M, Carpentier O, Sebag F, Palazzo FF, De Micco C, Mancini J, Henry JF, Mundler O, Taieb D (2011) Radiation doses to cohabitants of patients undergoing radioiodine ablation for thyroid cancer: poor compliance with radiation protection guidelines but low radiation exposure. Nuclear Medicine Communications 32 (9):829–833. doi:10.1097/MNM.0b013e328347f1c2

[55] Randolph GW, Daniels GH (2002) Radioactive iodine lobe ablation as an alternative to completion thyroidectomy for follicular carcinoma of the thyroid. Thyroid: Official Journal of the American Thyroid Association 12 (11):989–996. doi:10.1089/105072502320908321

[56] Alexander C, Bader JB, Schaefer A, Finke C, Kirsch CM (1998) Intermediate and long-term side effects of high-dose radioiodine therapy for thyroid carcinoma. Journal of Nuclear Medicine: Official Publication, Society of Nuclear Medicine 39 (9):1551–1554

[57] Kloos RT, Duvuuri V, Jhiang SM, Cahill KV, Foster JA, Burns JA (2002) Nasolacrimal drainage system obstruction from radioactive iodine therapy for thyroid carcinoma. The Journal of Clinical Endocrinology and Metabolism 87 (12):5817–5820. doi:10.1210/jc.2002-020210

[58] Burns JA, Morgenstern KE, Cahill KV, Foster JA, Jhiang SM, Kloos RT (2004) Nasolacrimal obstruction secondary to I(131) therapy. Ophthalmic Plastic and Reconstructive Surgery 20 (2):126–129

[59] Levenson D, Gulec S, Sonenberg M, Lai E, Goldsmith SJ, Larson SM (1994) Peripheral facial nerve palsy after high-dose radioiodine therapy in patients with papillary thyroid carcinoma. Annals of Internal Medicine 120 (7):576–578

[60] Vini L, Hyer S, Al-Saadi A, Pratt B, Harmer C (2002) Prognosis for fertility and ovarian function after treatment with radioiodine for thyroid cancer. Postgraduate Medical Journal 78 (916):92–93

[61] Handelsman DJ, Turtle JR (1983) Testicular damage after radioactive iodine (I-131) therapy for thyroid cancer. Clinical Endocrinology 18 (5):465–472

[62] Raymond JP, Izembart M, Marliac V, Dagousset F, Merceron RE, Vulpillat M, Vallee G (1989) Temporary ovarian failure in thyroid cancer patients after thyroid remnant ablation with radioactive iodine. The Journal of Clinical Endocrinology and Metabolism 69 (1):186–190. doi:10.1210/jcem-69-1-186

[63] van Santen HM, Aronson DC, Vulsma T, Tummers RF, Geenen MM, de Vijlder JJ, van den Bos C (2004) Frequent adverse events after treatment for childhood-onset differentiated thyroid carcinoma: a single institute experience. European Journal of Cancer 40 (11):1743–1751. doi:10.1016/j.ejca.2004.03.006

[64] Pawelczak M, David R, Franklin B, Kessler M, Lam L, Shah B (2010) Outcomes of children and adolescents with well-differentiated thyroid carcinoma and pulmonary metastases following (1)(3)(1)I treatment: a systematic review. Thyroid: Official Journal of the American Thyroid Association 20 (10):1095–1101. doi:10.1089/thy.2009.0446

[65] Demidchik YE, Demidchik EP, Reiners C, Biko J, Mine M, Saenko VA, Yamashita S (2006) Comprehensive clinical assessment of 740 cases of surgically treated thyroid cancer in children of Belarus. Annals of Surgery 243 (4):525–532. doi:10.1097/01.sla.0000205977.74806.0b

[66] Lazar L, Lebenthal Y, Steinmetz A, Yackobovitch-Gavan M, Phillip M (2009) Differentiated thyroid carcinoma in pediatric patients: comparison of presentation and course between pre-pubertal children and adolescents. The Journal of Pediatrics 154 (5):708–714. doi:10.1016/j.jpeds.2008.11.059

[67] Faggiano A, Coulot J, Bellon N, Talbot M, Caillou B, Ricard M, Bidart JM, Schlumberger M (2004) Age-dependent variation of follicular size and expression of iodine transporters in human thyroid tissue. Journal of Nuclear Medicine: Official Publication, Society of Nuclear Medicine 45 (2):232–237

[68] Patel A, Jhiang S, Dogra S, Terrell R, Powers PA, Fenton C, Dinauer CA, Tuttle RM, Francis GL (2002) Differentiated thyroid carcinoma that express sodium-iodide symporter have a lower risk of recurrence for children and adolescents. Pediatric Research 52 (5):737–744. doi:10.1203/00006450-200211000-00021